Recent Results in Cancer Research 63

Fortschritte der Krebsforschung
Progrès dans les recherches sur le cancer

Antitumor Antibiotics

Edited by
S.K. Carter H. Umezawa J. Douros Y. Sakurai

With 111 Figures

Springer-Verlag
Berlin Heidelberg New York 1978

U.S. Japan Joint Agreement on Cancer Research
3rd Annual Program Review Symposium on Antitumor Antibiotics May 12–13, 1977, San Francisco, California

Dr. S. K. CARTER, Director, Northern California Cancer Program, 1801 Page Mill Road, Bldg. B, Suite 200, Palo Alto, California 94304/USA

Professor HAMAO UMEZAWA, Head, Department of Antibiotics, National Institutes of Health, Kami-Osaki 2-10-35, Shinagawa-ku, Tokyo 1411/Japan

Dr. JOHN DOUROS, National Cancer Institute, Division of Cancer Treatment, Blair Bldg. Room 4A15, 8300 Colesville Road, Silver Spring, Maryland 20910/USA

Professor YOSHIO SAKURAI, Director, Cancer Chemotherapy Center, Japanese Foundation for Cancer Research, Kami-Ikebukuro 1-37-1, Toshima-ku, Tokyo/Japan

Sponsored by the Swiss League against Cancer

ISBN 3-540-08624-2 Springer-Verlag Berlin Heidelberg New York
ISBN 0-387-08624-2 Springer-Verlag New York Heidelberg Berlin

Library of Congress Cataloging in Publication Data. Program Review Symposium on Antitumor Antibiotics, 3d, San Francisco, Calif., 1977. Antitumor antibiotics. (Recent results in cancer research; 63) 1. Cancer—Chemotherapy—Congresses. 2. Antiobiotics—Congresses. 3. Antineoplastic agents—Congresses. I. Carter, Stephen K. II. Schweizerische Nationalliga für Krebsbekämpfung und Krebsforschung. III. Title. IV. Series. RC261.R35 no. 63 [RC271.A65] 616.9'94'008s [616,9'92'061] 78-2818

Printed in Germany.

Typesetting: William Clowes & Sons Limited, London, Beccles and Colchester/England
Printing and binding: Konrad Triltsch, Graphischer Betrieb, 87 Würzburg, Germany

2125/3140-543210

Table of Contents

List of Participants

ABE, M., Department of Radiology, Faculty of Medicine, Kyoto University, Shogoin Kawahara-cho, Sakyo-ku, Kyoto 606, Japan.

BENJAMIN, R. S., Department of Developmental Therapeutics, The University of Texas System Cancer Center, M. D. Anderson Hospital and Tumor Institute, 6723 Bertner Avenue, Houston, TX 77030/USA.

BONO, V. H., National Cancer Institute, Investigational Drug Branch, Bldg. 37, Room 6E22, Bethesda, MD 20014/USA.

CARTER, S. K., Northern California Cancer Program, 1801 Page Mill Rd, Bldg. B, Suite 200, Palo Alto, CA 94304/USA.

COMIS, R. L., Solid Tumor Oncology, Upstate Medical Center, 750 E. Adams St., Syracuse, NY/13210/USA.

CROOKE, S. T., Research and Development, Bristol Laboratories, P.O. Box 657, Syracuse NY 13210/USA.

DAVIS, H. L., National Cancer Institute, Division of Cancer Treatment, Clinical Investigations Branch, Landow Building, Room 8C03, Bethesda, MD 20014/USA.

DION: H. W., Antibiotics and Microbial Development, Parke-Davis Co., Joseph Campau at the River, Box 118, General Post Office, Detroit, MI 48232/USA.

DOUROS, J. D., National Cancer Institute, Division of Cancer Treatment, Blair Bldg., Room 4A15, 8300 Colesville Rd., Silver Spring, MD 20910/USA.

FRIEDMAN, M. A., Cancer Research Institute, University of California, 1276 Moffitt Hospital, San Francisco, CA 94143/USA.

FURUE, H., Department of Internal Medicine II, Teikyo University School of Medicine, Kaga 2–11–1, Itabashi-ku, Tokyo 173, Japan.

GOLDIN, A. National Cancer Institute, Division of Cancer Treatment, Building 31, Room 10A22, Bethesda, MD 20014/USA.

KIMURA, I., Department of Internal Medicine II, Okayama University School of Medicine, Shikata-cho 2–5–1, Okayama, Okayama Pref. 700, Japan.

KOYAMA, Y., National Medical Center Hospital, Toyama-cho 1, Shinjuku-ku, Tokyo 162, Japan.

LANGLYKKE, A. F., Frederick Cancer Research Center, P.O. Box B, Frederick, MD 21701/USA.

MATSUDA, A., Research Laboratories, Department of Anticancers and Antimicrobials, Nippon Kayaku Co. Ltd., Shimo 3-31-12, Kita-ku, Tokyo 115, Japan.

MIYAMOTO, T., Internal Medicine, National Institute of Radiological Science, Anagawa 4-9-1, Chiba, Chiba Pref. 280, Japan.

MUGGIA, F. M. National Cancer Institute, Division of Cancer Treatment, Bldg. 37, Room 6A17, Bethesda, MD 20014/USA.

NEIL, G. L., Cancer Research, The Upjohn Co., 301 Henrietta, Kalamazoo, MI 49001/USA.

ROSAZZA, J. P. N., University of Iowa, College of Pharmacy, Iowa City, IA 52240/USA.

SAKURAI, Y., Cancer Chemotherapy Center, Japanese Foundation for Cancer Research, Kami-IKebukuro 1-37-1, Toshima-ku, Tokyo, Japan.

SCHEIN, P. S., V. T. Lombardi Cancer Research Center, Georgetown University School of Medicine, 3800 Reservoir Road, Washington, D.C. 20007/USA.

SCHEPARTZ, S., National Cancer Institute, Division of Cancer Treatment, Bldg. 31, Room 3A51, Bethesda, MD 20014/USA.

SLAVIK, M., Georgetown University Hospital, Division of Medical Oncology, 3800 Reservoir Rd.,Washington D.C. 20007/USA.

UMEZAWA, H., Institute of Microbial Chemistry, Kamiosaki, 3-14-23, Shinagawa-ku, Tokyo 141, Japan.

VENDITTI, J. M., National Cancer Institute, Division of Cancer Treatment, Blair Bldg., Room 532-B, Silver Spring, MD 20910/USA.

YAMANAKA, N., Laboratory of Chemotherapy, Aichi Cancer Center Research Institute, Chikusa-ku, Nagoya 464, Japan.

Introduction

The scientific collaboration between the United States and Japan in the field of cancer goes back many years. In this successful international collaboration cancer chemotherapy has been one of the most productive areas. Pioneers such as YOSHIDA, UMEZAWA, SHEAR, and GOLDIN established firm links of mutual trust and respect in the period after the Second Great War. Japanese drugs, such as mitomycin C and bleomycin have become mainstays of clinical oncology in the U.S. and throughout the world. Many drugs developed in the U.S. have become established in Japanese cancer therapy. Within the cancer chemotherapy field the antitumor antibiotics rank as one of the most important groups. In the U.S.-Japanese collaboration this group of drugs has taken the paramount role. The Japanese, under the leadership of Umezawa, are considered to be among the most innovative and productive in this area which has also had great emphasis in the United States as part of the National Cancer Institute's drug development program and in the pharmaceutical industry. This extended collaboration in general oncology, and chemotherapy in particular, has received increased impetus by and support from the official U.S.-Japan Joint Agreement on cancer research, which was established in 1974 between the National Cancer Institute and the Japanese Society for the Promotion of Science.

One of the subsections of this agreement is cancer therapy with emphasis on chemotherapy. The chairman for Japan is Professor Yoshio Sakurai while I am chairman for the United States together with Dr. Franco Muggia of the NCI. Under the aegis of this agreement symposia have been held on cytosine arabinoside and cyclocytidine in Tokyo in 1975—and on the nitrosoureas and bleomycin in Kona, Hawaii, in 1976. On May 25–26 1977 a third symposium took place in San Francisco, California, sponsored by the Northern California Cancer Program. This symposium broadly concerned antitumor antibiotics and was designed to cover both the preclinical aspects of development and the clinical status of current and new drugs. It was organized by Dr. STEPHEN K. CARTER and Dr. JOHN DOUROS for the U.S. and by Professors HAMAO UMEZAWA and YOSHIO SAKURAI on the Japanese side. This publication contains the official papers of this symposium.

STEPHEN K. CARTER

Summary of Clinical Data on Antitumor Antibiotics in Japan

Y. Koyama

Several antitumor antibiotics are clinically used in Japan. Some have already been removed from clinical application—for example, sarkomycin and carzinophylin, and some, such as aclacinomycin A, have just entered the phase I study. The most widely used drugs are mitomycin C and bleomycin. Neocarzinostatin and adriamycin are used in rather limited cases at present.

The clinical data on solid tumors which will be presented here has been collected mainly from published papers in Japan. The data on single drug use is ten or more years old because the majority of antitumor drugs have recently been used in combination with chemotherapy, irradiation, and/or surgery. The criterion of the old clinical data was not as stringent as in current literature. In the old data, the decrease in size of tumors or the duration of remission were not recorded accurately.

Only the evaluable cases have been selected for the data presented here. The estimation has been made as closely as possible according to the NCI criterion. When the cases were evaluated according to Karnofsky's criterion, category I was selected. As a basis of clinical data, it should be considered that the death rate from gastric cancer has reached a summit and is slightly on the decrease. The death rate from lung cancer has increased markedly in the male. There is also a marked decrease in the death rate from uterine cervix cancer, and deaths from breast and colorectal cancer are slowly but steadily increasing in Japan.

Clinical Data on Single Use of Antitumor Antibiotics in Japan

Mitomycin C (MMC) was given i.v., i.m. or orally. The doses were 0.02–0.04 mg/kg daily; 0.08–0.12 mg/kg twice a week; 0.16–0.2 mg/kg once a week or every 2 weeks; and more than 0.3 mg/kg once every 3 or 4 weeks. When the number of evaluated cases was more than 20 (Table 1) [4, 24, 29, 39, 40, 70], the effectiveness of MMC was 27.6% for gastric cancer, 29.8% for colorectal cancer, 50% for breast cancer, 29.2% for malignant lymphoma, and 80% for chronic myeloid leukemia, CML. When administered by arterial infusion, MCC was 76% effective for uterine cervix cancer [18], and 70% for urinary bladder cancer [54, 66], after direct application of the dissolved drug into the cystic cavity. The side-effects of MMC are bone-marrow depression and gastrointestinal disorders—leukopenia, 30% (less than 3000); thrombocytopenia, 21.7% (less than 50,000); loss of appetite, 16%; nausea, 8%; vomiting 2%.

The clinical data on chromomomycin A3 (CHRM) from [Tsukagoshi, 1976] is shown in Table 2. In these cases, 0.01–0.02 mg CHRM/kg was administered i.v. The effectiveness was 35% for gastric cancer, 36% for colorectal cancer, 35% for hepatoma, 40% for bronchogenic cancer, 11% for breast cancer, 44% for uterine cervix cancer, 60% for ovarian cancer, and 73% for malignant lymphoma. The side-effects were loss of appetite (22%) and thrombophlebitis.

Table 1. Clinical data on mitomycin C

Site and type of tumors	No. of cases	Effective	
		Cases	%
Esophagus	12	2	17.0
Stomach	383	105	27.4
Colorectal	47	14	29.8
Liver	12	4	33.0
Pancreas	8	3	
Lung	70	27	38.5
Breast	26	13	50.0
Malignant lymphoma	48	14	29.2
C M L (i.v.)	15	12	80.0
(p.o.)	37	32	86.4
Reticulum cell sarcoma	18	10	55.0
Cervix (i.a.)	46	35	76.0 [18]
Urinary bladder (local)	27	19	70.4 [54.66]

Table 2. Clinical data on chromomycin A3 [From TSUKAGOSHI, 1976]

Site and type of tumors	No. of cases	Effective	
		Cases	%
Esophagus	17	2	11
Stomach	156	55	35
Colorectal	32	11	34
Hepatoma	20	7	35
Biliary tract	3	2	
Pancreatic	12	3	25
Head and neck	14	9	63
Bronchogenic	64	26	40
Breast	26	3	11
Uterine cervix	25	11	44
Ovary	38	17	44
Chrioepithelioma	12	8	67
Grawitz tumor	2	1	
Urinary Bladder	8	3	37
Prostate	1	1	
Skin	13	4	30
Brain tumors	14	6	42
Malignant lymphoma	45	33	73
Bone and soft tissue sarcoma	11	5	45

Table 3 shows the clinical data of bleomycin (BLM) [11, 14, 34, 50, 57, 58, 63, 64, 65, 70]. In most cases, the daily dosage was 0.2–0.6 mg/kg, given once or twice weekly. The effectiveness was 71% for maxillary cancer, 46% for pharyngeal cancer, 23% for lung cancer, 50% for esophagal cancer, 54% for skin cancer, 60% for urogenital cancer, 57% for uterine cervix cancer, 42%–58% for brain tumors, and 75% for reticulum cell sarcoma.
From the 486 cases recorded, the side-effects are, in order of frequency, fever (31%), loss of appetite (29.9%), alopecia (29.7%), sclerotic change in fingers and hands (26.7%), sclerotic change in toes and feet (22.8%), pigmentation (18.3%), changes in nails (17.3%), fatigue (15.8%), nausea and vomiting (9.8%), pulmonary fibrosis (3.6%), and leukopenia (0.8%).

Table 3. Clinical data on bleomycin

Site and type of tumors	No. of cases	Effective	
		Cases	%
Oral cavity	70	41	58.5
Tongue	12	8	66.7
Pharynx	12	7	58.3
Maxilla	63	45	71.5
Larynx	209	97	46.3
Lung squamous cell carcinoma	27	23	85.1
adenocarcinoma	18	10	55.6
others	9	4	
Lung	43	10	23.2
Esophagus	51	29	56.9
Skin	96	52	54.2
Malignant melanoma	8	2	
Urogenital	58	35	60.3
Cervix	91	52	57.2
Brain tumors	52	22	42.3
Brain tumors	67	39	58.2
Reticulum cell sarcoma	28	21	75.0
Lymphosarcoma	2	1	
Hodgkin's disease	7	6	
Malignant lymphoma	7	5	
Mycosis fungoides	5	5	
Total	935	514	

Recently, the long-acting new form of the BLM remedy has been clinically tested. This is the so-called oil-BLM. Oil-BLM is made up of 15 mg BLM, 10 mg aluminum monostearate and either yolk oil (A) or sesame oil (B) to give a total volume of 1 ml.

Fig. 1 [3] shows the blood levels of three kinds of BLM in cancer patients. Estimations were made in two to four cases for each type of remedy. The highest level was obtained soon after i.v. injection of BLM. This level drops rapidly. After the first hour, the level obtained from oil-BLM remains higher and longer than that of regular BLM.

In clinical tests [12, 22, 44, 55], 0.3 mg oil-BLM/kg was given i.m. once a week for 2-6 weeks (totaling 0.6-1.8 mg/kg). In cases of intratumor injection, 0.15-0.3 mg/kg was given twice a week (totaling 0.9-2.44 mg/kg) or, 0.3-0.6 mg/kg was given once a week for 3-5 weeks (totaling 0.18-5.8 mg/kg). Side-effects from oil-BLM are fever (highest in rating), fatigue, nausea, transitory pneumonitis, and pain, in descending order. The preliminary clinical data on i.m. oil-BLM shows five remissions out of six cases of reticulum cell sarcoma; three out of three in Hodgkin's disease; one out of two in malignant lymphoma; and none in lymphosarcoma, (Table 4). When oil-BLM is injected into the tumor, the response appears in all five cases of skin cancer [12], in one out of four cases of maxillary cancer, and in each case of cancer of the parotid gland and of the pharynx [55].

There is also another new type of BLM remedy, the solid-form BLM, developed by Professor Satoh of Tokyo University [53]. The remedy is based on polyethylene glycol and is kept in a thin, polyethylene tube of 2 mm outside diameter. A piece of solid-form BLM, containing 15 mg BLM, is inserted into the tumor using a needle of radon seed or the polyethylene tube itself.

Solid-form BLM has been clinically tested in ten cases of head and neck tumors [53] and in five cases of abdominal lymph node of esophageal cancer [69].

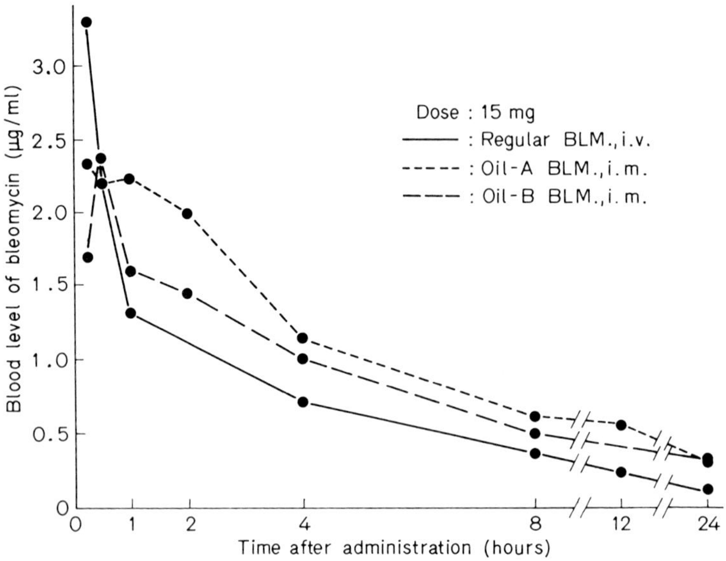

Fig. 1. Blood level of various types of bleomycin in cancer patients (after FUJITA [3])

Table 4. Clinical data on oil-bleomycin

Site and type of cancer	No. of cases	Remission		Effective	No change
		complete	partial		
Reticulum cell sarcoma	6	2	3		1
Hodgkin's disease	3	1	2		
Malignant lymphoma	2	1			1
Lymphosarcoma	1				1
Maxilla	4			1	3
Tongue	3				3
Parotid	1			1	
Pharynx	1			1	
Skin	5			5	
Total	26	4	5	8	9

Table 5 shows the clinical data on neocarzinostatin [1, 16, 23, 36, 51, 59, 61]. Neocarzinostatin (0.04–0.06 mg/kg i.v.) was given daily or every other day. A good response was obtained in 13 out of 324 cases of gastric cancer, three out of 70 cases of pancreatic cancer and in four out of 10 cases of adnex tumor. The side-effects from this drug, recorded from 323 cases, are: leukopenia (37%), loss of appetite (20%), thrombocytopenia (18%), nausea and vomiting (15%), and fever (15%).

Adriamycin (ADM) was given either i.v. or i.m.; 0.2 mg/kg on 4 successive days with weekly intervals or 0.6–0.8 mg/kg on 1 day with 3–4 week intervals. Table 6 shows the clinical data on ADM [2, 9, 13, 15, 35, 42, 43, 45, 48, 51, 71, 73]. In this table, the effectiveness means Category I by Karnofsky's criterion, except for lung metastasis of bone sarcoma, in which effectiveness was partial regression of tumor shadow on X-ray film [71].

Table 5. Clinical data on neocarzinostatin

Solid tumors

Site of tumor	No. of cases	Response		
		None	Slight	Good
Stomach	324	261	50 (19.4%)	13
Pancreas	70	59	8 (15.7%)	3
Adnex	10	1	5 (90%)	4
Cervix	12	3	8 (75%)	1

Acute leukemia

Type of leukemia	No. of cases	Remission		
		Complete	Partial	None
AML	29	4	4	21
APL	4	1	1	2
ALL	7	1		6
AMoL	11	3	4	4
Total	51	9 (17.6)	9 (17.6)	33

Table 6. Clinical data on adriamycin

Site and type of tumors	No. of cases	Effective	
		Cases	%
Lung	58	9	15.5
Esophagus	1	0	
Stomach	63	9	14.5
Colorectal	15	2	13.3
Liver	7	0	
Biliary tract	3	3	
Pancreas	4	1	
Breast	13	5	38.4
Ovary	4	1	
Cervix	4	1	
Bone and soft tissue sarcoma	15	3	20
Lung metastasis of bone sarcoma	12	8	66.6
Malignant chorioepithelioma	1	0	
Fibrosarcoma	1	0	
Leiomyosarcoma	1	0	
Total	202	42	20.8

The percentage effectiveness is 38% for breast cancer, 20% for bone and soft tissue sarcoma, and 15% for gastric and pulmonary cancer. Side-effects from ADM, in 82 recorded cases, show alopecia (73%) as the highest, then leukopenia (56%), thrombocytopenia (46%), stomatitis (33%), and ECG changes (32%).

In phase I study, 10–20 mg Aclacinomycin A were given i.v. twice a week, (totaling 200–500 mg). One case of breast cancer responded well. Two cases of gastric cancer, one case each of lung, uterine cervical cancers, and CML responded slightly (Table 7) [6]. The most frequent side-effect is nausea and vomiting (30%). Other side-effects are disturbance of liver function, anemia, and loss of appetite. Details will be presented in a separate thesis by Prof. H. Furue.

Table 7. Clinical data on aclacinomycin A

Site of tumors	No. of cases	Response		
		Effective	Slight regression	None
Stomach	7		2	5
Colon	1			1
Liver	1			1
Biliary tract	1			1
Lung	4		1	3
Breast	2	1		1
Cervix	3			3
Uterus	1			
Primary Region unknown	1			1
CML	1		1	
Total	22	1	5	16

Toxicity

Loss of appetite	4	Leukopenia	Less than 4000	4
Nausea, vomiting	7		Less than 3000	1
Salivation	2	Thrombocytopenia	$< 10 \times 10^4$	2
Fatigue	0		$< 7 \times 10^4$	1
Fever	0	Anemia	$<300 \times 10^4$	5
Epilation	1	ECG change		0
Disturbed liver function	5	None		7

A summary of clinical data on the single use of five antibiotics is shown in Table 8. The percentage of cases that responded to therapy are indicated by symbols. My conclusion from this table is that MMC has a broad spectrum, BLM a limited spectrum, and NCS a very limited spectrum. CHRM seems overrated and ADM is not yet widely used in Japan.

Clinical Data on Combination Chemotherapy in Japan

At present, more than 15 types of combined chemotherapy are used clinically [7, 8, 17, 21, 25, 28, 32, 33, 38, 41, 47, 51, 52, 62, 70, 72]. Table 9 shows the dosage and the schedule of the combination therapies.

Table 8. Summary of clinical data on single administration of antitumor antibiotics

Site and type of tumor	MMC	CHRM	BLM	NCS	ADM
Oral cavity			○		
Maxilla			○		
Esophagus	▲		○	▲	Δ
Stomach	Δ	•			
Colorectal	Δ	•			
Liver	•	•			
Pancreas	•	Δ			
Head and neck		○			
Lung	•	•	▲		
Breast	•				Δ
Uterine cervix		•	O	○	
Ovary	•	•			
Chorieopothelioma		○			
Grawitz tumor					
Utinary bladder		•			
Prostate					
Skin		•	○		
Brain tumors		•	•		
Bone and soft tissue sarcoma		•			▲
Malignant lymphoma	Δ	○	○		
Reticulum cell sarcoma	○		○		
Hodgkin's disease	○		○		
Lymphosarcoma	•				
CML	○				

○: >50%   •: 33%–50%   Δ: 25%–32%   ▲: 16%–24%.

Table 9. Doses (mg/kg) of drugs in combined chemotherapy

Type of chemotherapy	MMC	CQ	CHRM	CA	CPA	5FU	FT	TSPA	BLM	VCR	CC	Administration
MF	0.16–0.2					7.5						
MFT	0.04		0.02			10						1–2×/w
MFCT	0.08		0.02	0.4		10						2×/w
MFC	0.08			0.8		10						1–2×/w
FAMT	0.04		0.01		4	10						1–2×/w
FAM	0.08				4	10						1–2×/w
METT	0.04		0.01		2			0.2				q 4ds
FCQ		0.04–0.08		0.8		10						1–2×/w
FOBEM	0.08				8	5			0.3	0.02		1×/w
NeoMFC	0.08–0.12						16–24				12	p.o. 1×/w
MFtC	0.08			0.8			8–16					1–2×/w

FAMT: (5FU-CPA-MMC-CHRM); MFT: (MMC-5FU-CHRM); FAM: (5FU-CPA-MMC); MFC: (MMC-5FU-CA), CA: cytosine arabinoside; MFCT: (MMC-5FU-CA-CHRM); MFtC: (MMC-FT207-CA); FCQ: (5FU-CA-CQ), CQ: carbazilquinone; NeoMFC: (MMC-Ft207-CC), CC: cyclocytidine; FTPs: (5FU-CHRM-Ps), Ps: prednisolone; FOBEM: (5FU-VCR-BLM-CPA-MMC).

The usual dosage of MMC is 0.08 mg/kg but sometimes only a half of this amount is used. The dosage of CHRM is 0.01 or 0.02 mg/kg while that of cytosine arabinoside is 0.8 mg/kg, except in the case of MFCT where the dose is 0.4 mg/kg. The dosage of cytoxan is variable, 2-8 mg/kg. The usual dosage of 5FU is 10 mg/kg, that of FT207 is variable, and the dosage of BLM is 0.3 mg/kg.

There are two basic combinations used in solid tumors. One is FAMT [10, 39, 40, 62], which can be modified to MFT [5, 38] and FAM [31], and the other is MFC [10, 31, 33, 37, 41, 49, 51, 56], which can be modified to MFCT [30, 38] and MFtC [17]. FCQ [62, 68] is also induced from FMC by giving carbazilquinone instead of MMC. For oral use, NeoMFC was introduced for clinical test; this is a new combination just like FTPs [51] and FOBEM [19, 20].

Table 10 shows the results of combination chemotherapy in esophageal and colorectal cancer. In esophageal cancer, data is not available as too few cases were evaluated. For colorectal cancer, the most effective therapy was MFC (62%), followed by MFT. In gastric cancer, a high percentage is obtained using FAMT (41%), NeoMFC [46] (47%), and FTPs (42%). For cancer of the liver and biliary tract (Table 11), the highest percentage effectiveness was FMC and FAMT, followed by MFT and FCQ. In pancreatic cancer, MFC was effective in about 30% of cases, while in lung cancer, FAMT and MFT were most effective (30%), followed by FOBEM (Table 12). In breast cancer, only FAMT obtained 50% response. In ovarian and uterine cervix cancer (Table 13), FAMT also shows 50% response. MFC and FCQ show a higher percentage, but the number of recorded cases is too small to fully evaluate the data.

Side-effects from four types of combination chemotherapy are shown in Table 14 [62]. The results were obtained in our hospital and the number of cases is given in parenthesis. Incidence of side-effects is highest with FMC—both in gastrointestinal symptoms and bone marrow depression. Thrombophlebitis was induced by CHRM, and mucositis by cytosine arabinoside.

Table 15 summarizes combination chemotherapy. The spectrum of MFC is almost the same as that of FAMT, though the response differs.

Table 10. Clinical data on combined chemotherapy in colorectal and esophageal cancer

Type of chemotherapy	Colorectal		Esophagus	
	No. of cases	Effective cases	No. of cases	Effective cases
MFT	12	5 (42%)		
MFC	21	13 (62%)		
FAMT	9	2		
METT	6	1		
FCQ	6	2	1	0
MFCT	1	0	1	0
FAM	2	0		
MTPs[a]	1	0		
FTPs[a]	3	1	2	0
Ft T Ps[a]	4	1	4	1
FOBEM	2	1		

[a] Ps = prednisolone.

Table 11. Clinical data on combined chemotherapy in liver, biliary tract and pancreas cancer

Type of chemotherapy	Liver and biliary tract		Pancreas	
	No. of cases	Effective cases	No. of cases	Effective cases
MF	17	4 (23%)		
MFT	16	5 (31%)		
MFC	48	20 (41%)	12	4
FAMT	24	10 (41%)	1	0
FAM	6	2		
Neo MFC	1	1	2	1
MFCT	1	0	1	0
MFtC	10	2	3	1
FCQ	12	4	1	0
MTPs	1	0	1	0
FTPs	2	0	2	0
FtTPs	5	0	2	0
FOBEM	3	0	2	1

Table 12. Clinical data on combined chemotherapy in lung and breast cancer

Type of chemotherapy	Lung		Breast	
	No. of cases	Effective cases	No. of cases	Effective cases
MF	10	5		
MFT	25	8 (32%)	2	2
MFC	74	16 (22%)		
FAMT	72	25 (35%)	22	11 (50%)
Neo MFC	2	0		
METT	125	21 (20%)		
MFCT	4	2	1	1
MFtC	6	2		
FCQ	10	8	2	0
FOBEM	40	11 (27%)		

Table 13. Clinical data on combined chemotherapy in oviarial and cervical cancer

Type of chemotherapy	Ovarian		Cervical	
	No. of cases	Effective cases	No. of cases	Effective cases
MFT	5	2		
MFC	9	5	6	5
FAMT	12	6	12	6
METT	4	3		
FCQ	7	4	4	1
MFCT			1	0
FOBEM	1	0	2	0

Table 14. Side-effects of combination chemotherapy

Side-effects	FAMT (42)		MFT(90)		MFC (46)		FCQ (63)	
	No.	%	No.	%	No.	%	No.	%
Loss of appetite	11	26	30	33	33	72	28	44
Nausea	11	26	26	29	30	65	24	38
Vomiting	8	19	13	14	18	39	15	24
Diarrhea	6	14	20	22	8	17	9	14
Leukopenia								
< 3000	13	31	24	16	19	41	22	35
< 2000	5	12	15	17	11	23	8	13
Thrombocytopenia								
$< 5 \times 10^4$	9	21	20	22	14	30	16	25
$< 3 \times 10^4$	4	10	10	11	8	17	5	8
Fever					1		2	
Stomatitis	2		4		6	13	6	10
Exantheme	3		5		1		3	
Epilation	7	17	3		2		1	
Thrombophlebitis	6	14	20	22	5		2	
Hemorrhagic diathesis	1		4		1		3	

Table 15. Summary of clinical data on combination chemotherapy

Chemotherapy / Solid tumor	MFT	MFC	MFCT	FAMT	FAM	METT	FCQ	Neo MFC	MFtC	FTPs	FtTPs	FOBEM
Stomach	▲	•	▲	•	▲		Δ	•	Δ	•	▲	
Colorectal	•	○	▲	▲		▲	•					
Esophagus												
Liver,	Δ	•	•		•		•		▲			
Biliary tract						•						
Pancreas		•										
Lung	Δ	▲		•		▲	○		•			Δ
Breast				•								
Ovary	•	○		•			○					
Cervix		○		•								

○: >50% •: 33–50% Δ: 25–32% ▲: 16–24%

Controlled Clinical Trials With Antibiotics in Breast and Uterine Cervix Cancer

In 1959, national hospitals under the Ministry of Health and Welfare started the Cooperating Chemotherapy Research Committee on Cancer. Since then, seven cooperative studies have been carried out on a nationwide scale. The committee is composed of six cancer study groups: gastric, liver, pulmonary, breast, and uterine cervix cancers, leukemia, and lymphoma. In this paper, data from controlled trials in breast and cervix cancers will be presented.

The patients participating in the program were histologically diagnosed as having carcinoma. New patients who had never undergone chemotherapy were selected and control groups, without chemotherapy or with therapy using a known antitumor agent, were set up in each study. The Fisher-Yates' table of random numbers and the envelope method were used for randomization.

In the breast cancer study, patients in the age range from 30–59 were treated with radical surgery and postoperative irradiation of 4000 rad in each of the regions. Chemotherapy was started 1 week later and the relative survival rate was calculated. The schedule of chemotherapy is shown in Table 16 [27].

In the first study, 0.04 mg MMC/kg was administered i.v. every day for 1 month (totaling 0.8 mg/kg). This was the continuous chemotherapy program, and thio-TEPA was used as the control. The second study did not involve the use of antibiotics and will not be considered here. The third study employed intermittent drug administration, comparing MMC and

Table 16. Adjuvant chemotherapy to surgery and irradiation in breast cancer

Study	Drugs	Dosage					
		During surgery		Daily doses after surgery			Total
First	MMC	—		0.04	i.v.	1 month	> 0.8
	TSPA	—		0.1	i.m.		> 2
Second	TSPA	0.1	i.v.	0.1	i.m.	daily	> 1.4
	Control	—		—			—
Third	MMC	0.08	i.v.	0.08	i.v.	2×/wk	0.8–1.2
	CPA	6	i.v.	6	i.v.	2×/wk	60–100
	Control	—		—			—
Fourth	MMC	0.08	i.v.	0.04	p.o.		2–4
	CPA	6	i.v.	1.0	p.o.		60–100
	Control	—		—			—
Fifth	5FU	10	i.v.	10	i.v.	3×/wk 3—6wk	100
	FAM						
Sixth	5FU	10		10			70
	CPA	4	i.v.	4	i.v.	2×/wk 3-6wk	28
	MMC	0.04		0.04			0.28
Seventh	FT-207			16	p.o.	6 wk	672
	CPA			2	p.o.	12 wk	168

cyclophosphamide (CPA) to a control group without chemotherapy. The fourth study was the same as the third except that postoperative chemotherapy was administered orally. The fifth study was a comparison between single 5FU and combination therapy of FAM. The seventh study is now in progress, comparing FT-207 with CPA, administered orally without postoperative irradiation.

In the first study, the relative survival rate of premenopausal cases using MMC was slightly higher than using TSPA, but statistically insignificant. In the third and fourth studies, the survival rate using MMC was slightly higher in postmenopausal cases but this was also insignificant. In the fifth study, no difference was found among the three treatment groups (Figs. 2-4) [27].

The schedule of adjuvant chemotherapy in uterine cervix cancer is shown in Table 17. After surgery, a small dose of irradiation (1500 rad) was given in bilateral parametric regions. Chemotherapy was started during surgery and continued postoperatively for 4 successive days. In the second study, the protocol was the same as for the first study, but postoperative chemotherapy was prolonged by 8 days. In the fourth study, MMC was given intermittently, twice a week, until the total dosage reached 0.8 mg/kg. The control was without chemotherapy. In the fifth study, combination chemotherapy (FAMT) was used, and in the sixth and seventh studies, BLM was used for chemotherapy. Table 18 [27] shows the percentage survival after 2, 5 and 10 years. No differences were found among the treated group and the control group in these studies.

In stage III cases, chemotherapy was used as an adjuvant to radiotherapy. Irradiation (4000-5000 rad) was given at the bilateral points, A and B. Chemotherapy was started simultaneously with irradiation; chemotherapy schedules of the first through seventh studies

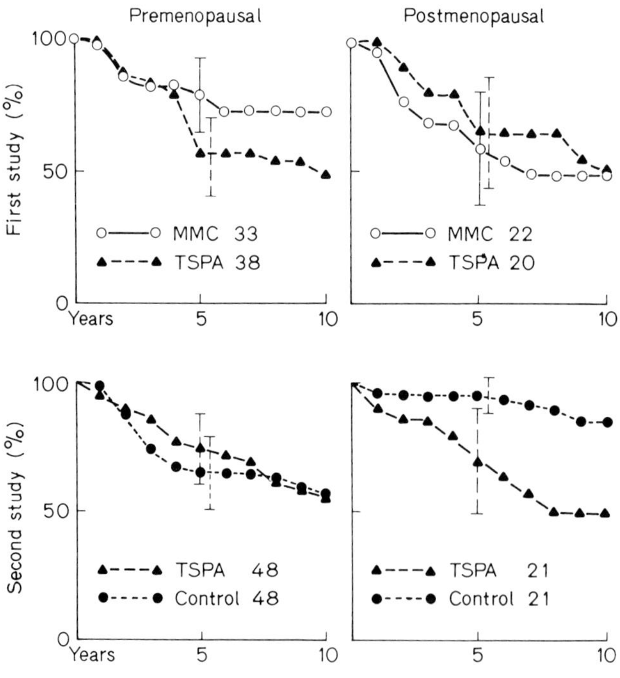

Fig. 2. Adjuvant chemotherapy to surgery and radiotherapy in breast cancer (the First and Second studies)

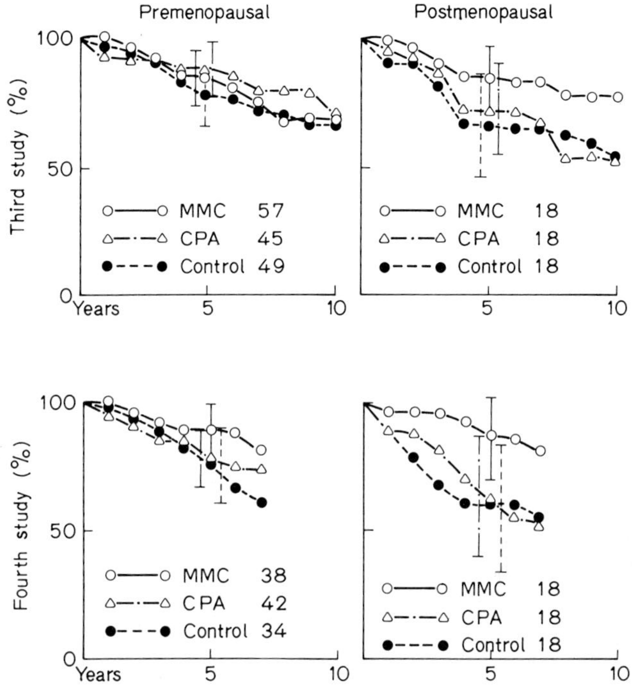

Fig. 3. Adjuvant chemotherapy to surgery and radiotherapy in breast cancer (the Third and Fourth studies)

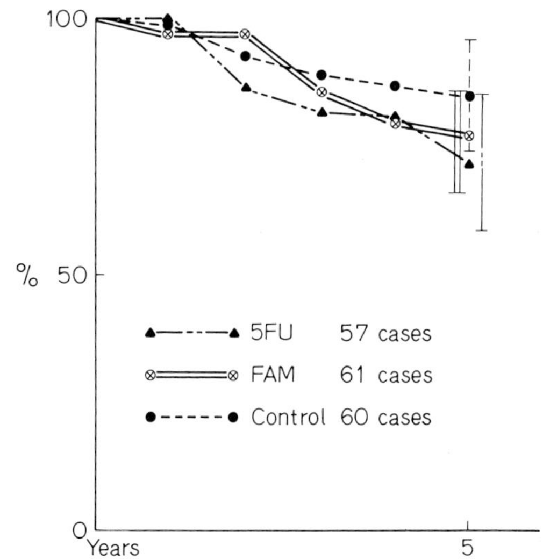

Fig. 4. Adjuvant chemotherapy to surgery and radiotherapy in breast cancer (Fifth study)

Table 17. Adjuvant chemotherapy in uterine cervix cancer: Stage II (T2b NX MO)

Study	Drugs	Dosage		
		During surgery	Daily doses after surgery	Total
First	MMC	0.08 i.v.	0.04 4× i.v.	0.24
	TSPA	0.2 i.v.	0.1 4× i.v.	0.6
	Control	—	—	—
Second	MMC	0.08 i.v.	0.04 8× i.v.	0.4
	TSPA	0.2 i.v.	0.1 8× .i.v.	1.0
	Control	—	—	—
Third	CPA	4.0 i.v.	4.0 preoperative 3×	4.0
	Control	—	— postoperative 6×	—
Fourth	MMC	0.12 i.v.	0.02 6× i.v. 2×/wk	0.84
	Control	—	—	—
Fifth	FAMT			
	5FU		5	40
	CPA		2	16
			8× i.v. 2×/wk	
	MMC		0.04	0.32
	CHRM		0.01	0.08
	Control		—	—
Sixth	BLM		0.3 10× i.m. 2×/wk	3
Seventh	Control		—	—

Table 18. Results of adjuvant chemotherapy to surgery and irradiation in uterine cervix cancer: Stage II

Study	Drugs	No. of cases	Survival rate		
			2 years	5 years	10 years
First	MMC	108	80.6	66.7	57.1
	TSPA	115	78.3	72.2	55.9
	Control	111	82.9	74.8	57.3
Second	MMC	92	78.2	68.3	35.4
	TSPA	97	83.3	68.2	42.1
	Control	85	85.5	76.0	51.2
Fourth	MMC	194	86.7	74.1	
	Control	178	87.2	79.0	
Fifth	FAMT	84	82.6	40.0	
	Control	104	82.4	57.1	
Sixth	BLM	26	88.5		
	Control	20	95.0		

are shown in Table 19 [27]. In the first two studies, MMC and TSPA are compared with the control group. In the third study, CHRM was compared with the control group. In the fifth study, the combination chemotherapy (FAMT) was compared with the control group. In the sixth and seventh studies, BLM was used as the chemotherapeutic agent.
Results of these trials are shown in Table 20 [27]. There are no differences between the control and chemotherapy groups.

Table 19. Adjuvant Chemotherapy in Uterine Cervix Cancer: Stage III (T3b NX MO)

Study	Drugs	Dosage (mg/kg)				
		Daily doses				Total
First	MMC	0.04-0.08	10-20×	i.m.	2-3×/wk	> 0.8
	TSPA	0.06-0.1	10-20×	i.m.	2-3×/wk	> 1.0
	Control		—			—
Second	MMC	0.04	20×	i.v.	2-3×/wk	> 0.8
	TSPA	0.1	20×	i.v.	2-3×/wk	> 2.0
	Control		—			—
Third	CHRM	0.02	20×	i.v.	3×/wk	0.4
	Control		—			—
Fifth	FAMT					
	5FU	5				40
	CPA	2				16
			8×	i.v.	2×/wk	
	MMC	0.04				0.32
	CHRM	0.01				0.08
	Control		—			—
Sixth	BLM	0.3	10×	i.m.	2×/wk	3
Seventh	Control		—			—

Table 20. Results of adjuvant chemotherapy to radiotherapy in uterine cervix cancer: Stage III

Study	Drugs	No. of cases	Survival rate		
			2 years	5 years	10 years
First and Second	MMC	69	47.5	34.5	14.9
	TSPA	68	49.7	32.8	16.4
	Control	71	53.7	26.6	8.6
Third	CHRM	151	53.9	37.1	
	Control	170	45.0	32.8	
Fifth and Sixth	FAMT	48	34.6		
	Control	55	36.2		
Sixth	BLM	29	55.2		
	Control	31	77.4		

Summary

In breast cancer, mitomycin C may be a useful drug as an adjuvent to surgery and radiotherapy.
The results indicate how difficult it is to obtain statistically significant results and that new ideas are necessary to advance the chemotherapy on solid tumors.

References

1. ANEHA, Y., KIKUCHI, K., KANNO, H.: Administration of high molecule antitumor agent "Neocarzinostatin" in gastric cancer patients. NIPPON-RINSHO (Jap. J. Clin. Med.) **32**, 870–874 (1974).
2. FUJIMOTO, M., HIRAO, S., MASADA, A., SAKAI, K.: Clinical trials of adriamycin, especially its intra-arterial use. GANN-NO-RINSHO (Jap. J. Cancer Clin.) **19**, 355–361 (1973).
3. FUJITA, H.: Pharmacokinetics of oil-bleomycin. GANN-TO-KAGAKURYOHO (Cancer & Chemother.) **4**, Suppl. 125–129 (1977).
4. FURUE, H., NAKAO, I., HATTORI, T., YAMANAKA, T., KUBO, A., KOIZUMI, H., YOKOYAMA, T., KIM, M., OHASHI, Y., FURUKAWA, K., KANKO, T., SUGIYAMA, N.: Clinical studies on antitumor drug administration. GANN-NO-RINSHO (Jap. J. Cancer Clin.) **16**, 896–909 (1970).
5. FURUE, H., NAKAO, I., KANKO, T., YOKOYAMA, T., FURUKAWA, K.: Chemotherapy of gastric cancer. GANN-TO-KAGAKURYOHO (Cancer & Chemother.) **2**, 351–359 (1975).
6. FURUE, H., FURUKAWA, K., NAKAO, I., HARASHIMA, S., YOKOYAMA, T., KANKO, T., FUJII, A.: Clinical information of Aclacinomycin A. GANN-TO-KAGAKURYOHO (Cancer & Chemother.) **4**, 75–79 (1977).
7. HARA, Y.: Combination chemotherapy malignant diseases. NAIKA (Internal Medicine) **29**, 1205–1211 (1972).
8. HARA, Y., TOBITA, Y.: Chemotherapy in cancer of the digestive organ. NIPPON-RINSHO (Jap. J. Clin. Med.) **33**, 1825–1832 (1975).
9. HARA, Y., KURITA, Y., HORIKAWA, K., TOBITA, Y., CHIHARA, S.: Clinical experiences of Adriamycin for malignant diseases. GANN-NO-RINSHO (Jap. J. Cancer Clin.) **18**, 336–340 (1972).
10. HARA, Y., KURITA, Y., TOBITA, Y.: Combined chemotherapy for solid tumors. GANN-NO-RINSHO (Jap. J. Cancer Clin.) **21**, 1057–1062 (1975).
11. IKEDA, S., HAMAMATSU, T., ISHIHARA, K.: Effect of Bleomycin on skin cancer. In: The GANN Monograph No. 19, Fundamental and Clinical Studies of Bleomycin, Carter, S. K., Ichikawa, T., Mathé, G., Umezawa, H. (eds.): Tokyo: University of Tokyo Press 1976, p. 235–254.
12. IKEDA, S., NAKAYAMA, T., HAMAMATSU, T., MIYASATO, H., IMAI, K., SEKI, M.: Local treatment of oil-bleomycin in dermatological diseases. YAKUBUTSU-RYOHO (Drug Therapy) **9**, 1237–1254 (1976).
13. INUYAMA, Y., OZU, R., HORIUCHI, M., NAKAJIMA, Y., ASAOKA, K., SAKAMOTO, Y., MATSUKAWA, J., HONMURA, Y., SHINKAWA, A.: Clinical trials with Adriamycin for malignant tumors of head and neck. GANN-NO-RINSHO (Jap. J. Cancer Clin.) **21**, 1301–1307 (1975).
14. IRIE, K., IKEJIRI, Y., FUJITA, K., SATO, H., YASUTAKE, K., TATSUMI, A., YAMADA, S., MAEDA, S.: Studies on the chemotherapy to malignant tumor with Bleomycin. HYOGOKEN-GANN-Center-KIYO (Hyogo Prefectural Cancer Center Bulletin) **7**, 7–22 (1974).
15. ISE, Y., OHTSUKI, H., SEKI, F.: Chemotherapy of malignant tumors in childhood (8th report).—Results of Adriamycin on malignant solid tumors—SHONIKA-SHINRYO (J. Pediatr. Practise.) **37**, 576–584 (1974).
16. ISHII, K., NAKAMURA, K.: Co-operative studies on chemotherapy for pancreatic cancer by "Neocarzinostatin". GANN-TO-KAGAKU-RYOHO (Cancer & Chemother.) **1**, 433–442 (1974).
17. KADONO, A., SAWAI, K., MISAWA, S., TAKINO, T., MASUDA, M., ABE, T., MORITA, M., KAWAI, K., NAKAMOTO, T., OKUDA, K., OHGAWARA, Y.: Combination chemotherapy with FT-207, Mitomycin C and Cytosine arabinoside. GANN-TO-KAGAKURYOHO (Cancer & Chemother.) **3**, 109–119 (1976).
18. KAWASHIMA, Y.: Chemotherapy of cervix cancer. RINSHO-TO-KENKYU (Jap. J. Clin. Exper. Med.) **49**, 93–100 (1972).
19. KIMURA, I., YASUHARA, S., URABE, Y., ONOSHI, T., SUGIYAMA, M., FUJII, M., OHSAWA, H., WATANABE, T., MACHIDA, K.: Combination chemotherapy with 5-Fluorouracil, Vincristine, Bleomycin, Cyclophosphamide and Mitomycin C for advanced cancer, GANN-TO-KAGAKURYOHO (Cancer & Chemother.) **2**, 655–659 (1975).

20. KIMURA, I., OHNOSHI, T.: Chemotherapy of lung cancer. GANN-TO-KAGAKURYOHO (Cancer & Chemother.) **2**, 995–999 (1975).
21. KIMURA, K.: Combination chemotherapy of cancer. GANN-NO-RINSHO (Jap. J. Cancer Clin.) **14**, 184–191 (1968).
22. KIMURA, K., NIITANI, H., SAKAI, Y., CHIKADA, C., SHIMOYAMA, M., SAKAI, T., IBUKA, T., MINATO, K., TAKENAKA, T., SASAKI, T., INOUE, T.: Antitumor agents, their cytocidal acting mode and the way of their administration. NIPPON-RINSHO (Jap. J. Clin. Med.) **33**, 1862–1872 (1975).
23. KITAJIMA, K., NAGAO, T., TAKAHASHI, I., KAMIMURA, O., TOKI, H., CHEM, P., NAITO, T., NAKANISHI, N., HAYASHI, H., NIIYA, K., MUGURUMA, M., SANADA, H.: Multicombination chemotherapy of acute leukemia with Neocarzinostatin and other conventional antileukemic agents. GANN-TO-KAGAKURYOHO (Cancer & Chemother.) **2**, 223–229 (1975).
24. KOYAMA, Y.: Cancer chemotherapy. NAIKA (Internal Medicine) **10**, 1029–1041 (1962).
25. KOYAMA, Y.: Chemotherapy of cancer, SHINDAN-TO-CHIRYO (Diagnosis and Treatment) **57**, 84–91 (1969).
26. KOYAMA, Y.: Criteria of clinical results of antitumor chemotherapy. NIPPON-RINSHO (Jap. J. Clin. Med.) **33**, 1794–1803 (1975).
27. KOYAMA, Y.: Clinical evaluation of chemotherapy in gastric, lung, breast, liver and cervix cancers and hematopoietic organ tumors. Annual report of the co-operative research committee on cancer chemotherapy in National Hospitals. Tokyo, 1976 (in press).
28. KOYAMA, Y., TAKEMASA, Y.: Chemotherapy of cancer. In: the RINSHO-YAKURIGAKU-TAIKEI (Encyclopedia of Clinical Pharmacol.) KUMAGAI, H., YOSHITOSHI, Y., ISHIKAWA, K., MASHIMO, K. (eds.): Tokyo: NAKAYAMA-SHOTEN 1973, Vol. I-B, p. 175–194.
29. KOYAMA, Y., TAKEMASA, Y., KIMURA, T.: Antitumor agents. SANKA-TO-FUJINKA (Obste. Gynecol.) **31**, 267–275 (1964).
30. KUBO, A., NAKAO, I., FURUE, H., FURUKAWA, K., KANKO, T., FUJII, A., HARASHIMA, S., OHKUBO, K., NISHI, I., YOKOYAMA, T., TAKEGOSHI, T., OHASHI, Y., KIM, K., SUGIYAMA, N., FUNADA, A., MASUDA, Y.: Clinical studies on combination therapy with special reference to use of Mitomycin C, 5-Fluorouracil, Cytosine arabinoside and Chromomycin A3 (MFCT therapy), GANN-NO-RINSHO (Jap. J. Cancer Clin.) **20**, 994–952 (1974).
31. KURIHARA, M., IZUMI, T., SHIRAKABE, H., NAMIHISA, T., HAYAKAWA, H.: Cancer chemotherapy of gastrointestinal tract. GANN-TO-KAGAKURYOHO (Cancer & Chemother.) **1**, 443–455 (1974).
32. MIYAMOTO, T., TAKABE, Y., WATANABE, M., TERASHIMA, T.: Drastic remission effect of a sequential combination of Bleomycin and Mitomycin C on advanced cervix cancer. GANN-TO-KAGAKURYOHO (Cancer & Chemother.) **4**, 273–291 (1977).
33. MURAKAMI, M.: Clinical study on multiple combination chemotherapy of solid tumors with special reference to prolongation of survival time. GANN-TO-KAGAKURYOHO (Cancer & Chemother.) **3**, 883–902 (1976).
34. NABEYA, K.: The use of Bleomycin in the treatment of carcinoma of the esophagus. In: The GANN Monograph No. 19, Fundamental and Clinical Studies of Bleomycin, CARTER, S. K., ICHIKAWA, T., MATHÉ, G., UMEZAWA, H. (eds.): Tokyo: University of Tokyo Press 1976, p. 177–186.
35. NAGAMATSU, S., NAKANO, A., NAGASHIMA, A., HIOKI, K., YAMAMOTO, M.: A clinical trial of Adriamycin in the cases of recurrent tumor. GANN-TO-KAGAKURYOHO (Cancer & Chemother.) **1**, 409–414 (1974).
36. NAGAO, T., KAMIMURA, O., TAKAHASHI, I., KITAJIMA, K., HIRAKI, K.: The induction chemotherapy of acute leukemia with a new antileukemic agent Neocarzinostatin. RINSHO-KETSUEKI (Jap. J. Clin. Hematol.) **14**, 925–930 (1973).
37. NAKAO, I., FURUE, H., FURUKAWA, K., KANKO, T., HARASHIMA, S., KUBO, A., HATTORI, T., KOIZUMI, H., YOKOYAMA, T., OHASHI, Y., KIM, M., FUNADA, A.: Multiple combined treatment in cancer chemotherapy. GANN-NO-RINSHO (Jap. J. Cancer Clin.) **18**, 138–143 (1972).
38. NAKAO, I., FURUKAWA, K., KANKO, T., YOKOYAMA, T., HARASHIMA, S., FUNADA, A., MASUDA, Y., FURUE, H., KUBO, A.: Combination chemotherapy in gastric cancer. GANN-TO-KAGAKURYOHO (Cancer & Chemother.) **2**, 377–384 (1975).
39. NIITANI, H.: Advance in chemotherapy of pulmonary cancer. NIPPON-RINSHO (Jap. J. Clin. Med.) **33**, 1833–1839 (1975).
40. NIITANI, H.: Chemotherapy of lung cancer. GANN-TO-KAGAKURYOHO (Cancer & Chemother.) **3**, 50–57 (1976).
41. NISHIMURA, M.: Combination chemotherapy for lung cancer. GANN-TO-KAGAKURYOHO (Cancer & Chemother.) **3**, 34–40 (1976).
42. NISHIMURA, S., KANO, M., MIKAWA, K., OHHAMA, I., SAKAMOTO, Y., SATOMI, M., OHNO, T., NISHIGAMI, T., SHIMOYAMA, T.: Clinical evaluation of antitumor effect of Adriamycin. GANN-TO-KAGAKURYOHO (Cancer & Chemother.) **2**, 679–691 (1975).
43. OGAWA, M.: Adriamycin. GANN-NO-RINSHO (Jap. J. Cancer Clin.) **21**, 1031–1036 (1975).

44. OGAWA, M., OHTA, K.: Clinical experiences of oil-bleomycin. YAKUBUTSU-RYOHO (Drug Therapy) **9**, 1255–1260 (1976).
45. OGAWA, M., KURITA, S., NISHIMURA, J., KAMEI, Y., ARIYOSHI, Y., MURAKAMI, M., OYAMA, A., SUGIURA, T., KATO, R., OHTA, K., NAKAMURA, A.: Clinical trials with Adriamycin. A new antibiotic, in treatment of malignant neoplasmas. GANN-NO-RINSHO (Jap. J. Cancer Clin.) **18**, 806–812 (1972).
46. OGAWA, M., KURIHARA, S., NISHIMURA, Y., KAMEI, Y., ARIYOSHI, H., MURAKAMI, M., OYAMA, J., SUGIURA, T., KATO, R., OHTA, K.: Clinical trial of oral MFC-treatment. GANN-NO-RINSHO (Jap. J. Cancer Clin.) **19**, 859–863 (1973).
47. OHTA, K.: Practice and evaluation of combination chemotherapy in cancer. CHIRYO (Treatment) **56**, 12–18 (1974).
48. OHTA, K.: Adriamycin. GANN-TO-KAGAKURYOHO (Cancer & Chemother.) **1**, 143–146 (1974).
49. OHTA, K., MURAKAMI, M.: Life prolonging effects of chemotherapy in solid cancers. NIPPON-RINSHO (Jap. J. Clin. Med.) **33**, 1804–1810 (1975).
50. OKA, S.: Treatment of lung cancer with Bleomycin. GANN-TO-KAGAKURYOHO (Cancer & Chemother.) **3**, 7–16 (1976).
51. SAITO, T., YOKOYAMA, M.: Treatment of solid tumors, mainly cancer of the digestive organ. NAIKA (Internal Medicine) **38**, 922–929 (1976).
52. SAKABE, T., YAMAGATA, S., FUNAHASHI, W., OKAMOTO, S., ITO, M., KOIKE, T., SAKAMOTO, T., YAMAGUCHI, O., SHIOSAKA, Y., KATAKURA, T.: Chemotherapy of cancer. NICHIDAI-IGAKUKAISHI (Nihon Univ. Med. J.) **29**, 352–366 (1970).
53. SATO, Y., MORITA, M., MIYAKAWA, K., INOUE, K., AKIDO, E., DOI, S.: Local sticktherapy with the solid Bleomycin, new treatment device for the recurrent foci of head and neck cancer. GANN-NO-RINSHO (Jap. J. Cancer Clin.) **21**, 1159–1166 (1975).
54. SHIDA, K., DOKUCHI, T., SHINOZAKI, T., SATO, H., TAKAHASHI, H., TAYA, M., KATO, N. URANO, E.: Clinical effect of Mitomycin C on urogenital tumors (First report). SHINRYO-TO-SHINYAKU (Med. Consult. & New Remed.) **3**, 121–129 (1966).
55. SHIMIZU, Y., OGASAWARA, H.: Recurrent head and neck cancers treated with oil-bleomycin. YAKUBUTSU-RYOHO (Drug Therapy) **9**, 1067–1072 (1976).
56. SUGA, S., HIROTA, Y., SHIMACHI, T., KOIDE, A., IWATA, T., NAKANE, M., KODAMA, M., MASUDA, T., YAMAMOTO, T., MIYAGI, Y., YOSHIDA, T., AIZAWA, N.: Chemotherapy of advanced gastric cancer, especially with Mitomycin C. 5-Fluorouracil and Cytosine arabinoside. GANN-NO-RINSHO (Jap. J. Cancer Clin.) **18**, 209–213 (1972).
57. SUZUKI, M., WATANABE, M., SATO, A.: Effect of Bleomycin on gynecological carcinoma. In: The GANN Monograph No. 19, Fundamental and Clinical Studies of Bleomycin. CARTER, S. K., ICHIKAWA, T., MATHÉ, G., UMEZAWA,H. (eds.): Tokyo: University of Tokyo Press 1976, p. 221–230.
58. SUZUKI, Y., MIYAKE, H., SAKAI, M.: Bleomycin treatment of maxillary cancer and the 5-year survival. In: The GANN Monograph No. 19, Fundamental and Clinical Studies of Bleomycin CARTER, S. K., ICHIKAWA, T., MATHE, G., UMEZAWA, H. (eds.: Tokyo: University of Tokyo Press 1976, p. 151–158.
59. TAKATA, M., KOIZUMI, K., OCHIAI, M., KAMEMORI, H.: Clinical studies on Neocarzinostatin in gynecological malignant tumors. GANN-TO-KAGAKURYOHO (Cancer & Chemother.) **1**, 801–812 (1974).
60. TAKEDA, K., SEGAWA, Y., AARAKAWA, T.: Therapeutic effect of Bleomycin for skin tumors. GANN (Cancer) **61**, 207–218 (1970).
61. TAKEMASA, Y.: Neocarzinostatin. GANN-TO-KAGAKURYOHO (Cancer & Chemother.) **2**, 515–517 (1975).
62. TAKEMASA, Y.: Clinical results and indication of multiple combination chemotherapy. NIPPON-RINSHO (Jap. J. Clin. Med.) **33**, 1873–1879 (1975).
63. TAKEMASA, Y., KOYAMA, Y.: Chemotherapy of solid tumors, SHINDAN-TO-CHIRYO (Diagnosis and Treatment) **57**, 1832–1840 (1969).
64. TAKEMIYA, S.: Evaluation of Bleomycin in the treatment of head and neck cancers in Japan. Otologia (Fukuoka) **22**, 77–88 (1976).
65. TAKEUCHI, K.: Effect of Bleomycin on brain tumors. In: The GANN Monograph No. 19, Fundamental and Clinical Studies of Bleomycin CARTER, S. K., ICHIKAWA, T., MATHE,G., UMEZAWA, H. (eds.): Tokyo: University of Tokyo Press 1976, p. 117–132.
66. TOMIYAMA, T.: Intracystic administration of antitumor agents to cancer of the bladder. NIHON-HINYOKIKA-GAKKAI-ZASSHI (Jap. J. Urol.) **63**, 497–518 (1972).
67. TSUKAGOSHI, S.: Chromomycin A3. GANN-TO-KAGAKURYOHO (Cancer & Chemother.) **3**, 778–781 (1976).
68. UCHINO, J., SAITO, Y., NOGATA, T., TAKAHASHI, H., KAWAMOTO, K., SHINADA, Y., IKEDA, Y.: Combination chemotherapy with Carbazilquinone, 5-Fluorouracil and Cytosine arabinoside for solid tumor. GANN-TO-KAGAKURYOHO (Cancer & Chemother.) **3**, 953–960 (1976).
69. WATANABE, H., IIZUKA, N., HIRATA, K., SUEMATSU, K.: Local chemotherapy with solid-form-

Bleomycin, supplemental to abdominal lymph node dissection in the surgery of cancer of the esophagus. GANN-TO-KAGAKURYOHO (Cancer & Chemother.) **3**, 485–494 (1976).
70. YAMAGATA, S., UZUKA, Y.: Chemotherapy of malignant diseases—cancer of the gastrointestinal tract—. CHIRYO (Treatment) **56**, 923–932 (1974).
71. YAMAWAKI, S., GOTO, M., CHIKAZAWA, M., SUKEGAWA, K., ISHII, S., SASAKI, T., USUI, M.: Clinical trials of Adriamycin in pulmonary metastasis from Osteosarcoma. GANN-NO-RINSHO (Jap. J. Cancer Clin.) **21**, 323–329 (1975).
72. YOKOYAMA, M., SAITO, T.: Evaluation of cancer chemotherapy from viewpoint of survival of patients with gastric cancer. GANN-TO-KAGAKURYOHO (Cancer & Chemother.) **2**, 367–375 (1975).
73. YOKOYAMA, M., HIMORI, T., UJIIE, S., SAITO, T.: Treatment of malignant neoplasms with Adriamycin. GANN-NO-RINSHO (Jap. J. Cancer Clin.) **20**, 536–544 (1974).

Role of Antitumor Antibiotics in Current Oncologic Practice

H. L. DAVIS, Jr., D. D. VON HOFF, J. E. HENNEY, and M. ROZENCWEIG

The antitumor antibiotics are a heterogeneous group of antineoplastic agents which share a common origin as fermentation products of microbial cultures. This brief review of selected agents will emphasize those agents that play a major role in current oncologic practice in the U.S.A. We are indebted to our Japanese colleagues for their vital role in the preclinical and clinical development of several of the agents in widespread use today. In the course of this discussion, we will present specific points to aid the future development in this important area. Table 1 lists the agents to be described and the areas in which they have exhibited a major impact in clinical practice.

Table 1. Antitumor antibiotics and their major impact in oncologic practice

Drug	Disease—Major impact
Actinomycin D	Trophoblastic disease, germinal tumors of testis and ovary, childhood tumors, Ewing's sarcoma, Kaposi's sarcoma
Mithramycin	Hypercalcemia of malignancy, testicular tumors
Chromomycin A_3	—
Daunomycin	Acute myelogenous leukemia
Adriamycin	Acute myelogenous leukemia, lymphomas, sarcomas, breast cancer
Bleomycin	Testicular, malignant lymphomas
Streptonigrin	—
Mitomycin C	—
Porfiromycin	—
Streptozoticin	Islet cell tumours

Mechanism of Action

The mechanisms of action of the antitumor antibiotics are varied. The actinomycins, mithramycin and chromomycin A_3, bind to DNA and inhibit DNA-dependent RNA synthesis [68, 34, 73, 31] while the anthracycline antibiotics, daunomycin and adriamycin, intercalate between base pairs and inhibit RNA and DNA synthesis [7].

Bleomycin is a peptide which reacts with DNA and uses strand scision [63] but alkylation is the predominant mode of action of streptonigrin, mitomycin C and porfiromycin [g 64]. Streptozoticin has a complex mechanism of action that may include alkylation [54].

The common feature in the mechanisms of action of the antitumor antibiotics seems to be their interaction with DNA. All of these drugs are also relatively non-cycle-specific.

Toxicity

The human toxicology of the antitumor antibiotics is of interest because of the variety of effects encountered.

Acute Toxicities

Myelosuppression is not generally encountered with chromomycin A_3, bleomycin and streptozoticin [35, 3, 58]. Selective myelosuppression, limited to the platelets, is encountered with mithramycin [32]. The problem of cumulative myelosuppression is most apparent with streptonigrin, mitomycin C and profiromycin [44, 41].

Other unusual toxicities include:

1. Hepatotoxicity—mithramycin [32]
2. Renal toxicity—chromomycin A_3 and streptozoticin [55, 6]
3. Hypocalcemia and/or decreased bone resorption—mithramycin and actinomycin D [32, 45]
4. Decreased glucose tolerance—streptozoticin [6, 30]
5. Fever and anaphylaxis—bleomycin [3, 4]

Chronic and Cumulative Toxicities

1. Interstitial pulmonary lesions—bleomycin [3, 4]
2. Arrythmias and EKG changes—daunomycin and adriamycin [72, 70]
3. Congestive cardiomyopathy—daunomycin and adriamycin [70, 37]

Thus, limitations of total cumulative dosage are currently imposed with bleomycin and anthracyclines [70, 36]. This minimizes the adverse effects but limits the duration of effective therapy and thus reduces the overall impact of these highly active agents.

In summary, the antitumor antibiotics present a wide range of toxicities which challenge the supportive facilities of the oncologist. It would seem logical to continue the search for analogues that minimize cumulative myelosuppression, cardiac damage, and pulmonary toxicity as a high priority for future developments in this highly active group of agents.

Overall Antitumor Activity of the Antibiotics

Table 2 outlines the general activity of these agents, grouped according to a general disease classification. The evaluation of activity is based on extensive data, both published and unpublished, on file in the Investigational Drug Branch, Cancer Therapy Evaluation Program, Division of Cancer Treatment. An agent is designated "#" if it had definite clinical activity, alone or in combination with other agents.

In some programs, cure may be possible. An agent is designated "+" if any responses were seen ("hints of activity"). The symbol "−" indicates no activity in at least 14 evaluable patients of the disease type. "NE" is used when the compound has not been tested in at least 14 patients, and includes studies deemed unevaluable for a variety of reasons.

The discussion to follow will emphasize those agents which are currently accepted as major therapeutic advances in selected tumor types. No attempt will be made to cover all investigational applications unless there are implications for the immediate future.

Acute Leukemia

The major accomplishment of therapy with daunomycin or adriamycin has been in acute nonlymphocytic leukemia (ANLL). The role of these agents in acute lymphocytic leukemia has been limited because of the proven value of other agents [24]. Studies incorporating these agents have focused on reinduction of remission or treatment of especially unfavorable stages [28]. Both daunomycin and adriamycin are highly active in acute myelocytic leukemia (AML) and are additive to combinations that include cytosine arabinoside [52]. There are programs in existence that project an overall gain in 2-year survival to 25%–30% [42].

Particularly active are the following induction programs:

Table 2. General activity of the antitumor antibiotics

Disease	Actinomycin D	Mithramycin	Chromomysin A3	Daunomycin	Adriamycin	Bleomycin	Streptonigrin	Mitomycin C	Porfiromycin	Streptozoticin
Acute leukemia	NE	NE	—	# [a]	# [a]	NE	NE	NE	NE	NE
Lymphomas	#	NE	NE	NE	#	#	# [b]	#	NE	#
Childhood solid tumors	# [c]	NE	NE	NE	# [c]	NE	NE	NE	NE	NE
Bone sarcomas	# [c]	+	NE	NE	# [c]	NE	NE	+	NE	NE
Soft tissue sarcomas	#	NE	NE	NE	#	NE	NE	NE	—	+
Kaposi's sarcoma	#	NE	NE	NE	NE	#	NE	NE	NE	NE
Melanoma	#	+	NE	NE	—	NE	NE	+	NE	+
Breast cancer	+	+	+	NE	#	NE	+	#	NE	+
Squamous head and neck, cervix, Esophagus	NE	NE	NE	NE	#	#	+	NE	#	NE
Gastrointestinal adenocarcinoma	NE	+	+	+	#	— / NE [gi]	NE	#	#	+
Endocrine (thyroid, adrenal, islet cell, carcinoid)	NE	NE	NE	NE	# [d]	NE	NE	NE	NE	# [e]
GU (kidney, bladder, prostate)	NE	NE	NE	NE	#	NE	NE	#	NE	NE
GYN (ovary, uterus)	#	NE	NE	NE	#	NE	NE	NE	#	NE
Germ cell (ovary testis)	# [f]	# [f]	NE	NE	+	#	NE	NE	NE	NE
Trophoblastic disease	# [f]	NE	NE	NE	NE	NE	NE	NE	NE	NE
Small cell lung	NE	NE	NE	NE	#	—	NE	+	NE	NE
Non small cell lung	—	+	NE	+	#	#	NE	+	NE	NE

[a] Major impact in acute myelogenous leukemia.
[b] In clinical trial in one group (Cancer and Leukemia Group B, CALGB).
[c] Potentially curative in combined modality treatment.
[d] Acrive in thyroid and carconoma.
[e] Islet cell carcinoma.
[f] May be curative alone or combined with other drugs.
[g] Negative in colon cancer.

= Definite activity.
+ = Hints of activity
— = Not active
NE = Not evaluable.

1. Daunomycyn, Cytosine arabinoside — "7 + 3" [52]
2. Daunomycin, Cytosine arabinoside, Thioguanine — "TAD" [20]
3. Adriamycin, Cytosine arabinoside, Vincristine, Prednisone — "AD-OAP" [42]
4. Daunomycin, 5-Azacytine, Cytosine arabinoside, Vincristine, Prednisone — "D-ZAPO" [1]

As in all programs containing anthracyclines, cardiotoxicity is presently avoided by total dose limitations. A pressing need for cirumventing this hazard is evident in an effort to prolong the period of drug administration.

Malignant Lymphomas

The MOPP combination is currently the therapeutic standard in the treatment of advanced Hodgkin's disease [16]. Bleomycin, in low dosage, is under trial as a nonmyelosuppressive addition to MOPP therapy (BLEO-MOPP). Preliminary reports indicate a higher response rate in direct comparison with MOPP [25]. A satisfactory regimen for patients who have failed MOPP has been developed by BONNADONNA and incorporates adriamycin and bleomycin with vinblastine and imidazole carboxamide [16]. This combination (ABVD) is not crossresistant with MOPP and represents a major therapeutic lead which may improve the rate of cure in this disease.

Likewise, adriamycin has improved the prospects of long-term control for the non-Hodgkin's lymphomas, notably the diffuse histiocytic subset. After six months of therapy, approximately 40% of patients may enjoy prolonged relapse-free survival and, potentially, cure [71]. The most successful current programs involve combinations of adriamycin with prednisone and vincristine (HOP) with the three drugs, plus cytoxan (CHOP, COPA), or the above plus bleomycin (BACOP, CHOP-BLEO) [59, 43, 18].

Childhood Solid Tumors

The most successful applications of antitumor antibiotic therapy have been in Wilms' tumor and embryonal rhabdomyosarcoma [18, 21].

After the original evaluation by Dr. SIDNEY FARBER, the widespread integration of actinomycin D into combined modality therapy has resulted in a cure rate of over 80% in children with localized disease, and up to 60% in patients with pulmonary metastases [14]. Adriamycin and vincristine are likewise highly active and are under investigation in patients with unfavorable presentations [14]. Combinations containing actinomycin D have likewise been highly successful in an aggressive attack on rhabdomyosarcoma of the embryonal variety in children [21].

Bone Sarcomas

Prior to the application of chemotherapy, the prognosis of Ewing's sarcoma was dismal. At least 90% of patients died from metastases. Studies combining actinomycin D, vincristine, and cytoxan (VAC) with aggressive radiation therapy have turned this around with up to 50% disease-free survival at 2 years [51]. Currently, adriamycin has been incorporated into this regimen (VAC-ADRIA) in a multidisciplinary intergroup study [46].

Adriamycin is active as palliative therapy in osteosarcoma and may be curative as adjuvant to amputation. It must be given aggressively. Studies by CORTEZ and HOLLAND have shown that major benefit accrues only to those patients who completed therapy according to doses specified; patients violating the protocol did only modestly better than historical controls [10].

In an effort to reduce the intensity of adriamycin therapy, it has been combined with high dose methotrexate [27] or multiple alkylating agents and vincristine [62]. Results of all these programs indicate a 2-year disease-free survival in excess of 50%.

Soft Tissue Sarcomas

Adriamycin is highly active (30%) in this refractory group of tumors [72, 47]. It has been extensively studied in combination with alkylating agents, vincristine and actinomycin D. However, it is not clear that the combinations are definitely superior to adriamycin alone; nevertheless, the duration of response may be prolonged through the use of multiple agents [22].

Kaposi's sarcoma is a special case. The major trials have been carried out at the Uganda Cancer Institute with comparisons of antinomycin D, actinomycin D with vincristine, and actinomycin D with vincristine and imidazole carboxamide (DTIC) [67, 69, 48]. Progressively better results occurred, culminating in a 94% complete response rate with the three drugs together [48]. The remissions were prolonged but relapse was frequent and the ultimate effect on survival is unknown. Recently, this group has reported 60% short term responses with bleomycin as a secondary therapy [68].

Germ Cell Tumors of Testis and Ovary

The chemotherapy of nonseminomatous testicular carcinomas has involved the use of antitumor antibiotics for years, and is best described in tabular form. Drugs of other origin play an important role, as seen in Table 3.

Certainly, the combination programs pose problems of enhanced toxicity. The number of actual "cures" is unknown at present, but it is reasonable to assume that it will be higher than the 5% cure rate obtained by actinomycin D, mithramycin, or triple therapy [8].

Germ cell tumors of the ovary have been less extensively studied, but triple therapy modifications have been associated with prolonged disease-free survival and probable cure [61].

Table 3. Chemotherapy of testicular carcinoma

Program	% Complete remission	Ref.
Actinomycin D	10+	[8]
Mithramycin	10	[8,10]
Actinomycin D, Chlorambucil, Methotrexate ("triple therapy")	12%	[39]
Vinblastine and Bleomycin	26%	[56]
Vinblastine and Bleomycin infusion	61%	[57]
Vinblastine, Bleomycin, cis platinum, Actinomycin D (VAB II)	48%	[53]
Cytoxan, Vinblastine, Bleomycin, Cis platinum (high dose) and Actinomycin D (VAB III)	63%	[13]
Vinblastine, Bleomycin, Cis platinum (Einhorn)	80%	[17]

Trophoblastic Disease

This entity was the first neoplasm to be cured by single-agent chemotherapy with methotrexate or actinomycin D [40, 49]. Refinements in technique have led to universal application of the biologic marker, human chorionic gonadotropin [63] associated with this disease, and to early treatment for virtually all patients at risk of dissemination[38].

Patients at high risk of death by virtue of markedly elevated (> 100,000 i.u) HCG titers, prolonged course of the disease, or unfavorable metastatic sites (liver, brain, or very extensive lung) are best handled by the immediate use of triple therapy consisting of actinomycin D, methotrexate, and cytoxan [23]. The overall cure rate ranges from 70% for high risk patients to 100% for nonmetastatic trophoblastic disease [38].

Breast Cancer

Adriamycin is the most active single agent for palliation yet uncovered [2, 72, 47] being noncrossresistant with other agents useful in this common tumor [2, 47]. A short duration of response coupled with potential cardiotoxicity limited its use as a single agent [26]; thus, it quickly moved into various combinations, principally with cytoxan, vincristine, and fluorouracil [29, 15, 53]. Response rates have been impressive in some series, but overall, there is no indication that adriamycin adds to duration of response in comparison with combinations not utilizing this agent [26, 65].

Malignant Islet Cell Tumors

The major therapeutic tool for metastatic or locally inoperable islet cell carcinoma is streptozoticin [58, 6]. This is especially true for insulinomas where the largest experience has accrued. Recently, gastronimas have been shown to respond to biochemically to streptozoticin [11]. The largest collected series, reported by BRODER and CARTER, indicates 64% biochemical and 50% measurable physiologic responses in 52 patients [6]. Survival of responders was doubled compared to nonresponders and historical controls.

Hypercalcemia of Malignant Disease

Mithramycin is clearly the agent of choice in hypercalcemia that is not associated with bone destruction by tumor, and is highly effective in steroid-resistant hypercalcemia associated with breast cancer and multiple myeloma [60, 50]. Success with mithramycin is independent of elevated parathormone levels.

Antinomycin D is likewise highly active but has received less investigation [45]. Both agents are active at relatively nontoxic doses and this effect is independent of antitumor activity.

Summary

The antitumor antibiotics have thus made a major impact on oncologic practice. The continued search for productive strains of these organisms should be encouraged. In addition, the activity and toxicity spectrum suggests the need for vigorous analog development. An active anthracycline devoid of cardiotoxicity; a bleomycin with no effect on pulmonary tissue; an analog of streptozoticin devoid of nephrotoxicity; these would be advances of inestimable benefit to the cancer patient of the future.

References

1. Baehner, R. L., Bernstein, I. O., Higgins, G., Mc Creadie, S., Chard, R. L., Hammond, D.: improved induction remission response in children with acute non-lymphocytic leukemia treated with daunomycin, 5-azacytidine, cytosine arabinoside, prednisone, and vincristine (D-ZAPO). Proc. Am. Assoc. Cancer Res. and Am. Soc. Cl. Oncology (in press) (1977).
2. Blum, R. H., Carter, S. K.: Adriamycin, a new anticancer drug with significant clinical activity. Ann. Intern. Med. **80**, 249–259 (1974).
3. Blum, R. H., Carter, S. K.: Agre, K.: A clinical review of bleomycin: a new antineoplastic agent. Cancer **31**, 903–913 (1973).
4. Bonadonna, G.;, De Lena, M., Monfardini: S., Bartoli, C., Bajetta, E., Beretta, G., Fossati-bellani, F.: Clinical trials with bleomycin in lymphomas and solid tumors. Eur. J. Cancer **8**, 205–215 (1972).
5. Bonnadonna, G., Zucilli, R., Monfardini, S., De Lena, M., Uslenghi, C.: Combination chemotherapy of Hodgkin's disease with adriamycin, bleomycin, vinblastine, and imidazole carboxamide versus MOPP. Cancer **36**, 252–259 (1975).
6. Broder, L. E., Carter, S. K.: Pancreatic islet cell carcinoma II: results of therapy with streptozoticin in 52 patients. Ann. Intern. Med. **79**, 108–118 (1973).
7. Calendi, E., Di Marco, A., Regiani, M., Et Al: On physico-chemical interactions between daunomycin and nucleic acids. Biochem. Biophys. Acta. **103**, 25–49 (1965).
8. Carter, S. K. Wasserman, T. H.: The chemotherapy of urologic cancer. Cancer **36**, 729–747 (1975).
9. Cohen, M., Shaw, M. W., Craig, A. P.: The effects of streptonigrin in cultured human leucocytes. Proc. Natl. Acad. Sci. USA **50**, 16–24 (1963).
10. Cohen, M. H., Hrushesky, W., Minna, J. D.: Chemotherapy response after initial treatment failure in small cell bronchogenic carcinoma. Proc. Am. Assoc. Cancer Res. and Am. Soc. Clin. Oncology **17**, 112 (1976).
11. Cortez, E. P., Holland, J. F., Wang, J. J., Sinks, L. F., Blom, J., Senn, H., Bank, A., Glidewell, O.: Amputation and adriamycin in primary osteosarcoma. N. Engl. J. Med. **291**, 998–1000 (1974).
12. Cvitkovic, E., Wittes, R., Golbey, R., Krakoff, I. H.: Primary combination chemotherapy (VAB II) for metastatic or unrespectable germ cell tumors. Proc. Am. Assoc. Cancer Res. and Am. Soc. Clin. Oncology **16**, 174 (1975).
13. Cvitkovic, E., Hayes, D., Golbey, R.: Primary combination chemotherapy (VAB III) for metastatic or unresectable germ cell tumors. Proc. Am. Assoc. Cancer Res. and Am. Soc. Clin. Oncology **17**, 296 (1976).
14. D'Angio, G. J. Evans, A. E., Breslow, N., Beckwith, B., Bishop, H., Feigl, P., Goodwin, W., Leapi, L. L., Sinks, L. F., Sutow, W., Tefft, M., Wolff, J.: The treatment of Wilms' tumor: results of the National Wilms' tumor study. Cancer **38**, 633–646 (1976).
15. De Lena, M., Brambilla, C., Morabito: A., Bonadonna, G.: Adriamycin plus vincristine compared to and combined with cyclo-phosphamide, methotrexate, and 5-fluorouracil for advanced breast cancer. Cancer **35**, 1108–1115 (1975).
16. De Vita, V. T., Canellos, G. P., Moxley, J. H., III: A decade of combination therapy of advanced Hodgkin's disease. Cancer **30**, 1495–1504 (1972).
17. Einhorn, L. H., Donohue, J. P.: Improved chemotherapy in disseminated testicular cancer. J. Urol. **117**, 65–69 (1977).
18. Farber, S.: Chemotherapy in the treatment of leukemia and Wilm's tumor. JAMA **198**, 826–836 (1966).
19. Frei, E., III: The clinical use of actinomycin. Cancer Chemother. Rep. **58**, 49–54 (1974).
20. Gale, R. P., Cline, J. J.: High remission induction rate in acute myeloid leukemia. Lancet **1977/I**, 497–499.
21. Ghavini, F., Exelby, P. R., D'Angio, G. J., Cham, W., Lieberman, P. H., Tam, C., Miki, V., Murphy, M. L.: Multidisciplinary treatment of embryonal rhabdomyosarcoma in children. Cancer **35**, 667–686 (1975).
22. Gottlieb, J. A., Baker, L. H., Burgess, M. A., Sinkovics, J. G., Moon, T., Bodey, G. P., Rodrigues, V., Rivkin, S. E., Saiki, J., O'Bryan, R. M.: Sarcoma chemotherapy. In: Cancer Chemotherapy. Chicago: Yearbook Medical Publishers 1975, pp. 445–454.
23. Hammond, C. B., Parker, R. T.: Diagnosis and treatment of trophoblastic disease; a report from the Southeastern Regional Center. Obstet. Gynecol. **35**, 132–143 (1970).
24. Holland, J. F., Glidewell, O.: Chemotherapy of acute lymphocytic leukemia of childhood. Cancer **30**, 1480–1487 (1972).
25. Hoogstraten, B., Chairman of the Southwest Oncology Group: Personal communication.
26. Hoogstraten, B., George, S. L., Samal, B., Rivkin, S. E., Costanzi, J. J., Bonnet, J. D.,

Thigpen, T., Braine, H.: Combination chemotherapy and adriamycin in patients with advanced breast cancer. Cancer **38**, 13–20 (1976).
27. Jaffee, N., Frei, E., III: Osteogenia sarcoma: advances in treatment. CA. **26**, 351–359 (1976).
28. Jones, B., Cuttner, J., Levy, R. N., Patterson, R. B., Kung, F., Pleuss, H. J., Falkson, G., Treat, C. L., Haurani: F., Burgert, E. O., Jr., Rosner, F., Carey, R. W., Lukens, J., Blom, J., Degnan, T. J., Wohl, H., Glidewell, O., Holland, J. F.: Daunorubicin (NSC-83142) versus daunorubicin plus prednisone (NSC-10023 versus daunorubicin plus vincristine (NSC-065) plus prednisone in advanced childhood acute leukemia. Cancer Chemother. Rep. **56**, 729–737 (1972).
29. Jones, S. D., Durie, B. G. M., Salmon, S. E.: Combination chemotherapy with adriamycin and cyclophosphamide for advanced breast cancer. Cancer **36**, 90–97 (1975).
30. Junod, A., Lambert, A. E., Stauffacher, W., Renold, A. E.: Diabetogenic action of streptozoticin: Invest. **48**, 2129–2139 (1969).
31. Kaziro, Y., Kamiyama, M.: Mechanism of action of chromomycin A_3 II: inhibition of RNA polymerase reaction. J. Biochem. (Tokyo) **62**, 424–429 (1967).
32. Kennedy, B. J.: Metabolic and toxic effects of mithramycin during tumor therapy. Am. J. Med. **49**, 494–503 (1970).
33. Kennedy, B. J.: Mithramycin therapy in advanced neoplasms. Cancer **30**, 755–766 (1970).
34. Kirk, J. M.: The mode of action of actinomycin D. Biochem. Biophys. Acta **42**, 167–169 (1960).
35. Kovach, J. S., Moertel, C. G., Ahmann, D. L., et al: Phase I study of chromomycin A_3 (NSC-58514). Cancer Chemother. Rep. **57**, 341–347 (1973).
36. Lefrak, E. A., Qitha, T., Rosenblum, S., Gottlieb, J. A.: Clinicopathologic analysis of adriamycin cardiotoxicity. Cancer **32**, 302–314 (1973).
37. Lenaz, L., Page, J. A.: Cardiotoxicity of adriamycin and related anthracyclines. Cancer Treat. Rev. **3**, 111–120 (1976).
38. Lewis, J. L., Jr.: Chemotherapy of gestational choriocarcinoma. Cancer **30**, 1517–1521 (1972).
39. Li, M. C., Whitmore, W. F., Golbey, R., Grabstadt, H.: Effects of combined drug therapy on metastatic cancer of the testis. JAMA **174**, 1291–1299 (1960).
40. Li, M. C., Hertz: T., Spencer, D. B.: Effect of methotrexate therapy upon choriocarcinoma and chorioadenoma. Proc. Soc. Exp. Biol. Med. **93**, 361–366 (1976).
41. Loo, R. V., Vaitkevicius, V. R., Reed, M. L., Vaughn, C. B.: Phase I trial of porfiromycin (NSC-56410). Cancer Chemother. Rep. **51**, 497 (1967).
42. Mc Credie, K. B., Hewlett, J. S., Kennedy, A.: The chemoimmuno-therapy of acute leukemia (CIAL), a cooperative group study. Proc. Am. Assoc. Cancer Res. and Am. Soc. Clin. Oncology **17**, 239 (1976).
43. Mc Kelvey, E. M., Gottlieb, J. A., Wilson, H. E., Haut, A., Talley, R. W., Stephens, R., Lane, M., Gamble, J. F., Jones, S. E., Grozea, P. N., Gutterman, J., Coltman, D., Jr., Moon, T. E.: Hydroxyldaunomycin (adriamycin) combination chemotherapy in malignant lymphoma. Cancer **38**, 1484–1493 (1976).
44. Moertel, C. G., Reitmeier, R. J., Hahn, R. G.: Mitomycin C therapy in advanced gastrointestinal cancer. JAMA **204**, 1045–1048 (1969).
45. Muggia, F. M., Heinemann, H. O.: Hypercalcemia associated with neoplastic disease. Ann. Intern Med. **73**, 281–290 (1970).
46. Nesbit, M.E.: Ewing's sarcoma. CA. **26**, 174–180 (1976).
47. O'bryan, R. M., Luce, J. K., Talley, R. W., Gottlieb, J. A., Baker, L. H., Bonadonna, G.: Phase II evaluation of adriamycin in human neoplasia. Cancer **32** (1), 1–8 (1973).
48. Olweny, C. L. M., Toya, T., Katongole-mbidde, E., Lwanga, S. K., Owor, R., Kyalwazi, S., Vogel, C. L.: Treatment of Kaposi's sarcoma by combination of actinomycin-D, vincristine and imidazole (NSC-45388): results of a randomized clinical trial. Int. J. Cancer **14**, 549–656 (1974).
49. Osathanondh, R. O., Goldstein, D. P., Pastorfide, G. B.: Actinomycin D as the primary agent for gestational trophoblastic disease. Cancer **36**, 1517–1521 (1972).
50. Perlia, C. P., Gubisch, N. J., Wolter, J., Edelberg, D., Dederick, M. M., Taylor, S. G., III: Mithramycin treatment of hypercalcemia. Cancer **30**, 389–394 (1970).
51. Pomeroy, T. C., Johnson, R. E.: Combined modality therapy of Ewing's sarcoma. Cancer **35**, 36–47 (1975).
52. Rai, K. R., Holland, J. F., Glidewell, O.: Improvement in remission induction therapy of acute myelocytic leukemia. Proc. Am. Assoc. Cancer Res. **16**, 265 (1975).
53. Ramirez, G., Weiss, A., The Central Oncology Group: A phase II study of adriamycin: 5 FU given weekly in the treatment of solid tumors. Am. Assoc. Cancer Res. and Am. Soc. Clin. Oncology **17**, 248 (1976).
54. Reusses, F.: Mode of action of streptozoticin. J. Bacteriol. **105**, 580–588 (1971).
55. Reynolds, R. D., Fisher, J. I., Jensen, P. A., Pajak, T. F., Bateman, J. R.: Phase I alternate-day dose study of chromomycin A_3. Cancer Treat. Rep. **60** 1251–1255 (1976).
56. Samuels, M. L., Hooloye, P. Y., Johnson, D. E.: Bleomycin combination chemotherapy in the

management of testicular neoplasia. Cancer **36**, 318–326 (1975).
57. SAMUELS: M. L., BOYLE, L. E., HOLOYE, P. Y., JOHNSON, D. E.: Intermittent versus continuous infusion bleomycin in testicular cancer: a comparison of response and survival in embryonal carcinoma (class 2) and teratocarcinoma (class 3 & 4). Proc. Am. Assoc. Cancer Res. and Am. Soc. Clin. Oncology **17**, 98 (1976).
58. SCHEIN, P. S., O'CONNELL, M. J., BLOM, J., HUBBARD, S., MAGRATH, I. T., BERGEVIN, P., WIERNIK, P. H., ZIEGLER, J. L., DE VITA, V. T.: Clinical antitumor activity and toxicity of streptozoticin (NSC-85998). Cancer **34**, 993-1000 (1974).
59. SCHEIN, P. S., DE VITA, V. T., HUBBARD, S., CHABNER, B. A., CANELLAS, G. P., BERARD, C., YOUNG, R. C.: Bleomycin, adriamycin, cyclophosphamide, vincristine and prednisone (BACOP): combination chemotherapy in the treatment of advanced diffuse histiocytic lymphoma. Ann. Intern. Med. **85**, 417–422 (1976).
60. SLAYTON, R. E., SHRUDER, B. I., ELIAS, E., HORTON, J., PERLILIA, C. P.: New approach to the treatment of hypercalcemia. The effect of short-term treatment with mithramycin. Clin. Pharmacol. Ther. **12**, 832–837 (1971).
61. SMITH, J. P., RUTLEDGE, F.: Advances in chemotherapy for gynecologic cancer. Cancer **36**, 669–674 (1975).
62. SUTOW, W. W., GEHAN, E. A., VIETTI, T. J., FRIAS, A. E., DYMENT, O. G.: Multidrug chemotherapy in primary treatment of osteosarcoma. J. Bone Joint Surg. (Am.) (5), 629–633 (1976).
63. SUZUKI, M., NAGAI, R., YAMAKI, H., TANAHA, N., UMEZAWA, H.: Mechanism of action of bleomycin: studies with growing culture of bacterial and tumor cells. J. Antibiot. (Tokyo) **21**, 379–386 (1968).
64. SZYBALSKI, W., EYER, V. N.: Crosslinking of DNA by enzymatically or chemically activated mitomycins and profiromycins, bifunctionally "alkylating" antibiotics. Fed. Proc. **23**, 946 (1964).
65. TRANUM, B., HOOGSTRATEN, B.: Adriamycin in combination for treatment of breast cancer. Am. Assoc. Cancer Res. and Am. Soc. Clin. Oncology **17**, 242 (1976).
66. UMEZAWA, H.: Principles of antitumor antibiotic therapy. In: Cancer Medicine. HOLLAND, J. F., FREI, E. (eds.) Philadelphia: Lea & Febiger 1973, pp. 817–826.
67. VOGEL, C. L., TEMPLETOM, C. J., TEMPLETON, A. C., TAYLOR, J. F., KYALWAZI, S. K.: Treatment of Kaposi's sarcoma with actinomycin-D and cyclophosphamide: results of a randomized clinical trial. Int. J. Cancer **8**, 136–143 (1971).
68. VOGEL, C. L., CLEMENTS, D., WANUME, A. K., TOYA, T., PRIMACK, A., KYALWAZI, S.: Phase II clinical trials of BCNU (NSC-409962) and bleomycin (NSC-125066) in the treatment of Kaposi's sarcoma. Cancer Chemother. Rep. **57**, 325–332 (1973).
69. VOGEL, C. L., PRIMACK, A., DHRU, D., BRIERS, P., OWOR, R., KYALWAZI, S. K.: Treatment of Kaposi's sarcoma with a combination of antinomycin D and vincristine. Cancer **31**, 1382–1391 (1973).
70. VON HOFF, D. D., ROZENCWEIG, M., LAYARD, M., SLAVIK, M., MUGGIA, F. M.: Daunomycin-induced cardiotoxicity in children and adults: a review of 110 cases. Am. J. Med. **62**, 200–208 (1976).
71. VON HOFF, D. D., ROZENCWEIG, M., SLAVIK, M.: Daunomycin: an antitumor antibiotic with activity in acute leukemia. Kanser **6**, 1–16 (1976).
72. WEISS, A. J., METTER, G. E., FLETCHER, W. S., WILSON, W. L., GRAGE, T. B., RAMIREZ, G.: Studies on adriamycin using a weekly regimen demonstrating its clinical effectiveness and lack of cardiac toxicity. Cancer Treat. Rep. **60**, 813–822 (1976).
73. YARBRO, J. W., BARNUM, C. P., KENNEDY, B. J.: Mithramycin inhibition of RNA synthesis. Cancer Res. **26**, 36 (1966).

Historical Overview of the National Cancer Institute Fermentation Program

S. A. Schepartz

In this report I will attempt to outline briefly the early history of the Chemotherapy Program of the National Cancer Institute (NCI) with particular emphasis on fermentation products. The detailed reports by Endicott in 1957 [1] and Zubrod et al in 1966 [3] discussed at considerable length the many factors that influenced the early development of the program. Although it is not possible to discuss those factors in detail here, I will attempt to present some of the highlights.

There were many early programs in cancer drug development in the United States, particularly the collaborative program under Shear [2] at NCI. It was not until after World War II, however, that several scientific discoveries occurred that greatly increased the interest in chemotherapy. First was the well-known accidental discovery of the effects of mustard gas on blood elements that led to nitrogen mustard and opened the entire field of alkylating agents. Second were the folic acid studies that resulted in the development of aminopterin and opened the field of antimetabolites. Third, was the rapid expansion in the antibiotic field and the discovery that some of the antibiotics, particularly the actinomycins, possessed antitumor properties. It thus appeared reasonable to conclude that new active drugs could be discovered. In the absence of sufficient knowledge to design drugs on a rational basis, a wide variety of chemical structures were screened in experimental tumor systems in order to select drugs for clinical trial. The testing capacity at the Sloan-Kettering Institute, where most screening was being done, was insufficient to cope with the demand. As a result of these and other needs, as recognized in both the scientific and public segments of the community, the Cancer Chemotherapy National Service Center (CCNSC) was created in 1955 to provide the following important services:

1. The establishment of experimental tumors for screening agents submitted by chemists who were specifically designing antitumor drugs, or who wished to have their compounds tested for other reasons.
2. The establishment of resources for preparing additional quantities of selected compounds for further testing in experimental systems, pharmacology and clinical studies.
3. A limited amount of new synthesis, concentrating on areas of specific program interest. It should be noted that the majority of synthetic efforts were, and still are, supported by research grants.
4. Development of resources for the preparation of clinical dose formulations.
5. The evaluation of endocrine materials in specialized systems and the development of agents of interest in those systems.
6. Toxicology and pharmacology studies on compounds intended for clinical trial.
7. Studies on the biochemical mechanisms of action of active drugs.
8. Development of clinical resources for the evaluation of new and old agents.

   Since the CCNSC had no laboratories of its own until the late 1960's (and even then only limited facilities), essentially all preclinical work was carried out by contracts with academic and other research institutions and with the chemical and pharmaceutical industry. Clinical studies were supported largely by grants.

From the very beginning of the program, new drugs for testing by CCNSC arose from a variety of sources:

1. Compounds synthesized by chemists on the basis of biochemical or other specific rationales.
2. Compounds synthesized as potential agents against other diseases.
3. Materials already showing activity in some other system whether rationally designed or not.
4. A wide variety of chemical structures with no prior biologic or biochemical rationale.
5. Fermentation, plant and other natural products developed as potential antitumor agents, or for other diseases.

Because of the outstanding success of fermentation products in the antibacterial field and the known antitumor activity of actinomycin D, fermentation products were recognized very early as potentially valuable sources of new active structures.

For legal reasons, it was not feasible at the beginning of the program to undertake comprehensive research and development contract programs with pharmaceutical companies. Therefore, the initial arrangements with those organizations involved the submission of crude broths for in vivo screening in one of the routine CCNSC contract laboratories. Bristol Laboratories was the first organization to submit broths, late in 1956, and was quickly followed by a large number of industrial and academic suppliers. In all cases, if reproducible activity was observed, the material was pursued by the supplier at his own expense, with the CCNSC continuing to provide in vivo testing capacity as a bioassay tool.

Such tests are, of course, exceedingly variable, timeconsuming, expensive, and require large amounts of test substance. A contract program was, therefore, initiated with the Upjohn Company and others to develop cell culture bioassays. They were highly successful in developing in vitro bioassay techniques, especially for the analysis of chromatographically separated fractions. The availability of such cell culture and other in vitro assay systems has greatly speeded up the rate of purification of active materials, although there have been some cases where only the in vivo activity could be used. In those cases, the time and effort required to obtain a pure material was indeed very long.

Although there was great interest on the part of the CCNSC collaborators in pursuing active leads, competition for resources, particularly in industry, prevented their devoting the manpower required for an aggressive effort so progress during the first few years was unfortunately rather slow. This situation was recognized and fortunately a change in the Government patent policy was approved specifically for this program, allowing industry to retain the rights to inventions made under research and development contracts. Comprehensive contracts, including fermentation, chemical isolation, pilot-plant production, and other necessary aspects of a total program were initiated, beginning with Upjohn early in 1959 and followed shortly afterward by Pfizer, Bristol and others.

Although many changes in approach have occurred since the late 1950's, the basic principles established at that time have continued to the present. They include (1) reliance on in vivo systems for selecting materials for clinical trials, (2) maximum possible use of in vitro assays, and (3) early elimination of duplicates. Through continued review of old methods, active search for new approaches, and the willingness to try new ideas, we hope to arrive closer to an optimal system or systems. We sincerely believe that an active interchange of ideas with other investigators, particularly the Japanese fermentation experts, will help us immeasurably in reaching that goal.

Summary

The background of the National Cancer Institute fermentation program is placed into the historical perspective of the entire NCI drug development program, which began as the Cancer Chemotherapy National Service Center and metamorphosed into the Chemotherapy Program and ultimately into the Division of Cancer Treatment.

References

1. ENDICOTT, K.: The chemotherapy program. JNCI **19**, 275–293 (1957).
2. SHEAR, M. J., HARTWELL, J. L., PETERS, V. B., DALTON, A. J., DUNN, T. B., HAUSCHKA, T. S., DILLER, I. C., MCCONNELL, J. R., OAKEY, R., REIMAN, S. P., REES, C. W., BECK, L. V., HOLLOMAN, A. L.: Some aspects of a joint institutional research program on chemotherapy of cancer: current laboratory and clinical experiments with bacterial polysaccharide and with synthetic organic compounds. In: Approaches to Tumor Chemotherapy. Moulton, F. R. (ed.) Washington, D.C.: Amer. Assoc. Advance. Sci. 1947, pp. 236–284.
3. ZUBROD, C. G., SCHEPARTZ, S., LEITER, J., ENDICOTT, K. M., CARRESE, L. M., BAKER, C. G.: The chemotherapy program of the National Cancer Institute: history, analysis, and plans. Cancer Chemother. Rep. **50**, 349–540 (1966).

National Cancer Institute's Fermentation Development Program

J. D. DOUROS

Summary

The present National Cancer Institute (NCI) fermentation antineoplastic development program is reviewed. The program regarding the isolation of microorganisms, their fermentation, screening productivity, antineoplastic structures of interest, and future plans follows.

NCI initiated its fermentation program in 1956 and, during the next four years, the primary organisms isolated and screened for their abilities to produce antineoplastic agents were fungi. Undoubtedly, the use of fungi was dictated by the early success of penicillin as an antimicrobial agent. [2] From 1960 to 1975, the isolation and fermentation of streptomycetes dominated the program. During this same period, *Streptomyces* were the most prolific organisms for the production of novel antimicrobial antibiotics, but this does not necessarily mean they would be the best producers of antineoplastic agents. During these years approximately 700 microbial metabolites, obtained by worldwide surveillance or by NCI sponsored research, were tested in various NCI in vivo screens (L1210, S180, Ca 755, Walker 256) While this research resulted in the discovery of several excellent antineoplastic antibiotics such as streptozotocin, mithramycin, adriamycin (Italian) and bleomycin (Japanese), it was decided that other unusual organisms might yield different, and possibly better, anticancer agents.

Streptomyces have been an excellent source of a number of antimicrobial antibiotics, however, under the test conditions previously used, these organisms have been a relatively poor source of antifungal or antiviral substances. [2] Results of the NCI program, during this period, indicated that the same agents were being rediscovered at a high rate. The program was redirected in late 1974. The emphasis was placed on obtaining a multitude of new organisms; to ferment them under unusual conditions, and to utilize more prescreens to obtain new types of structures. Hopefully, these efforts would increase the number of in vivo active beers and thus increase the total number of novel compounds isolated. Prescreens should conserve effort in that fewer fermentation broths would be subjected to in vivo testing. Prescreens may also identify new activities which might be caused by new chemical structures and simultaneously increase the efficiency of the in vivo tests.

The following data summarizes the current NCI contract research program. However, since the materials isolated during 1975 and 1976 have not yet reached clinical trials, it is too early to obtain a good measure of success of the overall program. Preliminary data indicates success in obtaining novel antineoplastic agents active against animal tumors.

Methodology

The first step in the NCI antineoplastic microbial metabolite program is to obtain a multitude of different types of microbes and to then evaluate their fermentations for the presence of anticancer agents (Table 1). Many known cultures are being grown on unusual carbon compounds, possibly under cometabolism conditions, and tested for their ability to biotransform compounds of interest to NCI. [14] The primary effort in obtaining cultures is to actually isolate them from various soils (collected worldwide) and other sources (Table 1). Isolation of organisms is primarily done using sprinkle-plate techniques and using varying environmental conditions, e.g., temperature (15°C–50°C), pH (2–9), and unique carbon and nitrogen sources (Table 2). Enrichment and percolation techniques are being used. The purification of these organisms is accomplished using standard microbial techniques. [21] Efforts have been initiated to isolate and evaluate new classes of organisms which are not typically evaluated by the pharmaceutical industry.

Organisms such as *Micromonospora*, *Microbiospora*, *Chainia*, *Actinomadura* and *Mycobacteriales* are being scheduled for evaluation of their fermentation potential and ability to produce antineoplastic compounds. In addition, a systematic evaluation of individual families of the microbial world is being conducted to identify their potential as producers of antineoplastic agents. Arthrobacter species (>100 cultures) are the first group of organisms undergoing systematic evaluation.

NCI scientists feel that the actinomycetales have been thoroughly evaluated for their ability to produce antineoplastic agents using common carbon sources and complex nondefined media for growth. For present studies, various carbon sources (as sole source of carbon) have been incorporated into our isolation and fermentation media (Tables 3 and 4). In addition, isoxazoles, n-methyl piperazine, etc. are being used as co-oxidation substrates (Tables 4–9).

The expense of testing numerous fermentation broths in vivo is high. Also, active materials often occur in only minute amounts in initial fermentations and only the most potent drugs in low concentrations, or those in largest amounts would be detected in typical in vivo tests. Some contractors recycle inactive fermentations and concentrates by lyophilization or by chemical extraction followed by lyophilization. This concentrates any active compounds which may then be retested and the activity of interest identified. Many of the most potent drugs are extremely cytotoxic and one feels that many worthwhile drugs are probably missed because they exist in such low and undetectable concentrations. The activity of a drug in the crude fermentation mixture may be masked by the presence of other toxic materials; alternatively the active compound itself may be rendered inactive by being bound to other substances.

With the above reasons as guidelines, NCI felt it would be prudent to identify worthwhile in vitro prescreens which could effectively monitor the isolation of new active chemicals of potential interest, even when present in low concentrations. Hopefully, the existing NCI animal tumor in vivo tests will correlate with the prescreen activities. If such correlation does not exist, additional meaningful tests would have to be added to the prescreens or to the in vivo test system.

The in vitro cell cytotoxicity tests to be used were KB (human epidermoid carcinoma of the nasopharynx), P388 mouse leukemia (PS), and L1210 mouse leukemia (LE). Broths have been manufactured which contain compounds which are selectively cytotoxic for the above mentioned cell lines. The infectious bronchitis virus (RNA) cilia test is another screen used to obtain antiviral agents. To date, this test has not been productive and will be dropped if no leads of note are obtained in the near future.

Enzyme screens are being used by scientists on our contract with the Institute of Microbial Chemistry (Japan) to find compounds with specific enzyme inhibitory properties. The enzymes used are proteases, cAMP phosphodiesterase, RNA-dependent DNA polymerase, and S-adenosyl methionine decarboxylase. In some cases, culture filtrates are being examined for their binding activity with microtubules to identify compounds possessing vincristine or maytansine-like activity.

Proteases are used because of their importance in membrane phenomena, cAMP phosphodiesterase because of its high concentration in brain tumors, RNA-dependent DNA polymerase because reverse transcriptase is necessary to make the RNA virus replicate and cause viral oncogensis. [22] S-adenosylmethionine decarboxylase is used because many scientists feel that the inhibition of methionine metabolism would kill certain tumor cells which require this amino acid. This reasoning is similar to the rationale which was used for asparaginase.

The expansion of new prescreen systems is being contemplated for use in the fermentation program; some of the systems being considered are listed in Table 5. Various contractors determine at different times whether the antineoplastic activity in fermentation broths is due to a known or novel compound. This timing, and the method used, varies from contract to contract. NCI has found that when contractors make a partial determination of the possible novelty of a compound early in the program flow, these researchers have the greatest success rate in obtaining new antineoplastic agents. This is because the limited resources of a contract can be concentrated on materials which seem novel and are not wasted in the isolation of known antineoplastic drugs. If novelty is determined late, a marked dilution of effort occurs in the microbiology and chemistry research effort, and also a greater cost is encountered per novel compound. It has been observed that certain types of antineoplastic agents have a particular antimicrobial spectrum, and this technique in conjunction with mutants (actinomycin D sensitive, etc.) can be used as one of the presumptive identifying tools of compound novelty. Highly qualified microbial taxonomists can often determine what group of compounds might be produced from a culture by identifying subtle cultural morphologic characteristics in the organisms. Finally, some simple extractions and preliminary paper or thin layer chromatography can often bracket a fermentation broth's active compound into a group such as the anthracyclines. One must be cautious, when a broth contains a known antibiotic, that the activity observed correlates with the chemical isolated. Sometimes, known antibiotics are found in a fermentation and have no antineoplastic activity. The antibiotic fermentation broth does contain antineoplastic activity therefore another interesting compound is in the broth.

A presumptive identification allows the chemist to more quickly determine whether the active compound is a novel antitumor agent or a known one. The final determination ultimately requires compound isolation, purification, and identification. Compounds which are already known antineoplastic agents or of a group NCI has found to be of no interest will be dropped or given a low priority. Cursory dereplication studies are accomplished first on fermentations showing good reproducible in vivo activity. Complete dereplication indicates the presence of a novel compound (Table 6). Results obtained in 1976 indicate that the present approach to obtaining new cultures which produce novel antineoplastic agents is bearing fruit. However, the final benefit of obtaining new drugs is to find a sufficient number which have clinical antineoplastic activity. The relative success of obtaining clinically valuable compounds using the above approach will probably require several years for proper evaluation (Table 7).

The increased number of novel compounds found by these methods compared to earlier methods is quite interesting. [10] While the results are not complete or comprehensive, it appears that certain substrates (terpenes and carboxylic acids) used in isolation and fermentation experiments are not yielding active fermentations. While amino acids are ideal carbon sources for culture isolation, they appear to be of little value as fermentation substrates for the production of anticancer active drugs (Table 8).

The major improvements, indicated by the 1976 statistics, are the greater number of presumed novel materials being assigned for chemical fractionation and the numbers of novel crystalline materials obtained for evaluation by the NCI tumor screens. These statistics do not include figures obtained through our biotransformation contract which has yielded five compounds of interest to date.

One contractor evaluated an antimetabolite screen and, while not overly productive in finding new leads, two of these leads progressed through the NCI program to Decision Network 2, a committee at NCI which determines if a compound should continue to toxicology, pharmacology and clinical trials. These compounds were isoxazoles which showed activity against the leukemias. One of these, NSC-163501 is being prepared in larger quantities for toxicologic evaluation (Fig. 1).

Cultures isolated	Antimetabolite activity detected	Confirmed in vivo	No. of new chemicals	Novel antineoplastic agents
11,600	585	12	8	2

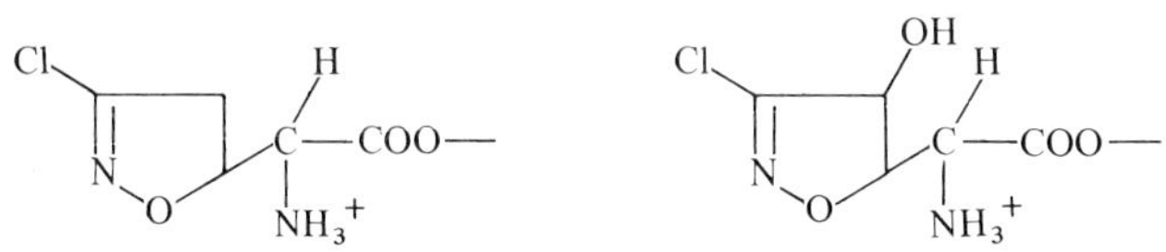

Fig. 1. Antimetabolite prescreen activity

Antimetabolite activity determined by HANKA [11] has been observed with 13 cultures obtained through our new isolation program. The antimetabolite activity was reversed by asparagine (2 cultures), glutamine (3 cultures), histidine (3 cultures), tyrosine (1 culture), fructose (3 cultures), and ribose (1 culture).

The reproducibility of fermentations of interest has been extremely good, and few problems have been observed while scaling up to fermentations of > 50 liters. Approximately 25 fermentation products (Table 9) are undergoing tumor panel testing and some have shown positive results in one test against the solid tumors (Table 10). These will be candidates for test formulation and toxicology if the retests are active.

Only about 20% of the organisms which reconfirm antineoplastic activity in their fermentations require fermentation-improvement studies. Typical methods used to increase the production potential of the organism are shown in (Table 11).

A fermentation facility has been developed at Ft. Detrick, Maryland which allows the NCI to take leads obtained at the shake-flask level by universities, etc. and scale-up production to 3,000 gal. In addition, many contractors (pharmaceutical companies) have capacities which include 20,000 gal fermentors to produce new agents for the NCI. This fermentation capacity will ensure that the natural-products chemists will obtain sufficient material to isolate adequate quantities of the compound for evaluating its activity and determining its structure. There should also be enough for the preparation of analogs which may enhance a compound's potential as an antineoplastic agent (Table 12). The pure compounds are evaluated as suggested in Step III of Fig. 4.

In addition to compounds obtained from NCI's research program, another 80–125 materials are added to the screen through a worldwide surveillance program. [11] These materials are obtained from outstanding scientists in industrial companies and research institutes. The compounds are obtained only when they fulfill the criteria indicated in Step II (Table 13). Several clinical and preclinical drugs have been evaluated by NCI through this surveillance program. Bleomycin, Adriamycin, Daunomycin, and others, represent clinically active drugs which were brought into the program by NCI. Aclacinomycin, Aphidicolin, Bleomycin PEP and PYP, Showdomycin, and others were obtained by surveillance and are at present in various stages of preclinical testing.

Results

Several compounds of interest to NCI but which are not yet clinically useful drugs are discussed.

Aclacinomycin. This drug is a cinarubin-like anthracycline which was originally obtained by the Japanese and reviewed by the NCI Anthracycline Committee. This drug is scheduled for testing to determine its degree of cardiac toxicity. The drug is quite active against animal tumors (Fig. 2).

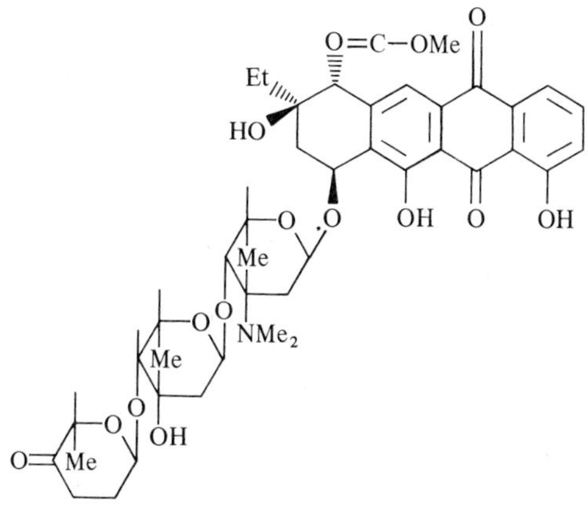

Fig. 2. Aclacinomycin—NSC-208734

Actinomycin PIP 1β. This compound is a peptide with a phenoxazine chromophore. The compound came out of the biotransformation program and has shown activity, in B16 in animals, that is superior to the present clinically used drug, actinomycin D. It is being considered for clinical trials but additional testing is scheduled (Fig. 3).

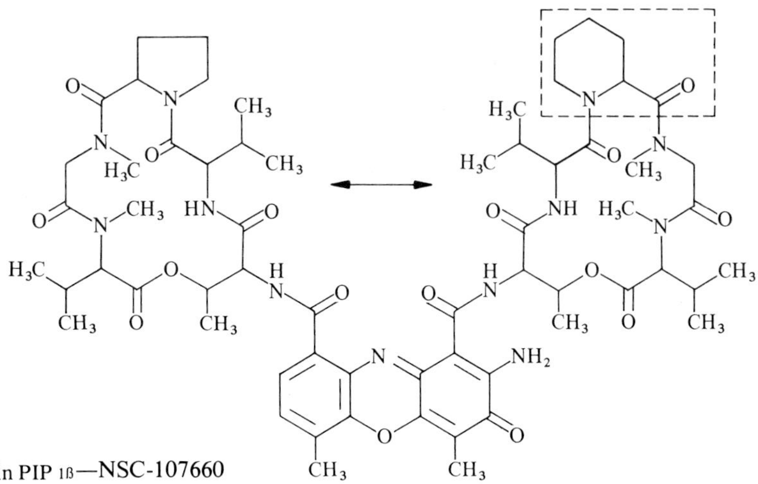

Fig. 3. Actinomycin PIP 1β—NSC-107660

Anguidine. This drug is a scirpinol which is of fungal (Fusarium) origin and it is similar to many mycotoxins. This antibiotic is underoing Phase II clinical studies (Fig. 4).

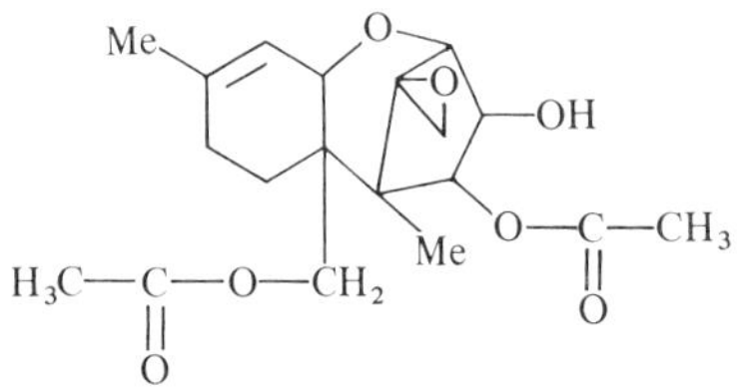

Fig. 4. Anguidine—NSC-141537

Aphidicolin. This tetracyclic diterpinoid obtained from England is scheduled for panel testing (Fig. 5).

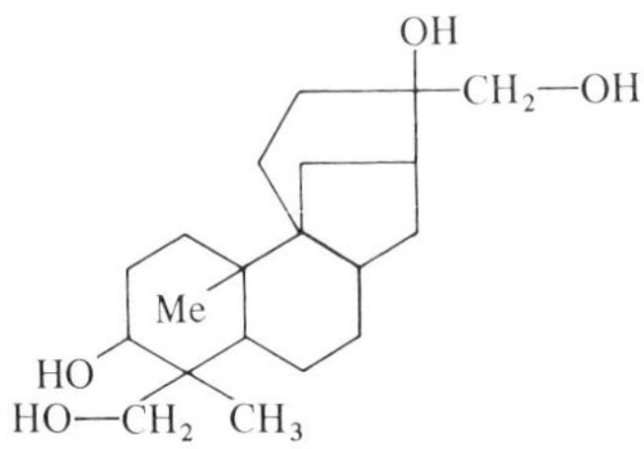

Fig. 5. Aphidicolin—NSC-234714

Bleomycin PEP. This Japanese-obtained peptide differs from bleomycin in the terminal amine group. This compound is scheduled for panel tumor testing (Fig. 6).

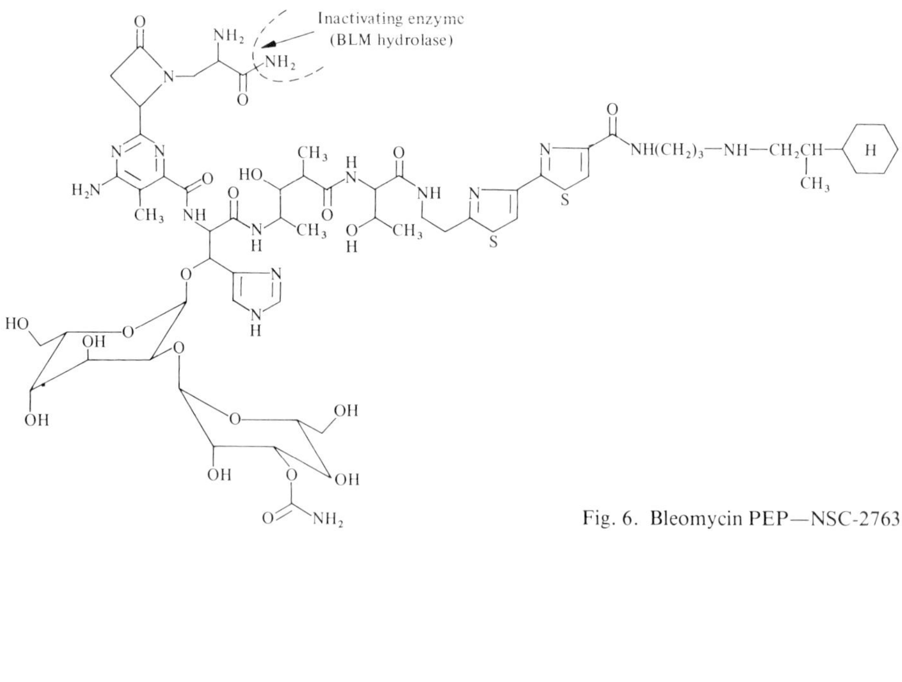

Fig. 6. Bleomycin PEP—NSC-276382

Bleomycin PYP. This is a Japanese-obtained peptide differing from bleomycin in the terminal amine group. This compound is scheduled for panel tumor testing (Fig. 7).

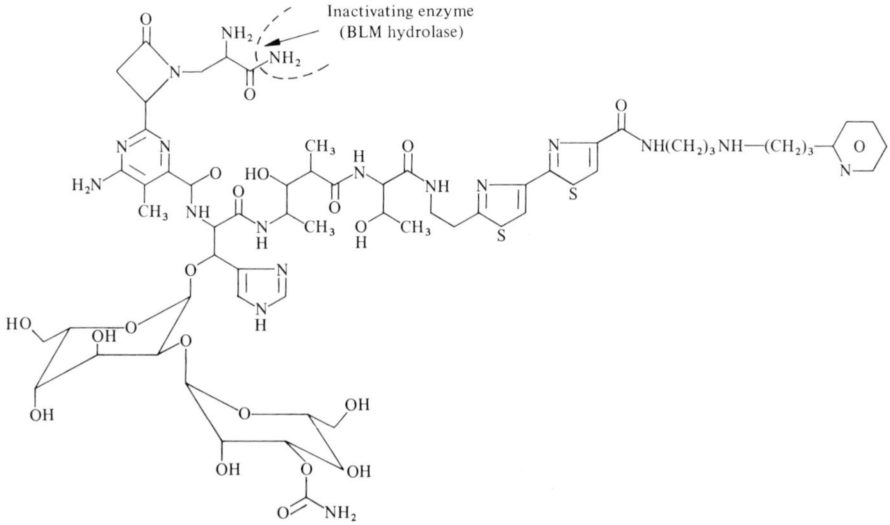

Fig. 7. Bleomycin PYP—NSC-276381

Chartreusin. This drug is a coumarin-like compound with a glycoside. While showing good in vivo activity in solid tumors, it is excreted too rapidly in the bile to be useful pharmacologically (Fig. 8). This is a candidate for biotransformation studies.

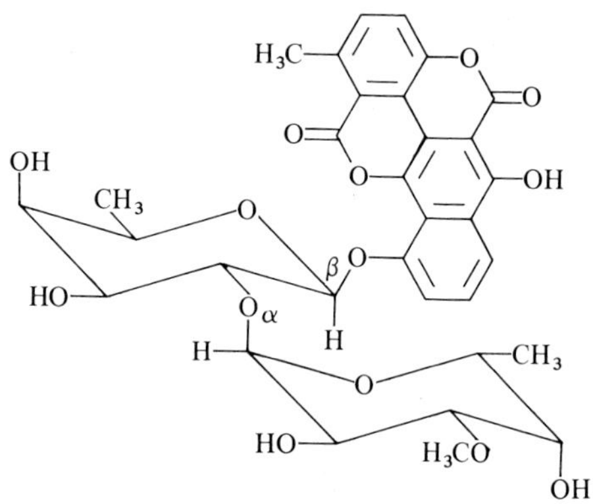

Fig. 8. Chartreusin—NSC-5159

Covidarabine (2′ deoxycoformycin). This is a deoxyriboside of an imidazodiazepine. This deaminase inhibitor is being considered for toxicology studies (Fig. 9).

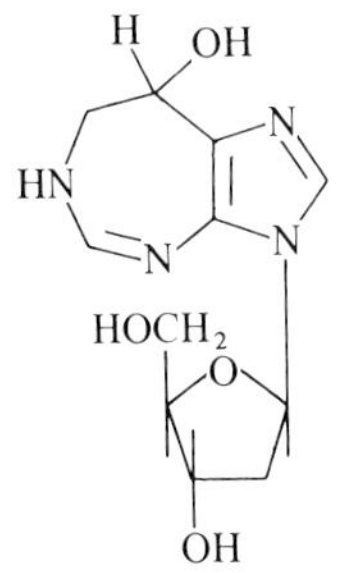

Fig. 9. Covidarabine—NSC-218321

Nogamycin. This is an anthracycline with a dioxobicyclononane fused to it. This compound, which was derived from the transformation program of one of our contractors, is scheduled for tumor panel (Fig. 10).

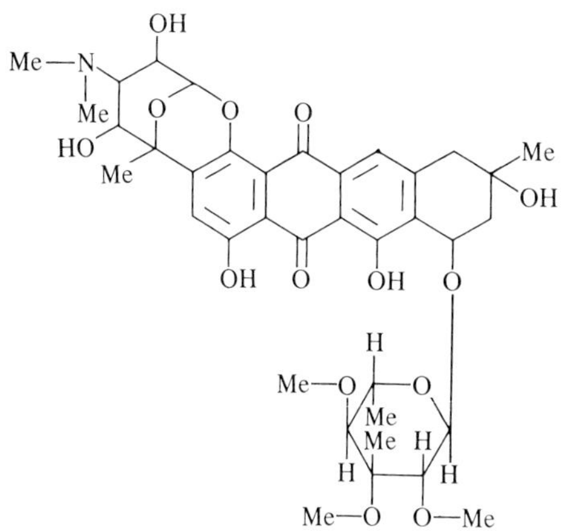

Fig. 10. Nogamycin—NSC-265450

Nogalamycin B. Same as above (Fig. 11).

Showdomycin. This antibiotic is maleimide with a ribofuranoyl residue. This compound is scheduled for tumor panel (Fig. 12).

Sterigmatocystin. This oxygen-containing fused heterocyclic produced by *Aspergillus* is highly toxic and carcinogenic. We will use this compound for a substrate to be biotransformed (Fig. 13).

T_2 *Toxin.* This scirpinol is similar to anguidine but showed more activity in animal tests and is scheduled for the complete tumor panel (Fig. 14).

Ten additional compounds which have not had their structures fully elucidated are also scheduled for advance testing. Michicarcin and lymphosarcin are undergoing formulation studies while the others are undergoing tumor panel testing (Table 14). NCI plans to maintain its rate of evaluating new cultures on various substrates and, if results so indicate, will increase its fermentation efforts in the more productive areas.

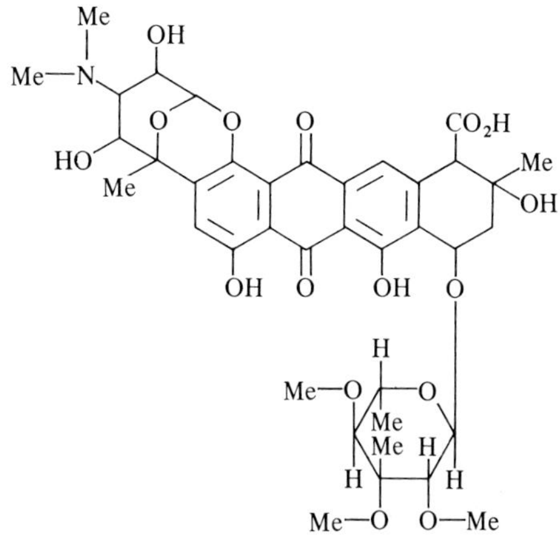

Fig. 11. Nogalomycin B—NSC-265449

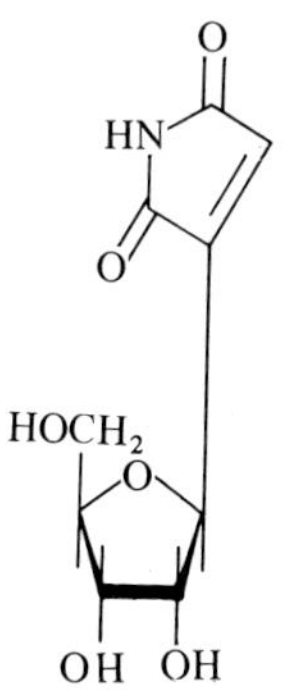

Fig. 12. Showdomycin—NSC-93047

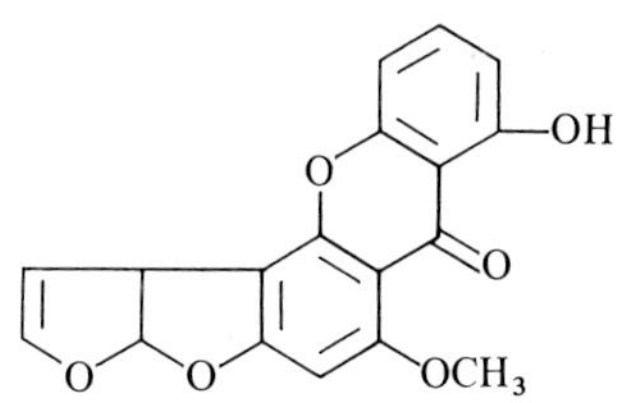

Fig. 13. Sterigmatocystin—NSC-204985

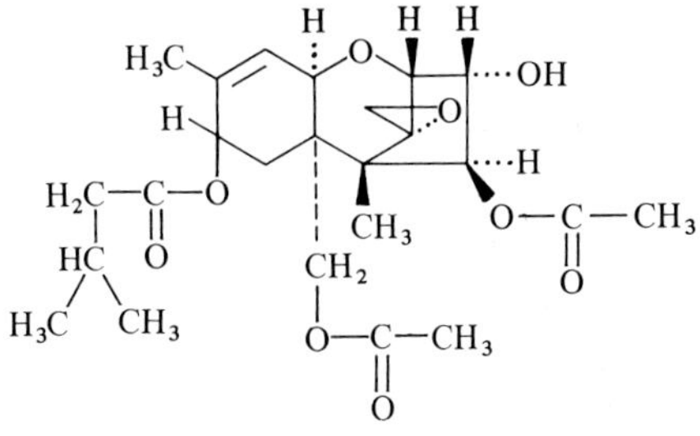

Fig. 14. T_2 toxin—NSC-138780

Discussion

Several prescreening techniques are being considered in the hope of identifying new compounds which have unique biochemical activities. The differentiation test, which has shown that Friend erythroleukemic cells could be differentiated to a more normal cell using dimethylsulfoxide (DMSO), is being considered as a screening tool. [17] Several of our newer leads (e.g., lymphosarcin and michicarcin), showed the same ability as DMSO. The test also can be used to show cytotoxicity. In the erythroblastic differentiation test, hemoglobin is measured using benzidine in a colorimetric method which has been adopted by Dr. Sartorelli's group at Yale University. Several studies with various cell lines using six antineoplastic agents and 12 cell lines indicate that drugs often selectively effect one type of cell and not another. This type of cell line battery could prove beneficial as an assay for guiding the isolation of antineoplastic agents, and as a "fingerprint" technique, similar to chromatography, to aid in identifying types of antineoplastic agents.

The possibility of using a spectrophotometric method to measure the effect of fermentation broths on the reactions of plant lectins on neoplastic cells is being considered. [16] This technique would simply show differences occuring on the surface of the cells due to the presence of some compound in a fermentation capable of causing slower or faster agglutination, larger aggregate formation, etc. Adriamycin is an example of an inducer of alteration of conconavalin A caused agglutination of S180 ascites cells. [13] Additional work by Sartorelli's group suggests that the changes in the cell surface induced by adriamycin may be involved, at least in part, in the antineoplastic actions of this drug. Adriamycin caused an increase in the lectin-induced cellular agglutination of S180 cells and shortened the time required for the agglutination process to begin. [16]

The use of a mutagen test as a prescreen has been considered. However, NCI would rather discover antineoplastic agents which are not mutagenic. A correlation between the potential for causing lysogenic induction and for causing cancer has been discussed for over a quarter of a century. Many of the drugs used today in combating cancer are mutagenic and thus, the use of lysogenic induction in a bacterial test might be worthwhile.

Various immunotherapy tests are being considered for use as prescreens. The model used by Hanna et. al. indicates the effect of a drug on established tumors that have metastasized. The drug is injected intratumorally. BCG caused line-10 hepatocarcinoma to regress and the regional lymph node metastases were eliminated. [12, 9]

Biotransformation and cometabolism are fermentation techniques which have just been adopted in NCI's program. We have received 12 compounds isolated from this work which are of interest.

Nine additional areas of fermentation are being contemplated as potential research programs for NCI in the future (Table 15). The potential of fermenting plant cells and animal cells is in its infancy and will be explored. Investigations have shown that the ability to produce alkaloids, amino acids, etc. using this technique is feasible. Unique organisms have not been thoroughly investigated for antibiotic production. Indications from our work of isolating unusual organisms from hydrocarbons, terpenes, etc. indicate this will be a profitable research area to exploit. The importance of developing more prescreens is self-evident. One can obtain different types of compounds with different mechanisms of action. Simple and sensitive prescreens can be used to monitor isolation of compounds, thus decreasing compound isolation costs, and expediting the isolation efforts.

Genetic exploitation of microbes has been a way to increase chemical yields by fermentation for decades and was the method used to obtain the new antineoplastic agent, adriamycin by Farmitalia. Many fermentation techniques have been developed through the years but have not been evaluated for their potential to produce new antibiotics or to increase yields. The cellophane bag technique, which can be adapted to scale-up by means of dialysis or ultrafiltration, was useful in toxin production and markedly increased the yield of these materials. This technique has never been fully exploited in fermentations outside of biologic warfare research.

The importance of biotransformations for modifying compounds as a potential for developing drugs was first recognized in steriod fermentations. The field of hydrocarbon fermentation identified other possibilities and recently this type of work has been undertaken with antineoplastic agents [19, 1, 20, 22].

Conclusion

In conclusion, 1976 was a banner year for NCI fermentation research in the obtaining of a multitude of new organisms, in increased cost effectiveness through prescreens, and in obtaining many new compounds. The final success of this work will not be fully determined until NCI discovers how many of these compounds are clinical candidates in the treatment of cancer.

Tables

Table 1. Culture acquisition

Knowns	Unknowns
World Federation of Culture Collections	Soil Isolates
Northern Regional Research Laboratories	a) Temperate
American Type Culture Collection	b) Tropical
Central Bureau Voor Schimmelcultures	c) Unusual organisms
Japanese Federation for Culture Collections	1) Microbiospora
Scientists (worldwide)	2) Myxobacteriales
	3) Chainia
	Leaves
	Marine

Table 2. Culture isolation

a) Various types of compounds as sole carbon sources in fermentation.
b) Techniques for isolation of novel microbes.
   1) Percolation
   2) Enrichment
   3) Sprinkle plate
c) Varied environmental conditions.
   1) pH
   2) Minerals
   3) Temperature
   4) Nitrogen sources
   5) Aeration

Table 3. Carbon sources for culture isolation and fermentation

Monosaccharides	*Polyhydroxy alcohols*
fructose	mannitol
galactose	sorbitol
mannose	ribitol
xylose	arabitol
rhamnose	glycerol
ribose	
erythrose	*Oligosaccharides*
	lactose
Glycosides	maltose
salicin	cellobiose
amydalin	trehalose
	melibiose
Substituted Sugars	raffinose
glucosamine	
gluconic acid	

Table 4. Carbon sources for culture isolation and fermentation

Terpenes	Miscellaneous	Miscellaneous (continued)
α pinene	corn meal	catechol
terpene hydrate	malt extract	phenylenediamine
citronellol	fish meal	3-hydroxy picolinic acid
	distillers solubles	2-(2 hydroxy ethyl) quinoline
Hydrocarbons	cotton seed	V8 juice
hexadecane	peptone	potato starch
decalin	n-methyl piperazine	chitin
adamantane	sodium formate	phenol
pristane	imidazole	
phenanthracene	isoxazoles	

Table 5. Prescreens in vitro

In use	Considered for future use
• KB cytotoxicity	• Inhibition of trans methylase
• L1210 cytotoxicity	• Cell differentiation
• P388 cytotoxicity	• Cell surface changes
• Infectious bronchitis virus	a) agglutinations of plant lectins
	b) binding of plant lectins
• Enzyme inhibition	• Immunogen stimulation
• Antimetabolite	

Table 6. Antibiotic dereplication methods

1. Cursory dereplication (after in vitro activity confirmed)[a]
   a) antimicrobial spectra
   b) use of drug resistant mutants
   c) cultural characteristics
   d) limited paper chromatography
2. Complete dereplication (after in vivo activity observed)
   a) paper chromatography (6–18 different standard solvent systems)
   b) bioautography
   c) microbiological spectrum
   d) column chromatography

[a] 88% reconfirmations.

Table 7. 1976 Fermentation program results

Cultures isolated	Active in vivo	Active in vitro	Undergoing chemical fractional	Novel antineoplastic agents isolated
2158 (contractor A)	319	64	15	9
846 (contractor B)	88	22	6	3
1425 (contractor C)	196	38	35	14
534 (contractor D)	160	38	18	4
4963	763 (15.3%)	162 (21.1%)	74	30

Table 8. Fermentation results on varied carbon sources[a]

Substrates	No. of isolates	In vitro actives	In vivo[b] actives
Unusual carbohydrates	241	60	9
Substituted sugars	23	6	2
Carboxylic acids	50	0	0
Amino acids	200	10	2
Fatty acids	179	35	11
Lipids	369	45	10
Hydrocarbons	99	23	1
Terpenes	10	0	0
Misc. organic compounds	254	17	3
Total	1425	196 (13.7%)	38 (19.4%)

[a] One company only for 1 year. Not complete for entire program.
[b] A number of in vivo evaluations still underway.

Table 9. Evaluation and processing of fermentation beers or crude concentrates

Basic screen
- Prescreens
- PS in mice (active ILS > 20)

Reconfirmation
- Duplication of original fermentation conditions
- Activity reconfirmed in original active systems (actives undergo dereplication)

Table 10. In vivo tumor panel testing compounds active in PS or Rationally selected

1. LE
2. Colon 26
3. B 16 (i.p., s.c.)
4. Lewis lung (i.v., s.c.)
5. Mammary CD
6. Xenografts

Table 11. Fermentation improvement parameters

1. Inoculum (spore, vegetative, etc.)[a]	5. Dissolved oxygen
a) Optimal growth time	
b) Optimal medium	6. CO_2 requirement
2. Carbon sources	7. Trace minerals
a) Growth	
b) Production	8. pH
3. Nitrogen sources	9. Temperature
4. Antifoam	10. Stirring rate

[a]Strain selection and mutation program sometimes initiated.

Table 12. Chemical fractionation and isolation of active fermentations

Sufficient active material obtained—scale-up (30–3000 gal)
Stability of material
In vitro assay development
Compound structure novelty
Pure compound
a) NSC No. assigned
b) In vivo testing
1 routine
2 rational bypass based on structure

Table 13. Selection and acquisition of fermentation compounds for screening

Step I	Step II	Step III
Acquire agents for screening	Criteria for screening	Test PS
Contracts	1. novel compound	Rational selection
a) isolate compounds which give activity in prescreens	2. deemphasize adequately studied classes or nonproductive classes	Other in vivo tests of interest
Literature surveillance	3. analogs of interesting compounds	B16
a) unusual organism	(preclinical or clinical stage)	colon
b) unusual structure	4. chemical has a biologic activity	mammary
c) various biological activities	of interest	Lewis lung
Outside organizations	a) inhibits an enzyme of interest	L1210
	b) differentiates cancer cells	xenografts

Table 14. Other fermentation leads

NSC-121341—BBRL Hedamycin-like
NSC-132346—Gelbecidine (chromomycin A_3-like)
NSC-270051—Chromomycin A_3 transformed product
NSC-208642—Lymphosarcin (large molecular.weight polyene)
NSC-191959—Michicarcin (glycoprotein)
NSC-219941—Musettamycin (anthracycline)
NSC-243047—Polypeptide containing high percent of sulfur
NSC-219877—Rachelmycin (peptide)
NSC-174951—Peptide
NSC-274540—Roridin-like

Table 15. Future fermentation research possibilities

- Growing plant cells in large fermentors and extract for new antineoplastic agents.
- Growing animal cells in large fermentors and extracts for new antineoplastic agents.
- Evaluate psychrophiles, thermophiles, and osmophiles as potential sources of new drugs.
- Develop more prescreens which measure new activities that might uncover new antineoplastic agents.
- Genetic manipulation of organisms.
- Evaluate various fermentation techniques:
  a) solid
  b) semisolid
  c) air lift
  d) continuous
  e) deep tank
  f) cellophane bag
- Microbes as immunologic stimulators.
- Evaluate marine, algae, lichens, and mixed culture fermentations.
- Co-metabolism.

References

1. Betts, R. E., Walters, D. E., Rosazza, J. P.: Microbial transformations of antitumor compounds. I. Conversions of acronycine to 9-hydroxyacronycine by *Cunninhamella echinulate*. J. Med. Chem. **17**, 599–602 (1974).
2. Brian, P. W.: Antibiotics produced by fungi. Botanical Rev. **17**, 357–430 (1951).
3. Dagley, S., Evans, W. C., Ribbons, D. W.: New pathways in the oxidative metabolism of aromatic compounds by microorganisms. Nature **88**, 560–566 (1960).
4. Davis, J. B., Raymond, R. L.: Oxidation of alky substituted cyclic hydrocarbons by a *Nocardia* during growth of N-alkanes. Appl. Microbiol. **9**, 383–388 (1966).
5. Douros, J. D., Jr.: Lower plants as a source of anticancer drugs. Cancer Treat. Rep. **60**, 1069–1080 (1976).
6. Douros, J. D., Jr., Frankenfeld, J. W.: Oxidation of alkylbenzenes by a strain of *Micrococcus cerificans* growing on n-pariffins. Appl. Microbiol. **16**, 320 (1968).
7. Douros, J. D., Jr., Frankenfeld, J. W.: Production of cinnamic acid from alkylbenzenes by soil microorganisms, effects of culture conditions on yield. Appl. Microbiol. **16**, 532 (1968).
8. Douros, J. D., Jr., Frankenfeld, J. W.: Fermentation Process for Preparing Cinnamic Acid and 5-phenyl valeric acid. U.S. 3,301,766.
9. Fidler, I. J., Budmen, M. B., Hanna, M. G., Jr.: Characterization of *in vitro* reactivity by BCG treated guinea pigs to syngeneic line-10 hepatocarcinoma. Cancer Immunology Immunotherapy **1**, 179–186 (1976).
10. Gordon, M. H.: A simulation study of the preclinical development of anticancer drugs. Cancer Chemother. Rep. Part 3 **5**, 65–78 (1974).
11. Hanka, L. J.: Proceedings of the 5th International Congress of Chemotherapy, Sec. B9/2 351–357 (1967).
12. Hanna, M. G., Jr., Peters, L. C.: The efficacy of BCG induced tumor immunity in guinea pigs with regional and systemic malignancy. Cancer Immunology Immunotherapy **1**, 171–177 (1976).

13. MURPHREE, D. S., CUNNINGHAM, L. S., HWANG, K. M., SARTORELLI, A. C.: Effects of adriamycin on surface properties of sarcoma 180 ascites Cells. Biochem. Pharmacol. **25**, 1227–1231 (1976).
14. RAYMOND, R. L., JAMISON V. W., HUDSON, J. O.: Microbial Hydrocarbon Co-Oxidation. I. Appl. Microbiol. **15**, 857–865 (1967).
measure plant lectin induced cell agglatination. Cancer Res. **34**, 3396–3402 (1974).
15. RAYMOND, R. L., JAMISON, V. W., HUDSON, J. O.: Hydrocarbon co-oxidation in microbial systems. Lipids **6**, 453–457 (1971).
16. SARTORELLI, A. C., MURPHREE, S. A., HWANG, K. M.: A quantitative spectrophotometric method to measure plant lectin induced cell agglutination. Cancer Res. **34**, 3396–3402 (1974).
17. SARTORELLI, A. C.: Preliminary Data Report to NCI (1976).
18. SEBEK, O. K.: Microbial conversion of antibiotics. Lloydia **37**, 115–133 (1974).
19. SMITH, R. V., ROSAZZA, J. P.: Microbial models of mammalian metabolism. Aromatic hydroxylation. Arch. Biochem. Biophys. **161**, 551–558 (1974).
20. SMITH, R. V., ROSAZZA, J. P.: Microbial systems for the study of drug biotransformations. Biotechnol. Bioeng. **17**, 785–814 (1975).
21. Society of American Bacteriologists: Manual of Microbiological Methods, New York: McGraw-Hill Book Co. 1957.
22. UMEZAWA, H.: Enzyme Inhibitors of Microbial Origin. Tokyo University: Tokyo Press 1972.

In Vivo Antitumor Evaluation of Antibiotics. Selected Results from the Drug Evaluation Program of the National Cancer Institute, U.S.A.

J. M. VENDITTI and R. K. JOHNSON

While we most often relate antibiotic chemotherapy to erradication of infectious foreign organisms, we must remain aware of the value of antibiotics (e.g. anthracyclines, bleomycin, actinomycin D, mitomycin C, mithramycin, L-asparaginase) as antitumor drugs [5, 12]. Moreover, fermentation products continue to represent a fruitful field for discovering new materials with clinical anticancer potential. During 1976, the Division of Cancer Treatment (DCT), National Cancer Institute (NCI) examined over 1000 fermentation broths for activity against one or more animal tumors. The yield of "active" materials from this in vivo screening program are presented elsewhere in this volume [2].

One purpose of this report is to summarize in vivo screening results for selected antitumor antibiotics in various stages of evaluation in our program. However, since the value of an animal screen depends ultimately on its ability to uncover clinically useful drugs, a brief description of our current screening practice and its objectives seems appropriate. A number of studies of the correlation between drug activity in animal screens and utility against human cancer [4, 12] had highlighted mouse leukemia L1210 as the animal model which best discriminated between clinically active and inactive drugs. However, these retrospective studies could be reasonably criticized because of the abiding—and sometimes exclusive—use of L1210 as a primary screen during the years when most clinically active drugs were selected. No prospective study of "animal-man" correlations had been attempted. The present DCT antitumor animal screening program represents one arm of such a prospective study; the other being the clinical trials of the drugs uncovered. In 1975, in order to provide the required preclinical data, we began to emphasize testing new synthetic compounds and "active" isolates from natural products against a spectrum of mouse tumors presumed to represent the major classes of human tumors (Fig. 1). These include transplantable colon, breast, and lung tumors of mice; human tumor xenografts of these tumor types grown in athymic mice; and mouse tumors of known value (e.g. L1210 and B16 melanoma). This decision to test materials of interest against all models comprising the "DCT Panel of Antitumor Screens" (Fig. 1) impacted seriously on many aspects of screening as it had been practiced. The greater effort required to test a material against most of the tumors in the spectrum—in contrast to the lesser effort to screen against L1210—plus the increase in the number of models, limited the number of materials that could be screened in the tumor spectrum to 500-1000 per year. Means of selecting these materials were needed. Having considered a number of alternatives (11), we determined that a reasonable and feasible plan would be to utilize, as an initial in vivo "prescreen," a model known to be sensitive to most classes of clinically effective anticancer drugs, but sufficiently restrictive to avoid overloading the spectrum. L1210 was considered to be too restrictive for a prescreen designed to minimize the probability of missing a material likely to show activity against one of the spectrum tumors. A comprehensive review of existing data [12] pointed to mouse leukemia P388 as an appropriate prescreen because its response to most useful drugs was qualitatively similar, but quantitatively greater than the response of L1210 [10, 12]. In accord with the present plan (Fig. 1) natural product isolates and synthetic compounds emerging from the P388 prescreen are tested against the entire tumor spectrum. Despite the necessity of using a prescreen, we

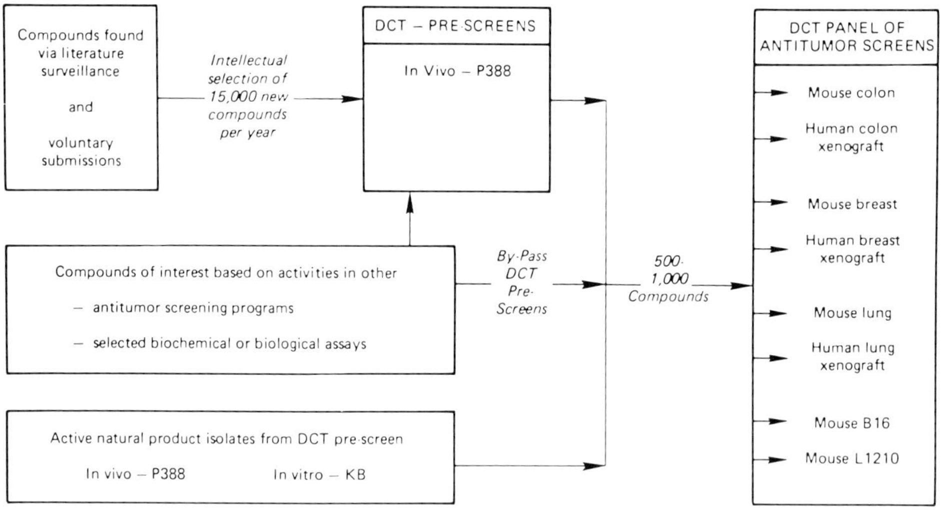

Fig. 1. Proposed flow of drugs through DCT screens

recognize that no single animal model is known to predict clinical utility perfectly. Therefore, the input to the spectrum is augmented with materials of interest based on activities in other screening programs and selected biochemical and biologic assays. Such a material is committed to spectrum testing regardless of its prescreen performance. Most synthetic compounds and crude plant extracts enter the screen without previous biologic data. In contrast, most fermentation products screened in vivo are selected from microbiologic or biochemical assays [2, 8] or are products of microbial biotransformation [9]. These materials, when purified, may be tested against the tumor spectrum regardless of their effects against P388. As materials emerging as active from any of the spectrum models are subjected to adequate clinical trial, this approach to screening should provide critical information on the value of the animal tumors used individually or in concert.

Tables 2-16 summarize in vivo screening results for selected fermentation products (Table 1) against mouse tumors in current use in our program. Protocols for screening against L1210 and P388 leukemias, B16 melanoma, and Lewis lung carcinoma (LL) have been previously published [3]. The origins and experimental methods for screening against the carcinogen-induced transplantable colon tumors 26 (Co/26) and 38 (Co/38) have been described by CORBETT, et al (1) and the spontaneous mammary carcinoma of CD8F1 mice (MC/CD) has been described by MARTIN, et al [7]. For screening against MC/CD, the first transplant generation from the spontaneous tumor is used.

In general, Tables 2-16 show, for each host-tumor model, the site of tumor implantation (day 0), the treatment route and schedule, and the degree of therapeutic activity at the optimal dose (OD). Drugs were administered at a number of dosage levels designed to range from an ineffective and nonlethal dose to a frankly lethal dose. Where increase in lifespan (ILS) is the parameter of response, the OD is that dose which produced the maximum percentage increase in mean or median survival time over controls. Where inhibition of tumor growth is the parameter of response, the OD is the nonlethal (LD_{10} or less) dosage that produced the greatest percentage tumor weight inhibition (TWI) from controls by a specific day. For an active treatment, results observed at the OD are shown. The notation "N" indicates lack of activity; i.e., a maximum ILS <25% or maximum TWI <50%. For an inactive treatment, the range of dosage levels employed is shown in parentheses. S/T denotes the number of longterm survivors over the total number of mice receiving the OD. For inactive treatments,

"T" is the number of mice per treatment group. All dosage levels are expressed as mg/kg/injection. Unless otherwise noted, drug treatment was i.p.

Anguidine (AGD, Tables 2 and 3) is in clinical trial on the basis of activity against P388, L1210, Co/38 and moderate activity against MC/CD. Activity against P388 or L1210 was independent of the route of drug administration. Against Co/38 the combination of AGD and 5-fluorouracil (FU) was clearly superior to treatment with either drug alone (Table 3). The treatments shown in Table 3 are LD_{10} or less dosage levels for the route and regimens used. In this study conducted by CORBETT, et al [1], i.v. treatment was delayed until the s.c. tumors had attained estimated weights of 100–300 mg. FU alone elicited a moderate increase in median survival time, but no tumor regressions. AGD alone produced >50% regression of tumor in six of ten mice, complete regression in three mice, and two longterm survivors. AGD plus FU produced complete tumor regression in nine of ten mice and eight longterm survivors.

Tables 4–6 summarize a series of experiments comparing PIP-1B and ACT-D against a number of mouse tumors. A comprehensive study of relative antitumor effectiveness among 34 ACT-D analogs, conducted by one of the authors (R. K. JOHNSON), showed only PIP-1B to have a small but reproducible superiority over ACT-D against a mouse tumor, B16 melanoma (Table 6). Comparison of the ODs for PIP-1B and ACT-D (Tables 4–6) suggests that PIP-1B is about eightfold less potent than ACT-D although the compounds displayed comparable degrees of therapeutic efficacy against L1210, P388, and Co/26.

The interesting activity of MCR (Tables 7–9) had been described previously [6]. Partially purified MCR preparations were moderately active against L1210 and P388 (Table 7) and very effective against i.p. implanted B16 (Table 8). While i.p. administered MCR was not effective against s.c. implanted LL, the latter tumor responded well to MCR injections directly into the site of tumor implantation (Table 9).

The remaining antibiotics presented in this report are in various stages of screening, and textual descriptions of results to date (Tables 10–16) would be redundant. Each has shown activity against at least one of the in vivo test systems, comprising the DCT tumor spectrum, as well as against P388. Thus, each is a potential candidate for consideration for development to clinical trial.

Summary

A summary is given of the in vivo screening results for selected antitumor antibiotics in various stages of the National Cancer Institute drug development program. In addition a brief description of general screening practices of the program is given. After long-term usage of leukemia L1210 as a primary screen, a new screening panel is being initiated with P388 leukemia as a prescreening system. Illustrative data on anguidine, actinomycin D, macromomycin, aclacinomycin, and other fermentation products are shown.

Tables

Table 1. List of fermentation products presented in this report

NSC number	Name	Organism	Source[a]
3053	Actinomycin D (ACT-D)	Streptomyces parvulus	Rutgers University Merck, Sharpe and Dohme
107660	Actinomycin-pip-1-beta (PIP-1B)	Streptomyces parvulus Streptomyces antibioticua	Georgetown University
141537	Anguidine (AGD)	Fusarium anguinoides	Bristol Laboratories
107105	Macromomycin (MCR)	Streptomyces macromyceticus	Kanegafuchi Chemical Company, Institute of Microbial Chemistry
191959	Michicarcin	Streptomyces sp.	Michigan Department of Health
208642	Lymphosarcin	Streptomyces murinus	Michigan Department of Health
208734	Aclacinomycin A	Streptomyces st. galileus	Sanraku Ocean, Institute of Microbial Chemistry
219877	Rachelmycin	Streptomyces sp.	Bristol Laboratories
219941	Musettamycin (Bristol C-36145)	Strepromyces sp.	Bristol Laboratories
269148	7-0-Methylnogarol	Chemical modification product of Nogalomycin (NSC-70845). Streptomyces nogalatin	Upjohn Company

[a]All materials were received from Dr. J. Douros, Natural Products Branch, Division of Cancer Treatment, National Cancer Institute.

Table 2. Anguidine (NSC-141537): Activity against mouse tumors

Tumor (site)	Treatment schedule	Optimal dose (mg/kg)	ILS (%)	TWI (%)	S/T
B16 (i.p.)	QD; Days 1-9, i.p.	1.0	31	—	0/10
MC/CD (s.c.)	Q7D; Days 1-29, i.p.	2.0	—	78	0/10
Co/26 (i.p.)	Q7D; Days 1, 8, 15, i.p.	(5.0-16)	N	—	0/10
Co/38 (s.c.)	Q7D; Days 2, 9, 16, i.p.	8.0	—	97	4/10
LL (i.m.)	QD; Days 1-11, i.p.	(0.5-16)	N	57	0/10
L1210 (i.p.)	QD; Days 1-13, i.p.	1.6	62	—	0/10
	QD; Days 1-13, s.c.	1.6	59	—	0/10
	QD; Days 1-13, p.o.	3.2	51	—	0/10
	QD; Days 1-13, i.m.	0.8	41	—	0/10
P388 (i.p.)	QD; Days 1-9, i.p.	3.0	93	—	0/10
	QD; Days 1-9, s.c.	1.0	70	—	0/10
	QD; Days 1–9, i.v.	1.0	63	—	0/10
	QD; Days 1-9, p.o.	2.0	90	—	0/10

Table 3. Anguidine (NSC-141537, AGD) plus 5-fluorouracil (NSC-19893, FU); Activity against advanced colon tumor 38[a]

Dose[b] days 17, 24, 31, 38 (mg/kg i.v.)	Median survival time[c] (days)	Tumor regression (number/10 mice) >50%	100%	Survivors
3.1 AGD + 77 FU	114	10	9	8
8.1 AGD	118	6	3	2
77 FU	67	0	0	0
Controls	44	0	0	0

[a] Corbett, *et al.* (1).
[b] Tumor size at beginning of treatment, 100–300 mg. There were no drug deaths.
[c] Dying mice only.

Table 4. Comparison of actinomycin D (NSC-3053, ACT-D) and actinomycin-PIP-1-beta (NSC-107660, PIP-1B) against mouse tumours

Tumor (implant site)	Treatment schedule	Drug	Optimal dose (mg/kg)	ILS (%)
Leukemia	Q4D; days 1, 5, 9	ACT-D	0.4	175
P388 (i.p.)		PIP-1B	1.2	118
Colon tumor	Q4D; days 2, 6, 10	ACT-D	0.5	56
26 (i.p.)		PIP-1B	5.0	53
Colon tumor	Once, day 2	ACT-D	(0.06–1.0)	N
26 (i.p.)		PIP-1B	(0.6–10)	N
Lewis lung	Q4D; days 1, 5, 9	ACT-D	(0.06–1.0)	N
(i.v.)		PIP-1B	(0.5–4.0)	N

Table 5. Comparison of actinomycin D (NSC-3053, ACT-D) and actinomycin-PIP-1-beta (NSC-107660, PIP-1B) against i.p.-implanted L1210

Treatment schedule	Drug	Optimal dose (mg/kg)	ILS (%)	S/T
		(Experiment 1)		
QD; days 1–9	ACT-D	0.05	200	1/8
	PIP-1B	0.2	125	0/8
Q4D; days 1, 5, 9	ACT-D	0.15	210	1/8
	PIP-1B	1.2	120	0/8
		(Experiment 2)		
QD; days 1–9	ACT-D	0.05	91	0/8
	PIP-1B	0.4	73	0/8
Q4D; days 1, 5, 9	ACT-D	0.2	82	1/8
	PIP-1B	1.8	77	1/8
Q4D; days 5, 9, 13	ACT-D	(0.11–0.45)	N	0/8
	PIP-1B	(0.9–3.6)	N	0/8

Table 6. Comparison of actinomycin D (NSC-3053, ACT-D) and actinomycin-PIP-1-beta (NSC-107660, PIP-1B) against i.p. implanted Big melanoma

Experiment no.	Treatment schedule	Drug	Optimal dose (mg/kg)	ILS (%)	S/T
1	QD; days 1-9	ACT-D	0.07	86	0/10
		PIP-1B	0.8	119	3/10
	Q4D; days 1, 5, 9	ACT-D	0.22	60	0/10
		PIP-1B	3.2	74	1/10
	Q4D; days 5, 9, 13	ACT-D	0.11	40	0/10
		PIP-1B	1.6	36	0/10
2	QD, days 1-9	ACT-D	0.05	50	0/10
		PIP-1B	0.4	66	0/10
	Q4D; days 1, 5, 9	ACT-D	0.15	55	0/10
		PIP-1B	2.4	82	0/10
	Q4D; days 5, 9, 13	ACT-D	0.11	16	0/10
		PIP-1B	1.8	32	0/10
3	Q4D; days 1, 5, 9	ACT-D	0.3	76	0/10
		PIP-1B	2.4	137	0/10

Table 7. Marcromomycin (NSC-170105): Activity against mouse leukemias L1210 and P388[a]

Tumor (site)	Treatment schedule	Dose[b] (mg/kg)	ILS (%)
L1210	Q2D; days 1, 5	48	37
(i.p.)	Q4D; days 1, 5, 9	8	33
	QD; days 1-9	8	22
P388	Once, day 1	16	37
(i.p.)	Q4D; days 1, 5, 9	8	68
	QD; days 1-9	8	68

[a]Lippman, *et. al.* [6]
[b]In each instance, the optimal dose was the highest in the range of dosage levels used. The possibility exists that higher dosages might have been more effective.

Table 8. Macromomycin (NSC-170105): Activity against i.p.-implanted B16 melanoma[a]

Dose range QD; days 1-9 (mg/kg)	Number of Mice	Responders[b] (no.)	Responders[b] (%)	Survivors
30-40	26	13	50	1
16-20	26	19	73	4
8-10	25	11	44	2

[a]Lippman, *et. al.* [6]
[b]Mice surveying beyond the range of survival of 95% of the untreated controls.

Table 9. Comparison of intratumor (i.t.) and intraperitoneal (i.p.) administration of macromomycin (NSC-170105) against s.c.-implanted Lewis lung carcinoma[a]

Drug route	Dose day 1 only (mg/kg)	Median survival time (days ± 1 standard error)
i.p.	16	21.5 ± 0.7
i.p.	8	17.0 ± 0.4
i.p.	4	20.0 ± 0.8
i.t.	16	32.5 ± 1.7
i.t.	8	29.0 ± 1.4
i.t.	4	22.5 ± 1.5
i.t.—Saline only		21.5 ± 2.1
Untreated control		20.5 ± 2.0

[a]Lippman, *et. al.* [6]

Table 10. Aclacinomycin A (NSC-208734): Activity against mouse tumors

Tumor (site)	Treatment schedule	Optimal dose (mg/kg)	ILS (%)	TWI (%)
B16 (i.p.)	QD; days 1-9	3	44	—
MC/CD (s.c.)	Q7D; days 1-57	3	—	95
L1210 (i.p.)	Q4D; days 2, 6	25	41	—
LL (s.c.)	QD; days 1-9	(1.5-6)	N	—
P388 (i.p.)	QD; days 1-9	5	108	—
	Q4D; days 1, 5, 9	9	103	—

Table 11. Rachelmycin (NSC-219877): Activity against mouse tumors

Tumor (site)	Treatment schedule,	Optimal dose (mg/kg)	ILS (%)
B16 (s.p.)	QD; days 1-9	1.2	87
L1210 (i.p.)	Q4D; days 2, 6	(0.2-1.6)	N
LL (s.c.)	Q8D; days 1,9	(0.2-1.6)	N
P388 (i.p.)	QD; days 1-9	1.6	98

Table 12. Lymphosarcin (NSC-208642): Activity against mouse tumors

Tumor (site)	Treatment schedule	Optimal dose (mg/kg)	ILS (%)	TWI (%)
B16 (i.p.)	QD; days 1-9	1.4	75	—
MC/CD (s.c.)	Q7D; days 1-57	1.0	—	85
CO/26 (i.p.)	Q4D; days 2, 6, 10	(3.0-13)	N	—
Co/38 (s.c.)	Q4D; days 2, 6, 10	2.8	236	—
L 0 (i.p.)	QD; days 1-9	(0.25-8.0)	N	—
LL (s.c.)	QD; days 1-9	(0.25-2.0)	N	—
P388 (i.p.)	QD: days 1-9	2.3	94	—

Table 13. Lymphosarcin (NSC-208642). Influence of treatment schedule on activity against mouse leukemia P388

IP treatment schedule	Optimal dose (mg/kg)	ILS (%)
Day 1 only	8.0	37
QD; days 1-9	2.3	94
Q4D; days 1, 5, 9	6.0	74
Q8D; days 1, 9	8.0	51
Q3Hr. X 8; day 1 only	1.5	82
Q3Hr. X 8; days 1, 5, 9	1.0	103
Q3Hr. X 8; days 1, 9	1.5	125

Table 14. Michicarcin (NSC-191959): Activity against mouse tumors

Tumor (site)	Optimal dose QD; days 1-9 (mg/kg)	ILS (%)
B16 (i.p.)	20.0	81
L1210 (i.p.)	(2.5-100)	N
P388 (i.p.)	20.0	95

Table 15. Musettamycin (NSC-219941): Activity against mouse tumors

Tumor (site)	Optimal dose QD; days 1-9 (mg/kg)	ILS (%)
B16 (i.p.)	1.8	64
L1210 (i.p.)	0.4	29
LL (s.c.)	(0.25-2.0)	N
P388 (i.p.)	1.6	161

Table 16. 7-0-Methylnogarol (NSC-269148): Activity against mouse tumors

Tumor (site)	Treatment schedule	Optimal dose (mg/kg)	ILS (%)
B16 (i.p.)	i.p.-QD; days 1-9	12.5	75
L1210 (i.p.)	i.p.-QD; days 1-9	12.5	82
P388 (i.p.)	i.p. day 1 only	50.0	97
	i.p.-QD; days 1-9	12.5	129
	p.o.-QD; days 1-9	12.5	43
	i.p.-Q4D; days 1, 5, 9	75.0	123

References

1. CORBETT, T. H., GRISWOLD, D. P., JR., ROBERTS, B. J., PECKHAM, J. C., SCHABEL, F. M., JR.: Evaluation of single agents and combinations of chemotherapeutic agents in mouse colon carcinoma. Cancer (in press).
2. DOUROS, J.: Present National Cancer Institutes Fermentation Development Program. (See Chapter 4 of this book.)
3. GERAN, R. I., GREENBERG, N. H., MACDONALD, M. M., SCHUMACHER, A. M., ABBOTT, B. J.: Protocols for screening chemical agents and natural products against animal tumors and other biological systems (Third Edition). Cancer Chemother. Rep. Part 3, **3** (2), 1-5 (1972).
4. GOLDIN, A., SERPICK, A. M., MANTEL, N.: A commentary. Experimental screening procedures and clinical predictability value. Cancer Chemother. Rep. **50**, 173-218 (1966).
5. HOLLAND, J. F., FREI, E. (Eds.): Cancer Medicine. Philadelphia: Lea and Febiger 1973. See UMEZAWA, H.: Principles of antitumor antibiotic chemotherapy, 817-826; DIMARCO, A., LENAZ, L.: Daunomycin and Adriamycin, 826-835; FRIEDMAN, P. A., CERAMI, A.: Actinomycin, 835-839; CAPIZZI, R. L., HANDSCHUMACHER, R. E.: Asparaginase, 850-859; GOLDIN, A., CARTER, S. K: Screening and evaluation of antitumor agents, 605-628.
6. LIPPMAN, M. M., LASTER, W. R., ABBOTT, B. J., VENDITTI, J. M., BARATTA, M.: Antitumor activity of Macromomycin B (NSC-170105) against murine leukemias, melanoma, and lung carcinoma. Cancer Res. **35**, 939-945 (1975).
7. MARTIN, D. S., FUGMANN, R. A., STOLFI, R. L., HAYWORTH, P. E.: Solid tumor animal model therapeutically predictive for human breast cancer. Cancer Chemother. Rep. Part 2, **5** (1), 89-109 (1975).
8. NEIL, G. L.: Detection and Assay of Antitumor Antibiotics. (See Chapter 2 of this book.)
9. ROSAZZA, J.: Antitumor Antibiotic Activation, Biotransformation and Derivation by Microbial Systems. (See Chapter 6 of this book.)
10. VENDITTI, J. M.: Forward in "Protocols for screening chemical agents and natural products against animal tumors and other biological systems (Third Edition). Cancer Chemother. Rep. Part 3, **3** (2), 1-5 (1972).
11. VENDITTI, J. M.: Drug evaluation branch program: Report to the screening contractors. Cancer Chemother. Rep. Part 2, **5** (1) 1-4 (1975).
12. VENDITTI, J. M.: Relevance of transplantable animal-tumor systems to the selection of new agents for clinical trial. In: Pharmacological Basis for Cancer Chemotherapy. Baltimore: Williams and Wilkins Co. 1975, pp. 245-270.

Antitumor Antibiotic Bioactivation, Biotransformation and Derivatization by Microbial Systems

J. P. N. Rosazza

Bacterial, yeast and fungal cells contain enzymes which perform highly selective metabolic transformation reactions with foreign organic compounds. In this paper, "Microbial transformations" will refer to reactions catalyzed by microbial enzymes, especially when desired and useful metabolites accumulate in fermentation media. Microbial transformations have tremendous potential for use in the development of new antitumor drugs. Concepts related to microbial transformations which may be relevant to the development of new agents will be discussed. The two areas which will be emphasized are:
1. The application of microbial transformations as a means of preparing potentially useful derivatives of antitumor agents;
2. The use of microbial transformations as models of mammalian metabolism.

Microbial Transformations

Microbial transformations have been widely used to accomplish selective chemical modification of many types of complicated organic compounds [6, 8, 15, 19, 22, 43-44, 49]. Single and specific chemical transformations have been achieved under extremely mild reaction conditions on substrates such as steroids, antibiotics and alkaloids. Microbial transformations were the basis of large-scale industrial syntheses of steroid hormone products which are difficult to synthesize. The technique has also been applied in the modification of some antibiotics. Systematic studies are most complete in the area of steroid bioconversions, but numerous recent reports document the use of microbial transformations with many types of substrates.

The role of microbial transformations in the development of new antitumor agents may be illustrated by comparing the structures of a few clinically useful drugs. The plant alkaloids, vinblastine (VBL) *1* and vincristine (VCR) *2*, differ only in the state of oxidation of the carbon attached to the vindoline nitrogen atom, while daunomycin *3*, and adriamycin *4* differ from one another only in the nature of the two-carbon side chain (see Fig. 1). The subtle differences in the structures of these similar molecules result in significant differences in their activity, toxicity and/or spectrum of antitumor activity. It is emphasized that microbial transformations are capable of causing similar subtle structural changes in other active antitumor compounds.

Extensive screening programs supported by the National Cancer Institute for many years now have provided us with numerous novel classes of highly active antitumor compounds from microorganisms, plant and other natural sources [40]. Some of the compounds have achieved clinical significance, including the Vinca alkaloids, the anthracycline antibiotics, and compounds like bleomycin and mitomycin. Others are highly active, but they are also quite toxic. Since most of the compounds uncovered through the NCI screening program are structurally complex, and difficult to synthesize or derivatize by chemical methods, they represent excellent candidates for chemical modification by microbial transformations.

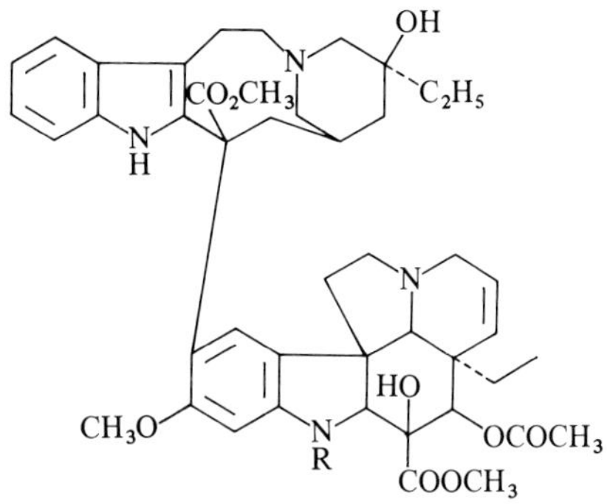

1 R=CH_3
2 R=CHO

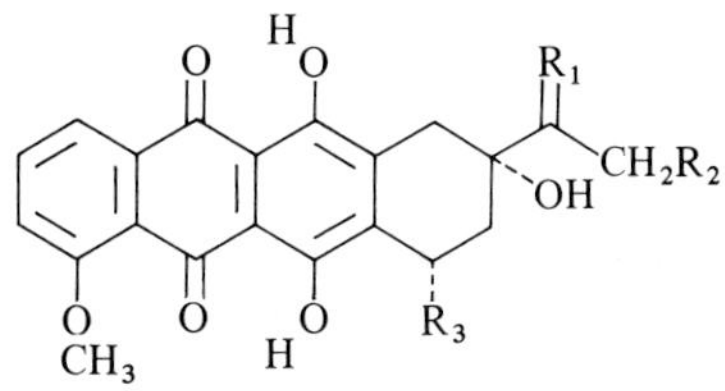

3 R_1=O, R_2=H, R_3=Daunosamine
3a R_1=H,OH, R_2=H, R_3=Daunosamine
3b R_1=O, R_2=H, R_3=H
4 R_1=O, R_2=OH, R_3=Daunosamine

Fig. 1. Structures of the Vinca alkaloids, vinblastine (1) and vincristine (2); and the structures of daunomycin (3), two of its microbial metabolites (3a) and (3b), and adriamycin (4)

Metabolism of Antitumor Compounds

The metabolism of antitumor agents by mammalian systems has been vigorously studied in recent years. The emphasis of this work has been to reveal how antitumor drugs may: a) become metabolically activated or deactivated; b) suffer changes in either the nature or spectrum of antitumor activity; and c) indicate how antitumor compounds may be converted into potentially toxic products responsible for adverse side reactions [7, 16, 30]. Although success has been achieved in studying the metabolic disposition of some antitumor antibiotics like adriamycin and daunomycin, little has been learned about the metabolism of compounds like VBL, VCR, thalicarpine and d-tetrandrine. This may be due to the low levels of metabolites formed by mammalian systems, but certainly also to the difficulties encountered in elaborating the structures of metabolites of these complicated molecules.

Microbial Models of Mammalian Metabolism

SMITH and ROSAZZA [45] described a concept which suggests that microbial transformations may be used to mimic many of the kinds of biotransformations of foreign organic compounds normally observed in mammals. In general, selected groups of microorganisms may be used to produce metabolites similar to those produced by in vivo or in vitro mammalian metabolizing systems. Microbial metabolism studies may be conducted at the same time that mammalian drug metabolism studies are performed, and metabolites which are produced by both metabolizing systems may be readily obtained in gram quantity by using routine fermentation scale-up techniques. Such metabolites would thus be available for: complete structure elucidation: biologic/toxicologic evaluation; and as analytical standards for further mammalian metabolism studies. The concept of microbial models of mammalian metabolism has been solidified by studies in comparative biochemistry which have shown that the pathways by which xenobiotics are altered by microbes and mammals are essentially the same [4, 13]. A recent successful application of this idea involved the alkaloid papaverine which undergoes 0-demethylations by rat and guinea pig microsomal preparations [41]. Microorganisms were used to obtain gram quantities of the 0-demethylated papaverine metabolites.

Microbial Transformations of Antitumor Agents

Microbial transformation experiments have been conducted with many antitumor compounds, and a number of examples are cited in Table 1. Not all of the compounds studied may be called antibiotics in the classic sense, since many of them are derived from higher plants. Some of the studies listed in Table 1 have been selected for expansion to illustrate how microbial transformations may be used in the development of new antitumor agents.

Bleomycin

The bleomycins are a group of structurally related antitumor antibiotics produced by strains of *Streptomyces verticillus.* The various bleomycins differ principally in the nature of the terminal amine moiety which attaches to the basic structure of all of the bleomycins, bleomycinic acid *5*. Microorganisms capable of selectively hydrolyzing bleomycin B_2 *5b* to *5* were sought since bleomycinic acid was considered to be a useful intermediate for the preparation of semisynthetic bleomycin derivatives (Fig. 2). Washed cells of *Fusarium anguioides* as well as cell-free enzyme extracts of the organism performed the desired reaction. The enzyme was characterized as an acylagmatine amidohydrolase, and was rather specific for the cleavage of the agmatine unit from bleomycin B_2 [48]. Bleomycin A_2, the main component of natural bleomycins was later shown to undergo chemical cleavage to bleomycinic acid [47], and by this chemical process new bleomycins were readily synthesized.

Anthracycline Antibiotics

The anthracycline antibiotics including adriamycin and daunomycin have become clinically important drugs. One major impetus for using microbial transformations was to convert daunomycin into less available antibiotics like adriamycin or carminomycin by hydroxylation

Table 1. Antitumor compounds which have been studied with microbial transformation systems

Antitumor Agent	Metabolite	Ref.
Acronycine	9-Hydroxyacronycine	[3, 5]
	3-Hydroxymethylacronycine	[5]
	3, 11-Dihydroxyacronycine	[5]
Actinomycin	Actinomycin monolactone	[39]
	Actinomycinic acid	[39]
Anthracyclines		
Daunomycin	Daunomycinol	[14, 28]
	7-Deoxydaunomycinone	[27, 28]
N-Acetyldaunomycin	N-Acetyldaunomycinol	[1]
Steffimycin	Steffimycinone	[27, 28]
Bleomycin	Bleomycinic acid	[48]
Mitomycin	Unknown metabolite	[17]
Mycophenolic Acid	Many metabolites	[20]
Papaverine	4'-0-Desmethylpapaverine	[41]
	6-0-Desmethylpapaverine	[41]
Rifamycin-B	Rifamycin-Y	[25]
Showdomycin	Isomer	[37]
d-Tetrandrine	N'-*Nor*-d-tetrandrine	[11]
	N-*Nor*-d-tetrandrine	[12]
Thalicarpine	(+)-Hernandalinol	[31]
Vinca Alkaloids		[34]
Vinblastine	Ether-derivative	[33]
	Phenol	[33, 34]
Vindoline	Numerous metabolites	[26, 32, 35, 33]
Withaferin-A	14-*Alpha*-hydroxywithaferin	[36]

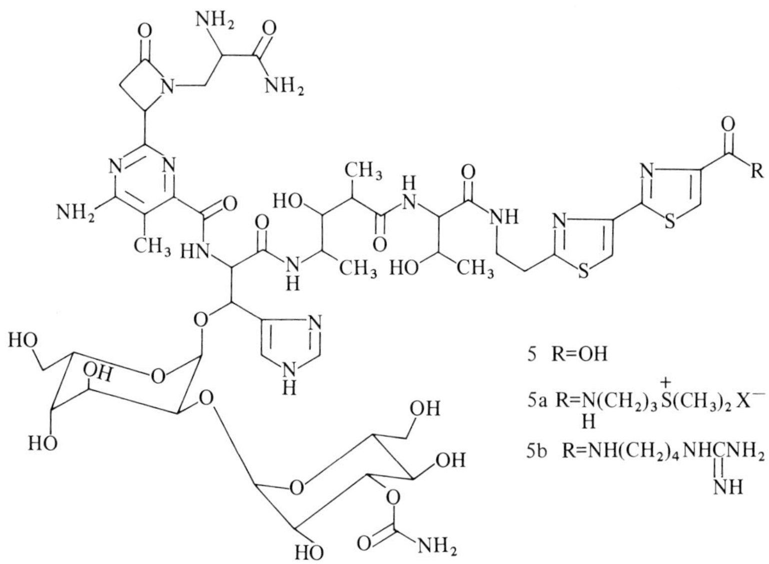

Fig. 2. Structures of bleomycinic acid (5), bleomycin A-2 (5a) and bleomycin B-2 (5b)

and O-demethylation respectively. The first report in this area described the reduction of daunomycin *3* to daunomycinol *3a* by several microorganisms [14]. Daunomycinol possesses in-vitro and in-vivo P-388 activity, and it was reported that the reduced derivative was a common mammalian daunomycin metabolite. Reduction of the side-chain ketone of the anthracyclines appears to be a common microbial and mammalian metabolic process [1, 2, 14, 21, 27, 28]. Daunomycinol produced by microorganisms is comparable in all stereochemical respects to the same metabolite produced by mammals [1]. Although they are active, it has been suggested that reduced metabolites like daunomycinol may have lower potential for use as drugs [2].

The reductive metabolism of several other anthracycline antibiotics has been studied in detail by several workers. Microaerophilically grown cultures of *Aeromonas hydrophila, Citrobacter fruendii* and *Escherichia coli* gave the 7-deoxyaglycones of a number of anthracyclines [27, 28]. Cell free extracts of *A. hydrophila* required NADH to accomplish the reductive glycoside cleavage. Apparently the transformation does not proceed through the aglycone first, followed by dehydration and subsequent reduction of the double bond. The same reaction occurs in mammals, but the reduction requires NADPH. These and other reactions with the anthracycline antibiotics reinforce the concept of microbial models of mammalian metabolism.

One attempt was made to use the glycosidization enzyme of a *Streptomycete* to prepare glycosides of daunomycinone [21]. The microorganism was known to glycosidize several anthraquinones. However, the microorganism only accomplished a reductuion of the side-chain ketone of daunomycinone, and no glycoside products were obtained.

Acronycine

Acronycine *6* is an acridone alkaloid found in members of the Rutaceae plant family. This compound demonstrated significant antitumor activity in several test systems, and it exhibited oral activity as well. Microbial transformation experiments were performed with this compound to prepare potentially more active derivatives and to determine its metabolic fate [3, 5]. Several microorganisms including a *Cunninghamella bainieri* strain produced several metabolites of the alkaloid. In a 4 g incubation with this culture, more than 1.3 g of the 9-hydroxyacronycine metabolite *6a* was isolated. The structure of the metabolite was fully determined by chemical and spectral methods, principally by pmr spectroscopy. Neither the metabolite nor its more soluble acetate ester derivative demonstrated significant antitumor activity in L-1210 or P-388 test systems [3]. This was probably due to the extreme insolubility of the compounds in aqueous media. Brannon and coworkers found other cultures which hydroxylated the gem-dimethyl group of the chromene ring of acronycine, and which gave the 11-hydroxylated derivative *6c* as well [5]. Neither of these metabolites were active in tumor test systems.

While the microbial transformation experiments were being conducted, a report appeared concerning the metabolism of acronycine in mammals [46]. The major mammalian metabolite of the alkaloid was 9-hydroxyacronycine *6a* which could be isolated in very small amounts, and which was not readily accessible by chemical synthesis. Other mammalian metabolites of the alkaloid included the 11-hydroxy-derivative, and the gem-dimethyl group hydroxylated product [46], the same kinds of metabolites produced by microorganisms.

D-Tetrandrine

D-Tetrandrine is a *bis*-benzyltetrahydroisoquinoline alkaloid *7* which demonstrated significant activity against the Walker-256 test system in the rat. Biotransformations of this compound occur primarily by means of N-demethylation reactions with microorganisms [11,

12]. It is possible to selectively cleave either the N-methyl or the N'-methyl group of d-tetrandrine simply by choosing the proper microorganism. For example, 50% yields of the N'-*nor*-d-tetrandrine derivative *7a* are obtained when *Streptomyces griseus* fermentations are used, while 20% yields of the N-nor-d-tetrandrine derivative *7b* are obtained with cultures of *Cunninghamella blakesleeana*. Chemical methods using methychloroformate as an N-demethylating reagent lead to complicated mixtures of all possible *nor*-d-tetrandrines [12].
The N'-*nor*-d-tetrandrine derivative *8a* is also known as cycleanorine, an alkaloid isolated in extremely small amounts from the plant *Cyclea peltata* by Kupchan and coworkers [24]. Interestingly, cycleanorine is inactive in the Walker-256 test system, and this suggests that the metabolic removal of the N'-methyl group of d-tetrandrine is responsible for the loss of activity of the alkaloid [18]. Since the N-methyl groups of compounds like d-tetrandrine are metabolically labile, and since there appears to be a connection between the presence of the N-alkyl group and antitumor activity, it will be worthwhile to prepare d-tetrandrine derivatives bearing various kinds of N-acyl and/or N-alkyl substituents which would be inert to metabolic N-Demethylation in mammals. This approach could provide d-tetrandrine derivatives with more desirable antitumor activity. The synthetic intermediates required for this work are being prepared by microbial N-demethylation of d-tetrandrine. The microbial N-demethylation is much more selective than the chemical demethylating procedure, and the *nor*-tetrandrines are obtained in higher yield [12]. We have both the N- and N'-*nor*-d-tetrandrine metabolites available for use as analytical standards for planned mammalian drug metabolism studies (Fig. 3).

Thalicarpine

Thalicarpine is a complex benzyltetrahydroisoquinoline-aporphine alkaloid *8*, and it possesses activity against the Walker-256 test system [23]. Like d-tetrandrine, this compound shows no activity in the L-1210 or P-388 leukemia systems. The alkaloid has been involved in Phase-I and Phase-II clinical trials. Although the general features of the mechanism of action of thalicarpine and d-tetrandrine have been described [9], little is known about the biodisposition of these compounds in mammalian systems [10, 38].
Microbial transformation experiments revealed an unusual type of biotransformation reaction where thalicarpine was converted into a metabolite identified as (+)-hernandalinol *8a* [31]. The metabolite was identified by spectral and chemical methods, and was prepared by chemical synthesis. (+)-Hernandalinol *8a* is formed when the aldehyde hernandaline *8b* is fed to cultures of *Streptomyces punipalus*, the organism which converts *8* to *8a*. Thus it was proposed that *Streptomyces punipalus* accomplishes an oxidative cleavage of the isoquinoline ring from thalicarpine to give *8b* which is subsequently reduced to the metabolite *8a*. It was suggested earlier that the active antitumor portion of the thalicarpine molecule resides in the aporphine moiety which must be connected to a part of the benzylisoquinoline moiety [29]. This conclusion was based on the finding that *8b* itself possesses cytotoxic activity. The possibility that thalicarpine may undergo metabolic conversion to hernandaline-like compounds in mammals is under investigation.

Vinca Alkaloids

The structural complexity of Vinca alkaloids such as vinblastine (VBL) and vincristine (VCR) has prevented their synthesis, and has also prevented complete structure-activity relationship studies. Workers at Eli Lilly have used microbial transformations as a means of preparing some derivatives of VBL [34]. The microbial transformation products were identified as

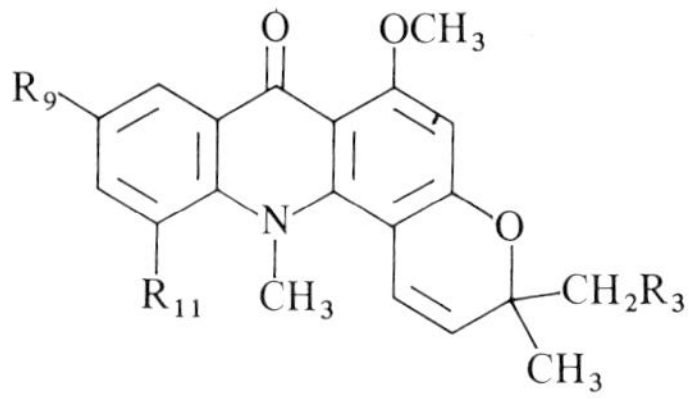

6 R_3=R_9=R_{11}=H
6a R_9=OH R_3=R_{11}=H
6b R_3= OH, R_9= R_{11}= H
6c R_3=R_{11}=OH, R_9=H

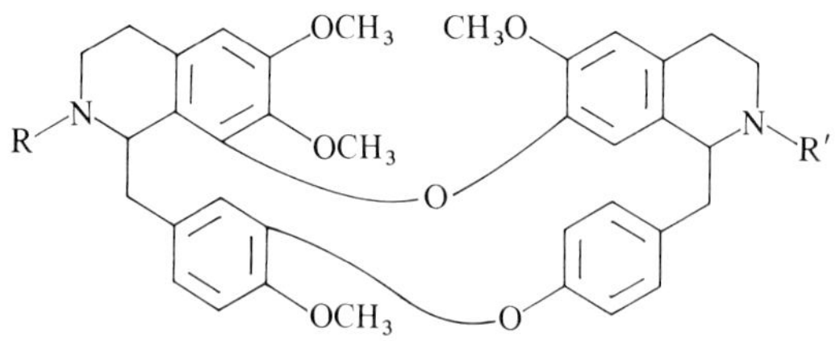

7 R=R′=CH_3
7a R′=H, R=CH_3
7b R′=CH_3,R=H

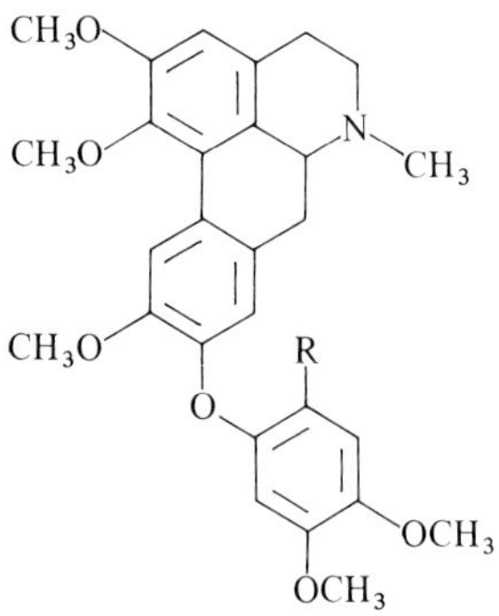

8 R=

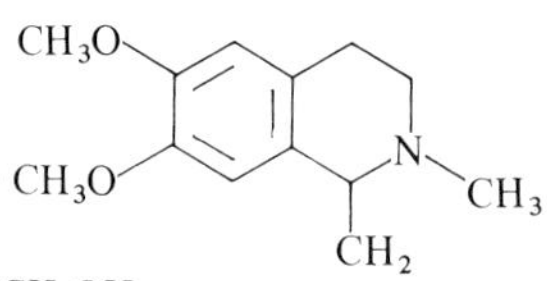

8a R=CH_2OH
8b R=CHO

Fig. 3. Structures of acronycine (6), d-tetrandrine (7), thalicarpine (8), and their microbial metabolites

VLB-ether, and hydroxy-VLB. Both metabolites were produced as a result of biotransformations occurring at the indolenine portion of VBL, while the vindoline moiety remained unaffected. The activities of the VBL metabolites have not been reported.

A series of microbial metabolites have been obtained with the vinca alkaloid vindoline [26, 32, 35, 33]. Vindoline *9* is one of the major alkaloids present in *Vinca Rosea* and it is present as one-half of the dimeric structure of VBL. The basic vindoline skeleton is also present in the structure of VCR. Microbial transformations of vindoline were performed to determine patterns of metabolism of this alkaloid. Streptomyces species were capable of producing several metabolites of vindoline identified as: des-N-methylvindoline, desacetylvindoline *9a*, dihydrovindoline ether (DHVE) *10*, desacetyl-DHVE *10a*, and acetonyl-DHVE *11*.

We investigated the metabolism of vindoline with a culture of *Streptomyces griseus* which produced DHVE, and one previously unidentified metabolite *12* [32]. The metabolite was characterized as a dimer of DHVE on the basis of C-13 nmr spectroscopy (50 carbons evident); high resolution mass spectrometry (908 m. wt. for $C_{50}H_{60}N_4O_{12}$); and pmr spectroscopy which enabled us to assign the points of attachment of the dimer as shown in *12* (Fig. 4).

The biotransformation achieved by *S. griseus* with vindoline is of interest for several reasons. First, the most active of the vinca alkaloids are all dimeric in nature. The biologic activity of the dimer 12 is being determined at present. Second, the structure of the dimer presents information regarding how this dimer, and indeed how some of the previously reported vindoline metabolites, may be formed by microbial metabolic systems. The dimer *12*, DHVE *10* and acteonyl-DHVE *11* most likely arise through the bracketed, enamine intermediate shown in Fig. 4. The respective metabolites would be obtained as follows: *12*, by joining one of each of the bracketed intermediates with the other; *10* by a reduction of a double bond; and *11*, by alkylation with an acetoacetate residue generated by the microorganism.

This work has demonstrated that vindoline-like molecules are capable of being metabolized to chemically reactive compounds by living systems. It is important to realize that the vindoline structure occurs nearly intact in antitumor active Vinca alkaloids like VBL and VCR, and that similar types of biotransformations can be rationalized for these alkaloids as well. We feel that this biotransformation reaction has provided valuable information concerning possible modes of mammalian biotransformation reactions of the Vinca alkaloids, and it has suggested certain chemical modifications of the Vinca alkaloids which may shed more light on structure-activity relationships.

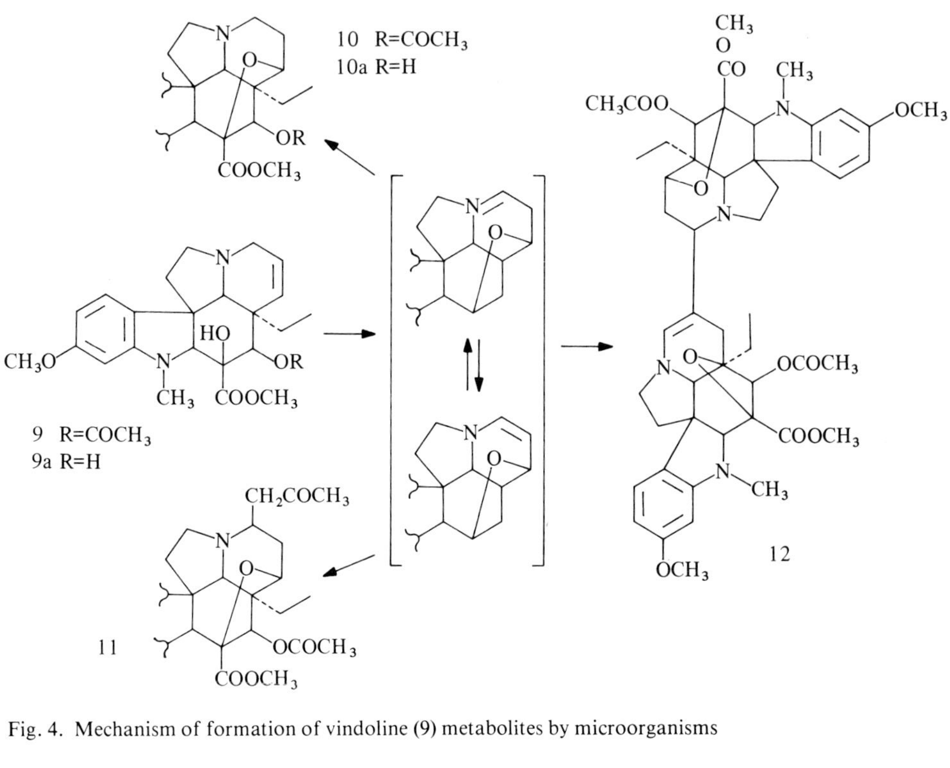

Fig. 4. Mechanism of formation of vindoline (9) metabolites by microorganisms

Conclusions

Microbial transformation experiments have been performed with several types of antitumor compounds to date. Most of the research described has required the interdisciplinary efforts of microbial chemists, pharmacologists and organic chemists. A true measure of the scope of efforts in this field will only become evident over the next several years as other workers publish their findings.

This tool has provided us with some insights as to how antitumor compounds undergo metabolic transformation in microbes and possibly in mammals as well. It has been useful for the production of minor, naturally-occurring compounds like cycleanorine. The results of such studies have provided new leads which may enhance our understanding of structure-activity relationships of complex antitumor agents. It should be emphasized that the examples cited in this brief review do not reflect the entire realm of metabolic reactions expected to occur with the antitumor compounds. Rather these have been selected to illustrate the scope and potential of microbial transformations in the development of newer antitumor agents.

Acknowledgements

The author wishes to recognize the outstanding efforts of several individuals who have been involved in research in his laboratory. These include Drs. P. J. Davis, T. Nabih, R. V. Smith, A. W. Nicholas, and M. Gustafson, S. Otten, R. Betts, L. Youel, M. A. Kammer. We also acknowledge financial support for some of the work through grant NCI-CA-13786.

Summary

Microbial transformations refer to reactions catalyzed by microbial enzymes, especially when specific and useful metabolites accumulate in fermentation media. These transformations have tremendous potential for use in the development of new antitumor drugs and these can also be used as models of mammalial metabolism. Microbial transformation experiments with antibiotics such as bleomycin, anthracyclines and with a variety of plant products are described.

References

1. Aszalos, A., Bachur, N. R., Hamilton, B. K., Langlykke, A. F., Roller, P. P., Sheikh, M. Y., Sutphin, M. S., Thomas, M. C., Wareheim, D. A., Wright, L. H.: Microbial reduction of the side-chain carbonyl of daunorubicin and N-acetyldaunorubicin. J. Antibiot. Tokyo **30**, 50–58 (1977).
2. Bachur, N. R., Steele, M., Meriweather, W. D., Hildebrand, R. C.: Cellular pharmacodynamics of several anthracycline antibiotics. J. Med. Chem. **19**, 651–654 (1976).
3. Betts, R. E., Walters, D. E., Rosazza: J. P.: Microbial transformations of antitumor compounds. 1. Conversion of acronycine to 9-hydroxyacronycine by *Cunninghamella echinulata*. J. Med. Chem. **17**, 599–602 (1974).

4. BOYD, D. R., CAMPBELL, R. M., CRAIG, H. C., WATSON, C. G., DALY, J. W., JERINA, D. M.: Mechanism of aromatic hydroxylation in fungi. Evidence for the formation of arene oxides. J. Chem. Soc. Perkin Transactions **1**, 2438–2443 (1976).
5. BRANNON, D. R., HORTON, H. R., SVOBODA, G. H.: Microbial hydroxylation of acronycine. J. Med. Chem. **17**, 653–654 (1974).
6. CHARNEY, W., HERZOG, H. L.: Microbial Transformations of Steroids, New York: Academic Press 1967.
7. CONNORS, T. A., PHILLIPS, B. J.: Screening for anticancer agents. The relative merits of *in vitro* and *in vivo* techniques. Biochem. Pharmacol. **24**, 2217–2224 (1975).
8. CRC: Handbook of Microbiology. Laskin, A. I., Lechevalier, H. A. (eds.) Cleveland, Ohio: CRC Press 1973, Vol. IV.
9. CREASY, W. A.: Biochemical effects of d-tetrandrine and thalicarpine. Biochem. Pharmacol. **25**, 1887–1891 (1976).
10. CREAVEN, P. J., ALLEN, L. M.: Thalicarpine (NSC-68075): Plasma decay and urinary excretion in man. Cancer Treat. Rep. **60**, 69–75 (1976).
11. DAVIS, P. J., ROSAZZA, J. P.: Microbial transformations of natural antitumor agents. 2. Studies with d-tetrandrine and laudanosine. J. Org. Chem. **41**, 2548–2551 (1976).
12. DAVIS, P. J., WIESE, D., ROSAZZA, J. P.: Microbial transformations of natural antitumor agents. 4. Formation of N-(2)-nor-d-tetrandrine by *Cunninghamella blakesleeana* (ATCC 8688a). Lloydia (In Press) (June 1977).
13. FERRIS, J. P., MACDONALD, L. H., PATRIE, M. A., MARTIN, M. A.: Arylhydrocarbon hydroxylase activity in the fungus *Cunninghamella bainieri*: evidence for the presence of cytochrome P-450. Arch. Biochem. Biophys. **175**, 443–452 (1976).
14. FLORENT, J., LUNEL, J.: Neue Vorfahren zur Herstellung des Antibiotikums 20, 789. Ger. Offen. 2,456,139. Chem. Abstr. **83**, 112355q (1975).
15. FONKEN, G., JOHNSON, R. S.: Chemical Oxidations with Microorganisms. New York: Marcel-Dekker 1972.
16. GILLETTE, J. R.: Formation of reactive drug metabolites as a basis of drug action and toxicity. Isr. J. Chem. **14**, 193–204 (1976).
17. GOUREVITCH, A., PURSIANO, T. A., LEIN, J.: Destruction of mitomycin C by *Streptomyces caespitosus* mycelia. Arch. Biochem. Biophys. **93**, 283–288 (1961).
18. HARTWELL, J. L.: Types of anticancer agents isolated from plants. Cancer Treat. Rep. **60**, 1031–1068 (1976).
19. IIZUKA, H., NAITO, A.: Microbial Transformations of Steroids and Alkaloids. State College of Pennsylvania: University Park Press 1967.
20. JONES, D. E., MOORE, R. H., CROWLEY, G. C.: Microbial modification of mycophenolic acid. J. Chem. Soc. (C) 1725–1737 (1972).
21. KARNETOVA, J., MATEJU, J., SEDANORA, P., VOKOURN, J., VANEK, Z.: Microbial transformation of daunomycinone by *Streptomyces aureofaciens* B-96. J. Antibiot. Tokyo **29**, 1199–1202 (1976).
22. KIESLICH, K.: Microbial Transformations of Non-Steroid Cyclic Compounds. New York: Wiley-Interscience 1976.
23. KUPCHAN, S. M., CHAKRAVARTI, K. K., YOKOYAMA, N.: Thalictrum alkaloids. I. Thalicarpine, a new hypotensive alkaloid from *Thalictrum dasycarpum*. J. Pharm. Sci. **52**, 985–988 (1963).
24. KUPCHAN, S. M., LIEPA, A. J., BAXTER, R. L., HITZ, H. L.: A new alkaloid and related artifacts from *Cyclea peltata*. J. Org. Chem. **38**, 1846–1851 (1973).
25. LANCINI, G. C., THIEMANN, J. E., SARTORI, G., SENSI, P.: Biogenesis of rifamycins. The conversion of rifamycin-B into Rifamycin Y. Experientia **23**, 899 (1967).
26. MALLETT, G. E., FUKUDA, D. S., GORMAN, M.: Microbial conversion of Catharanthus alkaloids. Lloydia **27**, 334–339 (1964).
27. MARSHALL, V. P., REISENDER, E. A., REINEKE, L. M., JOHNSON, J. H., WILEY, P. F.: Reductive conversion of anthracycline antibiotics. Biochemistry **15**, 4139–4145 (1976).
28. MARSHALL, V. P., REISENDER, E. A., WILEY, P. F.: Bacterial metabolism of daunomycin. J. Antibiot. Tokyo: **29**, 966–968 (1976).
29. MOLLOV, N. M., DUCHEWSKA, K. B., SILYANOVSKA, K., STOICEV, S.: Cytotoxic effect of alkaloids of *thalictrum minus ssp elatum* and their derivatives. C. R. Acad. Sci. (Bulg.) **21**, 605–608 (1968); Chem. Abstr. **69**, 58087 (1968).
30. MONTGOMERY, J. A., STUCK, R. F.: The relationship of the metabolism of anticancer agents to their activity. Prog. Drug Res. **17**, 322–409 (1973).
31. NABIH, T., DAVIS, P. J., CAPUTO, J. F., ROSAZZA, J. P.: Microbial transformations of natural antitumor agents. 3. Conversion of thalicarpine to (+)-hernandalinol by *Streptomyces punipalus*. J. Med. Chem. (In Press) (July 1977).
32. NABIH, T., YOUEL, L., ROSAZZA, J. P.: Microbial transformations of natural antitumor agents. 5. Studies with vindoline. Submitted for publication.

33. Neuss, N., Fukuda, D. S., Mallett, G. E., Brannon, D. R., Huckstep, L. L.: Vinca alkaloids XXXII. Microbiological conversions of vindoline, a major alkaloid from *Vinca Rosea* L. Helv. Chim. Acta **56**, 2418–2426 (1973).
34. Neuss, N., Mallett, G. E., Brannon, D. R., Mabe, J. A., Horton, H. R., Huckstep, L. L.: Vinca alkaloids. XXXIII. Microbiological conversions of vincaleukoblastine (VLB, Vinblastine) an antitumor alkaloid from *Vinca rosea.* Helv. Chim. Acta **57**, 1887–1891 (1974).
35. Neuss, N. Fukuda, D. S., Brannon, D. R., Huckstep, L. L.: Vinca alkaloids. XXXIV. Preparation of des-N-methylvindoline by microbiological conversion of vindoline, a major alkaloid of *Vinca Rosea* L. Helv. Chim. Acta **57**, 1891–1893 (1974).
36. Nicholas, A., Fyfe, L., Loebig, D., Rosazza, J. P.: Microbial transformations of withaferin-A, a Steroidal lactone. Abstracts 5th Internat. Fermentation Symp., W. Berlin, July 1976, p. 331.
37. Ozaki, M., Kariya, T., Kato, H., Kimura, T.: Microbial transformations of antibiotics. Part I. Isomerization of showdomycin by *Streptomyces.* Agr. Biol. Chem. **36**, 451–456 (1972).
38. Palm, P. E., Nick, M. S., Arnold, E. P., Yesair, D. W., Callahan, M. M.: Single- and repeated dose toxicity of thalicarpine (NSC-68075) in monkeys including physiological disposition studies. U.S. Dept. Commerce National Technical Information Service. PB Rep-201914, Chem. Abstr. **76**, 68093 (1971).
39. Perlman, D., Mauger, A. B., Weissbach, H. W.: Microbial metabolism of actinomycins and other heterodetic antibiotic peptides. Biochem. Biophys. Res. Commun. **24**, 513–518 (1966).
40. Proceedings of the 16th Annual Meeting of the Society for Economic Botany. Plants and Cancer. Cancer Treat. Rep. **60**, 973–1215 (1976).
41. Rosazza, J. P., Kammer, M., Youel, L., Smith, R. V., Erhardt, P. W., Truong, D. H., Leslie, S. W.: Microbial models of mammalian metabolism. O-Demethylations of papaverine. Xenobiotica **7**, 133–143 (1977).
42. Sebek, O. K.: Microbial conversion of antibiotics. Lloydia **37**, 115–133 (1974).
43. Sebek, O. K.: The scope and potential of antibiotic conversions by microorganisms. Acta Microbiologica **22**, 381–388 (1975).
44. Sih, C. J., Rosazza, J. P.: Microbial transformations in organic synthesis. In, Applications of Biochemical Systems in Organic Chemistry. Jones, B., Perlman, D., Sih, C. J. (eds). New York: Wiley 1976, Vol. IX, p. 69.
45. Smith, R. V., Rosazza, J. P.: Microbial models of mammalian metabolism. J. Pharm. Sci. **64**, 1737–1759 (1975).
46. Sullivan, H. R., Billings, R. E., Occolowitz, J. L., Boaz, H. E., Marshall, F. J., McMahon, R. E.: In vivo hydroxylation of the alkaloid acronine, an experimental antitumor agent. J. Med. Chem. **13**, 904–909 (1970).
47. Takita, T., Fujii, A., Fukuoka, T., Umezawa, H.: Chemical cleavage of Bleomycin to bleomycinic acid and synthesis of new bleomycins. J. Antibiot. (Tokyo) **26**, 252–256 (1973).
48. Umezawa, H., Takahashi, Y., Fujii, A., Saino, T., Shirai, T., Takita, T.: Preparation of bleomycinic acid: hydrolysis of bleomycin B-2 by a Fusarium acylagmatine amidohydrolase. J. Antibiot. (Tokyo) **26**, 117–119 (1973).
49. Wallen, L. L., Stodola, F. H., Jackson, R. W.: Type Reactions in Fermentation Chemistry. Peoria, Illinois: ARS Bulletin ARS-71-13, 1959.

Detection and Assay of Antitumor Antibiotics

L. J. Hanka, S. L. Kuentzel, D. G. Martin, P. F. Wiley, and Gary L. Neil

For over 20 years, The Upjohn Company has conducted research directed towards the detection, isolation, purification, characterization, and development of fermentation-derived antitumor agents—so-called "antitumor antibiotics." Most of this effort has been conducted in collaboration with, and with contract support from, the U.S. National Cancer Institute.

As is well known, fermentation broths have proven to be an excellent source of novel antitumor agents, and antitumor antibiotics have assumed a preeminent position in the armamentarium employed in the chemotherapy of human neoplasia. Unfortunately, even though fermentation broths may contain useful activities, the frequency of their occurrence is usually very low and, when they are present, they usually occur (at least initially) in extremely low concentrations. Consequently, we have concluded that in vitro detection (prescreening) methods are valuable (if not essential) tools in our attempts to find new antitumor antibiotics.

In vitro detection offers a number of advantages. First, it can reduce the total number of random samples submitted to a more definitive (but more expensive) in vivo screen by submitting only those samples whose probability of being active in the screen have been increased through application of this preselection process. Second, it is possible, by choosing an appropriate in vitro system, to select from a random-source pool, by relatively economic means, those compounds or activities that have defined and desired biologic or biochemical characteristics. Finally, the system employed in the in vitro detection of activity can, in many instances, be employed as an assay method to follow the activity during fermentation development studies and chemical and physical isolation work.

Over 20 years of Upjohn experience in the area of the discovery and development of antitumor antibiotics is summarized in Table 1.

Prior to 1958, the initiation of our contractual involvement with NCI, a number of Upjohn antimicrobial antibiotics were submitted to NCI for evaluation of potential antitumor activity. Among the antibiotics which showed significant antitumor activity were cycloheximide, chartreusin, streptovitacin A, and the streptovaricins. Since that time we have continued to evaluate, for antitumor activity, other antibiotics which had been isolated because of their antimicrobial activity. Among those showing significant antitumor activity have been: streptozocin, zorbamycin, porfiromycin, and the steffimycins. Streptozocin, an N-methyl, N-nitrosourea derivative of glucosamine has demonstrated significant activity in human cancer, specifically against malignant insulinoma. These examples represent antitumor antibiotics for which prior knowledge of antitumor activity (in vitro or in vivo) was not a consideration in their isolation and purification.

During the period prior to 1958, a number of randomly selected crude fermentation broths were also submitted to NCI for evaluation in vivo. Although several active broths were detected, our limited attempts at isolation of active components, involving the cumbersome in vivo assay, were totally unsuccessful. This lack of success and the advent of cell-culture technology led to our first attempts at the use of in vitro detection systems specifically designed to detect antitumor agents. Our efforts during the period of roughly 1958–1964 dealt

Table 1. Detection and assay of fermentation-derived antitumor agents by the Upjohn Company

Approximate dates	Detection systems	Assay method	Examples of antitumor agents isolated
Pre-1958	Antimicrobial	Antimicrobial	Cycloheximide Chartreusin (Streptovaricins) Streptovitacin A Streptozocin Porfiromycin (Steffimycins) Zorbamycin
1958–1964	Cell Culture (KB)	Antimicrobial/KB	Pactamycin Sparcomycin Tubercidin Nogalamycin
1965–1970	Antimicrobial (Antimetabolite)/ In Vivo	Antimicrobial	5-Azacytidine AT-125 Hydroxy-AT-125 AT-111
1971–1975	Cell Culture (L1210)/In Vivo	Cell Culture/ Antimicrobial/ In Vivo	CC-1014
1976–	Cell Culture/ Special Antimicrobial/ In Vivo	Cell Culture/ Antimicrobial	

with the development and adaptation of cell-culture methodology pioneered by Eagle and Foley [3] and others to an actual operational screening method applicable to fermentation broths. These methods, utilizing KB human epidermoid carcinoma cells, were elaborated by Smith, Grady, and others of our group [6, 11, 12]; and this prescreen was operated intermittently for about 6 years. For detection purposes, the KB cell-culture system was employed as a growth inhibition test in which inhibition of total cell protein was determined [12]. This assay and a related technique [6, 11] in which the biochemical integrity of the KB cells dispersed in an agar medium was determined by their ability to reduce a dye, proved valuable supplements to antimicrobial activity as assay methods for subsequent purification and isolation efforts. During this period of time, a number of important antitumor antibiotics were discovered. Among these were pactamycin, tubercidin, sparsomycin, and nogalamycin. Of these, however, only tubercidin proved effective in the treatment of human cancer.

During the mid-1960's, an in vitro microbial system for the detection of materials possessing antimetabolite activity was developed [8]. This prescreen was based on the observation that known antimetabolites inhibited the growth of susceptible microorganisms much more strongly when these organisms were grown in limited, chemically defined (or synthetic) media, rather than in the commonly used, fully supplemented, complex media, e.g., nutrient agar. This prescreen, operated roughly from 1966–1970, offered the additional advantage in that it allowed one, at the initial crude broth evaluation stage, to derive some information concerning the mechanism of action of the active component and even some hints as to its structural class. This specific antimicrobial activity also proved very useful for monitoring activity in subsequent work up and isolation.

About 1970, we developed an in vitro prescreen based on the ability of test samples to inhibit growth of L1210 mouse leukemia cells in suspension culture—the so-called "in vitro L1210 cytotoxicity" prescreen [1]. This technique was originally employed as the initial step of a cell-cycle phase-specificity prescreen [4]. In the early evaluation of the phase-specificity approach, we found that materials preselected on the basis of in vitro L1210 cytotoxicity alone, regardless of phase-specific cytotoxicity, yielded a relatively large number of in vivo active leads. This prescreen was employed from about 1971–1975. The assay methodology employed included both cell culture and antimicrobial systems and, in a few instances, in vivo evaluation.

Our experiences with the antimetabolite and in vitro L1210 cytotoxicity prescreens, employed for roughly comparable periods of time, is compared in Table 2.

Table 2. Summary of two in vitro prescreens

	Antimetabolite	L1210 in vitro *"cytotoxic cultures"*
Total number of broths tested	11,600	3294
In vitro actives	585 (5%)	624 (19%)
Confirmed in vivo actives	12 (2%)	174 (28%)
Number of *new*, significant antitumor agents	3	2+

The throughput (number of broths tested) with the antimetabolite prescreen was considerably higher than that for the L1210 cytotoxicity prescreen. The latter is, of course, more technically demanding and more time consuming (2–3 days, compared to 8–16h). The yield of in vitro actives with the antimetabolite prescreen (5%) was considerably lower than that (20%) for the cell culture prescreen. However, because the activity criteria in both cases are somewhat arbitrary, this is not particularly meaningful. The yield of in vivo actives from the antimetabolite prescreen was quite low (2% of the in vitro active leads). In spite of this, three new antitumor antimetabolites were isolated (Table 1). The first, 5-azacytidine (also known as ladakamycin), has proven useful in the clinical treatment of acute myelocytic leukemia. Two related amino acid antimetabolites, AT-125 [(αS,5S)-α-amino-3-chloro-4, 5-dihydro-5-isoxazoleacetic acid; NSC-163501] and its 4-hydroxy derivative also originated from this prescreen. AT-125 is currently undergoing preclinical evaluation at NCI. In addition, a senfolomycin-related antibiotic with antitumor activity (U-43,120; AT-111) and a number of new antimetabolites which proved to have little in vivo antitumor activity were also isolated.

The yield of in vivo actives with the L1210 cytotoxicity prescreen was extremely high—28% of the in vitro active broths proved active in the P388 in vivo system employed during this period of time. We are, of course, still involved very much in the follow-up of these materials. As discussed in detail in another paper in this symposium [2], "dereplication" (the processes of determining the presence of a known agent in a candidate broth) is a necessary component of antibiotic discovery. This process has proved to be of particular importance for this group of leads. Well over half of the 174 lead cultures have been shown to produce a known agent. In addition, we have suspended efforts on a number of these cultures because of miscellaneous difficulties with the fermentation or because isolation efforts have been unsuccessful. Roughly 30 of these cultures are currently of interest to us, and isolation and purification studies are in progress. We have, to date, isolated two pure, apparently novel, antitumor agents. One of these, CC-1014 (U-53,948), has been partially characterized [13]. It is a polypeptide of molecular weight 1217 containing 10–12 amino acid residues, a number of which have been identified. It has moderate activity against P388 leukemia at doses of less than 1 mg/kg/day.

One characteristic shared by U-53,948 (see above) and other leads of current interest is their potency. With one of our current leads, activity in vivo has been observed at doses less than 10 μg/kg/day. This tendency of the cell-culture prescreen to select highly potent and toxic agents (and other considerations) persuaded us to examine in considerable detail some aspects of our general prescreening and screening methodology which may be limiting our attempts to detect and isolate novel antitumor activities. In our laboratories, and probably in many others, the samples of which critical, initial prescreening and screening evaluations are conducted, are usually crude liquid fermentation broths or reconstituted lyophilized solids obtained from these broths prior to any purification attempts. We have, for a number of years, been concerned about the wisdom of this approach. We had a particularly enlightening experience with AT-125 [9]. Our experience during the isolation and purification of this agent is summarized in Table 3.

Table 3. Detection and antitumor activity of AT-125 (NSC-163501) in fermentation broths

Sample	Purity %	Maximum dose employed mg/kg	Dose required for 25% ILS mg/kg	Result[a]
Lyophilized crude broth	~0.013	600	3850	Inactive
First purification fraction	0.2	600	250	Active
Pure AT-125	100	>0.5	0.5	Active

[a] P388 or L1210, QD, D1-9.

The activity of AT-125 in crude fermentation broths was detected in the antimetabolite prescreen described above. Larger quantities of broth were prepared and crude lyophilized solids were submitted to NCI for in vivo evaluation. At that time, such screening was carried out by a separate contractor and it was approximately 6 months from the time of sample submission until the in vivo test data were received. During this time, studies of the antimetabolite characteristics of the fermentation broth were carried out and, because of a rather specific reversal pattern, attempts at crude fractionation were initiated. These attempts were in progress when the in vivo data were received. The in vivo results were negative (Table 3). The crude fermentation broth was inactive. In retrospect, we calculate that the purity of that initial crude lyophilized broth was approximately 0.01%. The maximum daily dose employed for evaluation of crude fermentation broths was 600 mg/kg. Based on data obtained later with pure material, we can calculate that a dose of at least 3850 mg/kg (over six times that employed) would have been required to observe activity with this crude material.

Since partial purification of the antimetabolite activity (approximately 20-fold) had already been achieved, this fraction was submitted for in vivo evaluation (in spite of the negative data with the crude broth solids). To our delight (and surprise), the fraction proved active and we eventually obtained pure AT-125. If in vivo activity of crude broths had been a necessary criterion for further development, and it hadn't been for this serendipitous delay in the testing and transmittal of results, it is quite possible that AT-125 would never have been isolated.

Based on this experience, an analysis was made of the ability of our cell-culture prescreen (Table 4) and in vivo screening systems (Table 5) to detect fermentation antitumor agents in crude broths.

It is assumed (based on considerable experience) that a typical streptomyces fermentation broth submitted for first evaluation contains approximately 20 mg solids/ml and that the active material is present at a level of 0.1% (or 20 μg/ml). Using the criterion currently employed for cell-culture activity (i.e., $ID_{50} < 100 \mu g$ solids/ml, equivalent to 0.1 μg/ml of the active component), and the ID_{50} values for a number of pure antitumor antibiotics, these antibiotics can be grouped into three classes with respect to the ability of the prescreen to detect their activity (Table 4). On this basis, the L1210 in vitro cytotoxicity prescreen would

Table 4. Can a cell culture prescreen detect fermentation-derived antitumor agents in crude broths?

"Detectable"	Maybe	"Not detectable"
ID_{50}<0.05 μg/ml	ID_{50} 0.05–0.20 μg/ml	ID_{50} >0.20 μg/ml
Actidione	Mitomycin C	Streptozocin
Actinomycin D	Porfiromycin	
Adriamycin	Sparsomycin	
5-Azacytidine	AT-125	
Cinerubins A or B		
Cirolemycin		
Daunomycin		
Levomycin		
Muconomycin		
Nogalamycin		
Pactamycin		
Tubercidin		
Xanthomycin		

Assumptions:
1. Test broth has 20 mg solids/ml containing 0.1% (20 μg/ml) active component.
2. The criterion for cell-culture activity is an ID_{50} (50% growth inhibitory concentration) of <100μg solids/ml = 0.1 μg/ml active component.
3. Activities are "detectable" in crude broths only where the active component has an ID_{50} <1/2 the criterion and "not detectable" where it is >2 the criterion.

Table 5. Can a mouse tumor screen detect fermentation-derived antitumor agents in crude broths?

"Detectable"	Maybe	"Not detectable"
LD_{10}<0.5 mg/kg	LD_{10} 0.5–2 mg/kg	LD_{10} >2 mg/kg
Actinomycin D	Adriamycin	Actidione
Cirolemycin	Cinerubins A or B	5-Azacytidine
Levomycin	Daunomycin	Porfiromycin
Muconomycin	Mitomycin C	Streptozocin
Xanthomycin	Nogalamycin	Bleomycin
Mithramycin	Pactamycin	Azaserine
	Sparsomycin	
	Tubercidin	
	AT-125	

Assumptions:
1. Test broth has 20 mg solids/ml containing 0.1% (20 μg/ml) active component.
2. Maximum dose employed is 500 mg/kg solids = 0.5 mg/kg active component.
3. Testing involves daily i.p. injections for 9 days.
4. Activity is only observed at doses greater than 1/2 the LD_{10} dose on that schedule.

detect most of these antitumor antibiotics. Only one, streptozocin, has an ID_{50} value >0.2 μg/ml; and only four would be borderline. It is of considerable interest that, of the streptomyces fermentation broths leads obtained with this prescreen approach which have been dereplicated as producing known antibiotics, 80% of them have been shown to contain cinerubins, actinomycins, quinomycins, or xanthomycins. These agents are particularly cytoxic (all with ID_{50} values <0.01μg/ml).

Analysis of the in vivo tumor screen is presented in Table 5 Another assumption is made concerning the maximum dose employed for in in vivo evaluation. If one assumes further that activity would not be observed at doses below roughly half the LD_{10} dose, one can again make groupings similar to those for the in vitro evaluation. Again, members of three of the four "nuisance" antibiotic classes (the actinomycins, quinomycins, and xanthomycins) fall in the "detectable" class. The other, the cinerubins, *might* be detectable. Most interesting, and of most concern, was that, based on this analysis, in vivo evaluation of crude fermentation broths would not detect such important (although less potent) antitumor antibiotics as 5-azacytidine, porfiromycin, streptozocin, bleomycin, or azaserine (all of which have demonstrated clinical utility).

Based on this analysis, a number of approaches to the solution of this problem were considered. Because of the high degree of effort involved (and the associated costs), it was felt that preliminary fermentation development purification attempts for all cultures prior to in vivo evaluation were not justified. Instead, a pilot study was conducted in which cultures producing broths that were active in vitro in the cell-culture prescreen but inactive in vivo (and nontoxic at the highest dose tested) were "recycled." Recycling involved simple attempts at preliminary purification (e.g. butanol extraction at three pHs, resin extraction, ultrafiltration) [10] and determination of activity enrichment using the cell-culture assay. Where five fold enrichment (by in vitro assay) was achieved, that procedure was employed to process a larger quantity of broth for subsequent reevaluation in vivo. The results of this pilot study are displayed in Table 6.

Table 6. "Recycled" cytotoxic cultures[a]

		Number of cultures
Enrichment unsuccessful		6
Enrichment successful but again inactive in vivo		42
Enrichment successful and now active in vivo		19
—Dereplicated as knowns	14	
—Dereplication survivors	6	
Total		67

[a] Active in vitro, inactive (but nontoxic at the highest dose tested) in vivo.

Of 67 cultures submitted to these simple procedures, 61 (91%) were enriched over five fold in their in vitro activity and were reevaluated in vivo. Of these 61, 19 (31%) showed in vivo activity on reevaluation (recall that original broths were all inactive). Most of these 19 [13] have been dereplicated as producing known materials (as one might expect) but six cultures are under active investigation and, at this stage, must be considered successfully "salvaged." We were sufficiently encouraged by this result to include this recycling process in our regular screening effort.

About 1 year ago, we introduced the prescreen approach we are currently employing at Upjohn. In designing this "multiendpoint" prescreen (Table 7) we analyzed and considered the relative advantages and disadvantages of antimicrobial and cell-culture techniques as detection and assay systems.

As a detection system, our experience (see, e.g., Table 2) suggests that the cell culture technique performs well. However, antimicrobial systems, by virtue of their speed, economy, ease of use, and adaptation to chromatographic (bioautography) techniques are definitely superior for assay and dereplication purposes. Consequently, we have attempted to design a prescreen assay system which combines the advantages and minimizes the disadvantages of

Table 7. Current Upjohn multiendpoint prescreen for fermentation-derived antitumor agents

Cell culture:	L1210 growth inhibition		("cytotoxicity")
Antimicrobial:	Gram-positives	(2)	Complex and synthetic media
	Gram-negatives	(2)	
	Streptomyces	(1)	
	Yeasts	(2)	
in vivo:	P388 with recycling		

these two approaches. Full details have been presented elsewhere [7]. Briefly, broths, produced by cultures obtained under a wide variety of unusual conditions are being evaluated both for inhibition of growth of L1210 cells in culture and for activity against a carefully selected group of microorganisms. Included are organisms and conditions (media) designed to detect specific types of antimetabolite activity (e.g., sugars, certain amino acids, and nucleic acid precursors) which we believe hold some promise, and a particular strain of *Streptomyces* which, in our experience, has frequently proven to be sensitive to agents which do not affect many other microorganisms. Also included will be a yeast, *Saccharomyces cerevisiae* FL200 and its mutant (FL 599-1B) developed by F. Lacroute (Laboratory of Physiological Genetics, Institute of Molecular Biology, Strasbourg, France) and studied by Gause [5]. The mutant, possessing a distorted cell membrane, appears to be selectively inhibited by antibiotics with antitumor activity. Based on activity in these systems, broths will be selected for evaluation in vivo after application of simple procedures designed to dereplicate a few commonly occurring "nuisance" antibiotics. Recycle techniques, similar to those described above, will be applied to appropriate cultures. Although we have just initiated this approach, a number of interesting leads have been generated, and we are confident that significant new antitumor agents will result from these efforts.

Summary

Cell culture techniques and antimicrobial systems can be used as detection systems for new antibiotic structures. Antimicrobial systems by virtue of their speed, economy, ease of use, and adaptation to chromatographic (bioautographic) techniques are definitely superior for assay and for dereplication purposes. A prescreen assay system which combines the advantages and minimizes the disadvantages of the two approaches is described.

References

1. Buskirk, H. H.: Assay of cytotoxic agents with L1210 cells. Proc. Tissue Culture Assoc. **20**, 23 (1969).
2. Dion, H.: Fingerprint methods used to identify known antineoplastic agents in culture filtrates. (see Chapter 8 of this book)
3. Eagle, H., Foley, G. E.: The cytotoxic action of carcinolytic agents in tissue culture. Am. J. Med. **21**, 739-749 (1956).
4. Fonken, G.S.: *In vitro* phase-specificity screening: an interim report. Cancer Chemother. Rep. Part 3, **3**, 7-12 (1972).
5. Gause, G. F., Laiko, A. V., Selesneva, T. I.: Yeast mutants with distorted cell membranes as tests in the screening for antitumor antibiotics. Cancer Chemother. Rep. **60**, 637-638 (1976).
6. Grady, J. E., Lummis, W. L., Smith, C. G.: Tissue culture bioautographic system. Proc. Soc. Exp.

Biol. Med. **103**, 727–730 (1960).
7. Hanka, L. J.: A multiendpoint *in vitro* system for detection of new antitumor drugs. Proc. Int. Congr. Chemother. (in press).
8. Hanka, L. J.: *In vitro* screen for antimetabolites. Proc. 5th Int. Congr. Chemother. **139**/2 351–357 (1967).
9. Hanka, L. J., Martin, D. G., Neil, G. L.: A new antitumor antimetabolite, (αS,5S)-α-amino-3-chloro-4,5-dihydro-5-isoxazoleacetic acid (NSC-163501): Antimicrobial reversal studies and preliminary evaluation against L1210 mouse leukemia *in vivo*. Cancer Chemother. Rep. **57**, 141–148 (1973).
10. Hanka, L. J., Martin, D. G., Wiley, P. F., Neil, G. L.: Problems related to the detection of activity of antitumor antibiotics. Chemotherapy **7**, 303–308 (1976).
11. Perlman, D., Lummis, W. L., Geiersbach, H. J.: Differential agar-diffusion bioassay for cytotoxic substances. J. Pharm. Sci. **58**, 633 (1969).
12. Smith, C. G., Lummis, W. L., Grady, J. E.: An improved tissue culture assay. I. Methodology and cytotoxicity of antitumor agents. Cancer Res. **19**, 843–846 (1959.
13. Wiley, P. F.: Unpublished results, these laboratories

Fingerprint Methods used to Identify known Antineoplastic Agents in Culture Filtrates

R. H. BUNGE, D. E. MCCREADY, L. A. BALTA, B. D. GRAHAM, J. C. FRENCH, and H. W. DION

In the search for novel antineoplastic agents in culture filtrates, several techniques have been used for detection or assay purposes. Some of these methods have involved a microbial or antimetabolite prescreen [7], or tissue culture cytotoxicity assay systems [6], prior to testing of the culture filtrate in animals. In the program that will be discussed here, all fermented beers are screened initially against the L1210 and KB9 cell lines for cytotoxic activity, and the "actives" are refermented in shake-flasks for confirmation of cytotoxicity. The confirmed active leads are then screened by a series of fingerprint methods designed to eliminate most of the more common antitumor agents prior to testing in animals. We have found that the use of this screening technique to eliminate knowns as quickly as possible in the early stages of the program has been very successful; it has increased the efficiency of our overall program. The purpose of this paper is to present some of the details of our "fingerprint" techniques.

We presently use seven fingerprints to help us identify known antineoplastic agents in culture filtrates. These are listed below in the usual order of actual practice.

Antimicrobial spectrum
Culture characterization
Paper chromatography—System 83/101
Thin-layer chromatography
Ultraviolet spectrum
Expanded yeast spectrum
High performance liquid chromatography

The identification scheme consists of the set method of processing all active cancer leads through the first three prints mentioned above. The results and deductions from these will dictate the feasibility of using any or all of the four remaining prints to identify the particular antineoplastic agent(s) in a culture filtrate. A detailed accounting of the three critical fingerprint methods is presented below and several work examples of the four remaining techniques will follow.

Antimicrobial Spectrum

In the early phases of our antitumor program, all of the known antitumor antibiotics in our library of compounds were tested at a concentration of 50 μg/ml against a large number of organisms using the standard agar trays and paper-disc, agar-diffusion method (12.7 mm disc) [5]. This was done in order to devise some type of antimicrobial screen that would allow us to classify known antitumor agents according to their antimicrobial activities. The above work led us to using the following organisms in our screening method:

Primary Spectrum

Escherichia coli 04863 (Ec) on glycerol asparagine agar (CIM 41)
Escherichia coli 04863 (Ec) on mycin agar (MYC)
Bacillus subtilis 04555 (Bs) on mycin agar
Sarcina lutea 05064 (Sl) on Penassay seed agar (PAS)
Torulopsis albida M1390 (Ta) on ADM 102

Secondary Spectrum

Compounds or beers exhibiting any *E. coli* activity are tested against the following G- pathogens:

a) *Escherichia coli* CIM 41 actives
Pseudomonas aeruginosa 05111 (Pa), *Salmonella typhimurium* 05063 (St), and *Klebsiella pneumoniae* 05114 (Kp) all on CIM 41 agar.
b) *Escherichia coli* mycin actives
Pseudomonas aeruginosa 05111 (Pa, *Proteus vulgaris* 05112 (Pv), *Salmonella typhimurium* 05063 (St), *Shigella sonnei* 05113 (Ss), and *Klebsiella pneumoniae* 05114 (Kp), all on mycin agar.

The data obtained from the screening of known antitumor agents against the above microbial spectrum showed that these antitumor antibiotics could be grouped according to their antimicrobial activity in ten distinct classes as shown in Table 1.

Table 1. Antitumor antibiotics grouped according to antimicrobial activity

Class	Antimicrobial activity
I.A.	Active *vs.* G- (Ec), G+ (Bs or S1) and yeast (Ta)
I.B.	Active *vs.* G- (Ec), (Bs or S1), inactive[a] *vs.* yeast (Ta)
I.C.	Active *vs.* G- (Ec) and yeast (Ta), inactive *vs.* G+ (Bs and S1)
I.D.	Active *vs.* G- (Ec), inactive *vs.* G+ (Bs and S1) and yeast (Ta)
II.A.	Active *vs.* G+ (Bs or S1) and yeast (Ta), inactive *vs.* G- (Ec)
II.B	Active *vs.* G+ (Bs and S1), inactive *vs.* G- (Ec) and yeast (Ta)
II.C.	Active *vs.* G+ (Bs), inactive *vs.* G- (Ec), G+ (S1) and yeast (Ta)
II.D.	Active *vs.* G+ (S1), inactive *vs.* G- (Ec), G+ (Bs) and yeast (TA)
III.	Active *vs.* yeast (Ta), inactive *vs.* G- (Ec), G+ (Bs and S1)
IV.	Inactive *vs.* G- (Ec), G+ (Bs and S1) and yeast (Ta)

[a] Inactive = inactive (0) or slightly active (sl.).

Space does not allow a complete listing of all of the antitumor agents in the various classes but examples of some of our data are presented in Table 2; the diameters of the zones of inhibition are reported in mm.
Upon confirmation of cytotoxicity against L1210 and KB9, the shake-flask beers are screened against the primary antimicrobial spectrum and tested whether *E. coli* active against the appropriate secondary spectrum. The resulting data are used to classify the antitumor lead in one of ten groups. Obviously, this fingerprint alone cannot identify a particular antitumor agent in a beer but it allows us to narrow down the possibles. Moreover, many culture filtrates that contain two or more antitumor agents exhibit different antimicrobial activities, and for this reason it may be impossible to classify the particular lead, or it may be classified erroneously.

Table 2

Class IC: Active *vs. E. coli* and *T. albida*
Inactive *vs.* the Gram-positive bacteria

	Ec Mycin	Ec CIM 41	Bs Mycin	Sl PAS	Ta ADM 102
AT 125	0	52	0	0	37
Formycin	0	26	0	0	30
Tubercidin	0	22	0	0	18/25

Class ID: Active *vs. E. coli*
Inactive *vs.* the Gram-positive bacteria and *T. albida*

	Ec Mycin	Ec CIM 41	Bs Mycin	Sl PAS	Ta ADM 102
5-Azacytidine	0	30	sl[b]	0	0
593-A	0	16p	0	0	0
Lenamycin (cellocidin)	0	25	0	0	0
Psicofuranine	0	20i[a]	0	0	0

Class IIA: Active *vs.* one or both gram-positive bacteria and *T. albida*
Inactive *vs. E. coli*

	Ec Mycin	Ec CIM 41	Bs Mycin	Sl PAS	Ta ADM 102
Kanchanomycin	0	0	18	17	18
Trienine	0	0	0	15	17

Class IIB: Active *vs.* the Gram-positive bacteria
Inactive *vs. E. coli and T. albida*

	Ec Mycin	Ec CIM 41	Bs Mycin	Sl PAS	Ta ADM 102
A649	0	0	22	20	0
Actinomycin F	0	0	27	27	0
Actinomycin P_2	0	0	21	16	0
Aureolic acid	0	0	25	28	0
BA 181314	0	0	16	15	0

[a] i = ingrown; [b] sl = slight.

In our fingerprint operations, we work on the tacit assumption that the antitumor activity correlates with some antimicrobial activity. Through our many years of experience in the antitumor field, we have found that this assumption is valid about 75%–80% of the time. In recent years, 65% of the shake-flask leads processed through our identification scheme exhibited sufficient antimicrobial activity so that they could be handled in our fingerprint method. Approximately 20% of the leads exhibited such weak activity that paper chromatograms could not be bioautographed, and the remaining 15% were completely inactive in our primary antimicrobial spectrum. In several cases, however, solvent extraction, carbon adsorption, or use of certain yeasts solved the bioautography problem and allowed the chemists to detect and classify the antitumor agent in the culture filtrate.

Culture Characterization

The second fingerprint used in the identification scheme is culture characterization. Cultures producing confirmed in vitro active antitumor beers are examined macroscopically and identified as actinomycetes, bacteria, or fungi using the classical taxonomic methods [3-4, 8, 9, 10, 12]. Using physiologic and morphologic data and the antimicrobial spectrum data from above, experienced microbiologists are able to recognize certain "keys" which allow them to accurately identify microorganisms that frequently produce the more common antitumor antibiotics in culture filtrates. In other cases, the microbiologists are able to classify some cultures as "first of its kind" types of lead, or in certain groups such as the xanthomycin, or actinomycin, or rhodomycin, or mithramycin, etc. producers. The data from the first two fingerprints usually lead to a preliminary classification, a suggestion, or a tentative identification of a particular antitumor agent produced by the culture. All of the information collected up to this point is forwarded to the chemists for preliminary chemical examination.

Paper Chromatography—System 83/101

All of our antitumor leads exhibiting antimicrobial activity are chromatographed descendingly on Whatman #1 paper pretreated with 1 *M* Na_2SO_4 at pH 3 using our primary solvent system 83/101 which consists of methanol: water: acetic acid: 25% aqueous sodium chloride (160 : 56.5 : 20 : 5.5).

For coding purposes, each antitumor lead is chromatographed side by side with a pool of seven antibiotics, namely neomycin B, paromomycin, J245 (P-D antibiotic), streptothricin, streptomycin, actinobolin, and Chloromycetin®. After exposure to ammonia or a pH 7 spray, the developed chromatogram is bioautographed using one or two organisms which are particularly sensitive as indicated by the antimicrobial spectrum of the antitumor lead. According to the mobility of the antimicrobial component relative to the standards in the antibiotic pool, a code number, estimated to the nearest 0.1 of a unit, is assigned to the antitumor lead. This method has proved to be very reliable for us because the relative R_f values obtained are not dependent on day to day chromatographic variations. In order to explain the above procedure, a typical chromatogram of the pool is given below (Fig. 1) and an explanation of the assignment of a code number follows.

Neomycin and any other antibiotic which does not move well from the origin in 83/101 is assigned a code number of 1.0; paromomycin or any other antibiotic with the same mobility is assigned a code number of 2.0, and in a like manner J245 is assigned a code number of 3. Chloromycetin[0] which is the seventh and fastest moving compound in the pool is assigned, in a like manner, a code number of 7.0. Antibiotics migrating farther than code 7 are assigned values of 7 + 1, 7 + 2, 7 + 3, etc; the plus number indicates the number of centimeters the antibiotic moved beyond 7. Any compound moving between two of the standards is given a code number with a decimal value such as 5.5 which indicates it moves exactly halfway between streptomycin and actinobolin. Using the same approach, a compound moving only 1/5 of the distance between these two standards is assigned a code number of 5.2.

Upon chromatography of each antitumor beer or concentrate therefrom, the lead is assigned a code number. A comparison of this code number with those in our catalog system containing over 250 antitumor antibiotics gives a valuable clue to possible identities of the unknown. The code number in 83/101 is also very useful in predicting a concentration

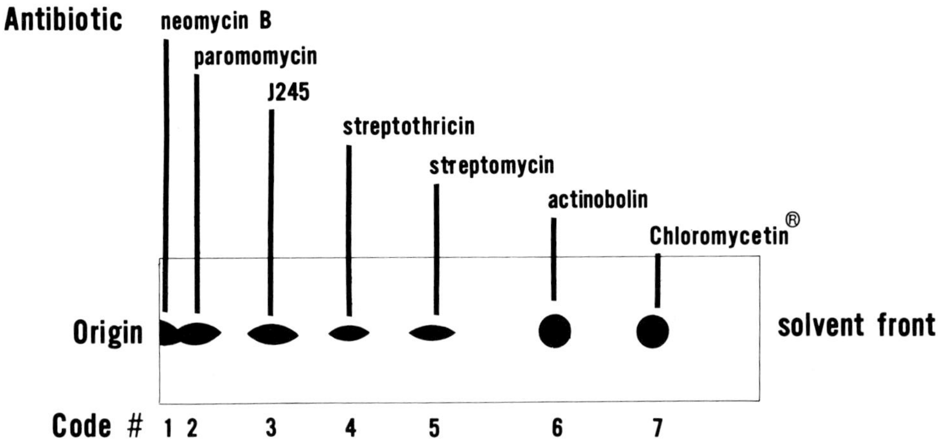

Fig. 1. Paper chromatography of the antibiotic standard pool in system 83/101

scheme for a particular antitumor agent. A lead with a code number of about 6.0 or greater should be extractable from the beer with butanol and one with a code number greater than 6.5 should be extractable with ethyl acetate. Leads with code numbers 1-6 can be concentrated by means of ion exchange resins or by carbon adsorption and subsequent elution with aqueous acetone or alcohol. In Table 3, we have listed the code numbers of several of the more commonly encountered tumor agents.

After a cancer lead has been processed through the first three fingerprints, it may be dropped if all data concerning the identity correlate, but in practice, we usually employ one more fingerprint to give us a more positive identification. The four remaining techniques in our identification scheme are thin-layer chromatography (TLC), ultraviolet absorption (UV), expanded yeast spectrum, and high-performance liquid chromatography (HPLC). These techniques are self-explanatory and need no detailed accounting here. We will merely cite specific examples of their practical use.

Table 3. Code numbers in system 83/101

Antineoplastic agent	Code no.
Gougerotin	4.0
Bleomycin A_2	4.4
Doxorubicin	4.7
Zorbamycin	5.3
Daunorubicin	5.4
Formycin	5.5
Tubercidin	5.8
AT 125	5.9
Azaserine	5.9
Gliotoxin	6.5
Iyomycin B	6.5
Echinomycin	7.0
Sarkomycin	7.0
Cinerubin A	7 + 1
Mithramycin	7 + 3

Example 1: Thin-Layer Chromatography

Cancer lead (CL) 248 and CL-812 exhibited identical antimicrobial spectra. Culture characterization indicated that both were possible xanthomycin producers, and chromatography in the 83/101 system gave slightly different code numbers in the 6.2–6.3 region; the code number for standard xanthomycin is 6.3. Since the code number is above 6.0, butanol extraction of both beers yielded active concentrates which were then chromatographed side by side with xanthomycin on silica gel plates using the solvent system ethyl acetate:methanol (2:1) and bioautographed on *B. subtilis*. Both leads, CL-248 and CL-812, gave the identical patterns in the above TLC system as standard xanthomycin, i.e., two main zones with a trace of antibiotic remaining at the origin. This example demonstrates the value of TLC comparisons with standards. In actual practice, two or three TLC systems are usually used in order to confirm the identify of a particular lead.

Example 2: TLC and UV Absorption

The antibacterial spectrum and culture characterization of CL-770 indicated that it might be a "first of its kind" type lead but with some similarity to the iyomycin B-producing culture. Paper chromatography of a beer extract in 83/101 gave a code number of 6.8, which is the code of iyomycin B. The yellow concentrate was chromatographed on a silica gel plate using chloroform : methanol : formic acid : water (35 : 25 : 3 : 5) and gave the same two major zones as obtained with our standard sample of iyomycin B. The UV spectrum was qualitatively identical to iyomycin B. (λ max 242, 268, 422 with a shift to λ max 252, 330, 538 in alkali.) Thus, we identified CL-770 as an iyomycin B producer and it was dropped from our program.

Over the years, we have developed an extensive classification system of known antibacterial, antiviral, and antitumor antibiotics based on ultraviolet absorption. This UV catalog has been of tremendous value in giving us an initial clue or a positive identification of a particular antibiotic lead. With many of our leads, we have no good clue as to their identity after processing through the first three fingerprints. In these cases, we attempt to prepare a concentrate either by extraction or carbon adsorption depending on the 83/101 code number. The UV of the concentrate is determined and reference to our UV catalog file sometimes yields our first solid hint for identification.

Example 3: TLC and UV Absorption

One of our leads, CL-350, exhibited only *T. albida* activity in the antibacterial spectrum, culture characterization suggested cycloheximide, and the 83/101 code was 5.5. Standard cycloheximide has a code of 7. Perusal of our chromatography code catalog indicated that a number of *T. albida* active antibiotics exhibited a code of about 5.5, namely formycin, tubercidin, sangivamycin, and toyocamycin. Carbon treatment of 30 ml of beer and subsequent elution with aqueous acetone yielded a concentrate which exhibited a maximum in the UV at λ 294 with a shift in base to λ 300. Reference to our UV file indicated that this portion of the spectrum was identical to that of formycin. TLC on silica gel using butanol : ethyl acetate : heptane : ethanol : water (10 : 50 : 20 : 30 : 10) confirmed the identification.

Example 4: Expanded Yeast Spectrum and TLC

Periodically, we process cancer leads that exhibit such weak antimicrobial activity that they cannot be bioautographed. We allow these type leads to accumulate to a dozen or so and then they are screened against our expanded yeast spectrum which consists of 46 different organisms. Many times, the results of this screen allows us to classify the leads on the basis of activity but more important it occasionally gives us a susceptible yeast which can be used for plating of chromatograms and as a guide to preliminary isolation studies. We have one example where a series of seven leads were grouped together on the basis of culture characterization data. These leads exhibited only slight zones against our primary spectrum, but against one of the 46 yeasts in the expanded yeast spectrum, *Candida stellatoidea* M1521, they exhibited zones of 28–37 mm. The data are presented in Table 4.

Table 4. Microbial spectrum of CL-leads. Zone diameters in mm (12.8 mm disc)

Lead	*E. coli* Mycin	GAA	B. subtilis	S. lutea	T. albida	Candida stellatoidea
CL-555	15	0	0	0	0	32
CL-657	0	19	0	18	0	32
CL-671	0	20	0	20	0	37
CL-708	0	18	0	0	0	30
CL-751	0	0	0	14	0	33
CL-597	0	15p	0	16	0	28
CL-835	0	0	0	14	p	32

Using the above data, the 83/101 chromatograms of all the above seven leads were bioautographed on plates of *Candida stellatoidea*; a code number of 6.5 was obtained for all the leads. TLC of concentrates from these leads on silica gel using benzene : ethyl acetate (1 : 1) indicated that all seven leads were identical. As a result of the above, one lead was picked as representative of the group and submitted for P388 evaluation in animals.

Example 5: High Performance Liquid Chromatography (HPLC)

The antibacterial spectrum and culture characterization of cancer lead CL-511 suggested several possible pigmented leads. Paper chromatography of the beer in 83/101 gave a streak from code 1 to 7 +, whereas a butanol extract of the beer gave a fairly sharp zone at 7 +. TLC of the concentrate on silica gel using chloroform : methanol : formic acid (55 : 45 : 4) yielded a purple streak from the origin to ~ R_f 0.75. From our experience, this type of chromatographic data is obtained with certain anthracycline-type compounds such as the rhodomycins. Mild acid hydrolysis of the CL-511 organic concentrate, and subsequent TLC yielded several distinct red zones, one of which compared with rhodomycin A. HPLC of a CL-511 concentrate using a μ Bondapak C_{18} column (Waters Assoc.) with a paired ion PIC Reagent B-5) yielded a major peak by UV detection with the identical retention time (4.6 min) as standard rhodomycin A. In our hands, HPLC is rapidly developing as one of our most useful and highly specific fingerprints for the identification of antitumor leads at the shake-flask level.

In summary, the rapid elimination of known antitumor antibacterial antibiotics in culture filtrates arising from a soil screening program can be accomplished by a variety of techniques. We have presented the seven fingerprint methods which have been effective in our hands. There are other approaches that can be used but the most important ingredients in all of these techniques are reliable reference data and the necessary experience in the antibiotic field to interpret the data. An experienced scientist in the antibiotic isolation work will recognize the tell-tale signs of the particular shape of zone on a chromatograph, or an ingrown zone, or a streak in a particular system, or the way a certain antibiotic is eluted from carbon; all of the above seemingly trivial details are significant in the hands of an experienced scientist. The availability of reference materials, catalog systems for isolation and chromatographic data, classification of antibiotics, whether on an activity basis or physical property basis such as UV, are all critically important for the overall efficiency of any antibiotic program. While new techniques and instrumentation have enhanced the science of antibiotic identification and isolation, the experience gained from years of actual practice is still most important.

References

1. BARNETT, H. L.: Illustrated Genera of Imperfect Fungi, 2nd ed. Minneapolis: Burgess Publishing Co. 1955–1960.
2. BENEKE, E. S.: Medical Mycology Laboratory Manual. Minneapolis: Burgess Publishing Co. 1957.
3. BUCHANAN, R. E., GIBBONS, N. E.: Bergey's Manual of Determinative Bacteriology, 8th ed. Baltimore: Williams and Wilkins Co. 1974.
4. GILMAN, J. C.: A Manual of Soil Fungi. Ames Iowa: Iowa State College Press 1957.
5. GROVE, D. C., RANDALL, W. A.: Assay Methods of Antibiotics, A Laboratory Manual. New York: Medical Encyclopedia Inc. 1955, pp. 192–193.
6. Lymphoid Leukemia L1210 (Protocol 1.100) and KB Cell Culture Screen (Protocol 1.600). Cancer Chemother. Rep. Part 3, **3** (2) (1972).
7. SCHABEL, F. M., Jr., PITTILLO, R. F.: Screening for biological characterization of antitumor agents using micro-organisms. Adv. Appl. Microbiol. **3**, 223–256 (1961).
8. SHIRLING, E. B., GOTTLIEB, D.: Methods for characterization of streptomyces species. Int. J. Systemic Bacteriol. **16**, 313 (1966).
9. SKERMAN, V. B. D.: Society of American Bacteriologists, Manual of Microbiological Methods, New York: McGraw-Hill Co. 1957.
10. SKERMAN, V. B. D.: A Guide to the Identification of the Genera of Bacteria. Baltimore: Williams and Wilkins Co. 1967.

Microbial Process Translation—Laboratory to Pilot Plant at the Frederick Cancer Research Center*

A. F. Langlykke

In June 1972, the Frederick Cancer Research Center (FCRC) began operations under contract arrangements with the U.S. National Cancer Institute (NCI). Since then the Center has grown to its present size, diversity, and importance. In 1973, the Chemotherapy Fermentation Laboratory (CFL), which was to include an intermediate scale production unit or pilot plant, was first proposed for installation at FCRC as a service operation in support of the Division of Cancer Treatment (DCT) of the NCI.

The Need for a Pilot Plant

While the DCT supported a substantial program in natural products discovery and development, it was apparent that there was a need for a production unit which could quickly supply newly discovered drugs in substantial quantity. With more than 400 antitumor substances produced by microorganisms [5], many active screening or search programs underway, many promising leads under study and the frequently expressed needs of cancer scientists for large volumes of experimental materials, a pilot plant or producing unit was clearly desirable. With such a unit serving the purposes of the DCT, promising new drugs could be expedited in production so as to minimize the delivery time of a new drug to the laboratory scientist and the clinical investigator.

Though the need for a pilot plant to expedite the course of development from discovery to availability may be obvious, the figures shown in Table 1 are offered to illustrate the increasing requirements for quantities of a new drug as development progresses. These figures are based upon estimates of labor, materials, and overheads for the preparation of products at each stage. Under the conditions assumed, the costs of materials only become significant when the volume of fermentation liquor exceeds 1000 liters. As requirements increase, economy dictates the use of pilot scale production equipment.

In the earliest stage of development, the total estimated cost of material is low, though the cost per g of active agent is very high, reflecting, particularly, the cost of laboratory effort in the conduct of flask-scale fermentation. If a substance is found which shows acceptable activity in the search process, the requirements for larger quantities of substance immediately begin to develop. Early in the course of study, fermentations which are first conducted in flasks will be translated to stirred-jar and fermentor operation to satisfy the needs of the chemist engaged in isolation and characterization studies.

As demand increases, and as costs justify, fermentations will be carried out on progressively increasing scale and recovery will also be conducted in large-volume pilot plant equipment. Also depending on volume requirements and escalating costs, strain selection, as well as fermentation and recovery improvement programs, will be undertaken to raise the overall

* Program sponsored by NCI under contract #NO1-CO-25423 with Litton Bionetics, Inc.

Table 1. Development of a hypothetical antitumor agent produced by fermentation: Requirement and costs

Stage of development	Requirements		Cost of product	
	Product g	Fermentation liquor, liters	Per g. $	Total $
Search process	0.015 (crude)	3.0	33,000	500
Chemical isolation, assurance of novelty	0.500 (crude) 0.050 (90% pure)	40.0	2640	1320
Extended testing, various tumor systems	10	2000[a]	820	8200
Pharmacology, toxicology and and experimental therapy	50	4000[b]	330	16,500
Clinical investigation				
Phase 1	50	3000[c]	100	5000
Phase 2	200	10,000	50	10,000
Phase 3	2000	80,000	40	80,000

[a] At this stage, strain development yields five-fold improvement in fermentation yields. Recovery, pure material = 10%.
[b] At this stage, recovery improved to 25%.
[c] As demand increases, continual improvement is expected in yields and recoveries.

efficiency of the production process. The reasonable extent of developmental study must be based on cost-benefit analysis; for greatest economy, the cost of development must not exceed the savings realized in production costs.

Though the figures in Table 1 probably underestimate likely experience, in our hypothetical case a successfully developed drug will be made available at ever lower costs. This is, indeed, the logical expectation and the justification for our pilot plant installation.

The Overall Plan

As its focal point, the concept of the CFL embraced a pilot plant of such size as to meet eventual needs for the production of natural products in amounts adequate to supply all the needs of clinical trials.

Design of the pilot plant emphasized the fermentor assembly which was designed and furnished by Fermentation Design, Inc., of Bethlehem, Pennsylvania, a division of the New Brunswick Scientific Co., Inc. It comprised two 30-gallon (gal) fermentors, two 300-gal fermentors and one 3000-gal fermentor, all closely similar in design and all geometrically similar in all dimensions. Total design of the pilot plant included certain recovery equipment of kind and capacity estimated to be adequate for a presumed process for adriamycin production [1, 2]. It should be emphasized, however, that the pilot plant was, from the beginning, intended to be a versatile installation, capable of application to the production and recovery of any conceivable product regardless of its chemical and physical characteristics. The FCRC pilot plant (Fig. 1) was delivered to the CFL in April, 1976. Since then, its program has included operability trials, installation of equipment to attain greater versatility, training of an operating crew, and a variety of general small scale processing operations.

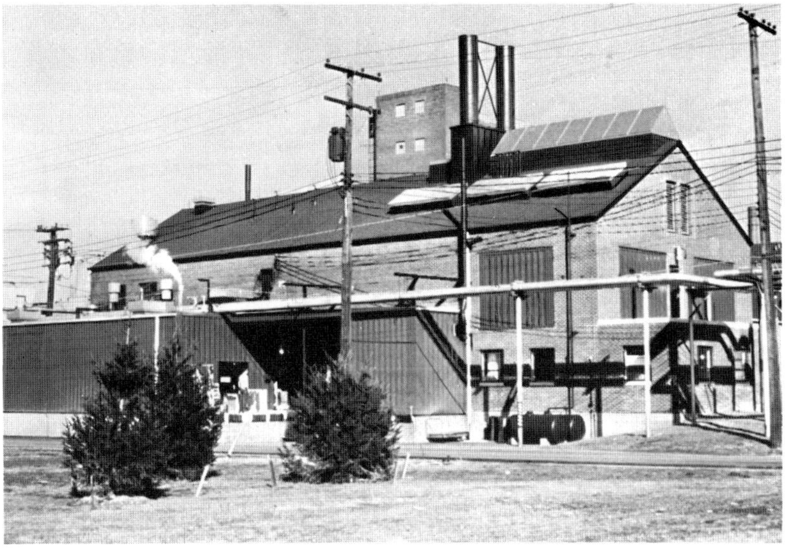

Fig. 1. Pilot plant, Frederick Cancer Research Center

Program of the CFL

The CFL pilot plant is responsible for the development and production of natural products to satisfy the needs of many investigators. In general, these natural products are fermentation products or products which can be elaborated in deep or submerged culture. The development program will be applied to fermentation products originating in other laboratories as well as to products generated internally. However, the unique recovery facilities can also be applied to the extraction of products derived from botanical or animal sources.

The CFL laboratory sections fill a necessary supporting role for the pilot plant. Processes to be introduced into the pilot plant must be adapted to the installed equipment. The microbiology laboratories serve the pilot plant with supplies of inoculum, basic laboratory-scale operating procedures and with biologic assay definition and service. The Chemistry laboratories similarly provide process details as well as analytic methodology and service and, when volumes are reduced to manageable proportions, the chemical laboratories will also conduct the final steps in recovery and purification.

The laboratories are also engaged in research programs to support the continuity of the pilot plant program. A screening program designed to uncover unique organisms and novel antitumor compounds produced by such organisms has already revealed more than 20 agents which are active in vivo and which are progressing to pilot plant assignment.

Resulting from research in microbial transformations, several conversions of daunorubicin have been described with one which proves to be novel. However, the product, N-acetyldaunorubicin-13-ol, appears to be less promising than the parent compound [3] and therefore, large scale production of this product is not now planned.

Process Translation: Laboratory to Pilot Plant

The translation of laboratory process to the pilot plant for the production of fermentation products involves both fermentation and recovery phases. The fermentation process as carried out in laboratory flasks must be converted to a different mode utilizing tank-type fermentors. Recovery processes as carried out in the laboratory, must also be adapted to large scale equipment with the associated advantages and limitations.

Fermentation Process

Laboratory-scale fermentations, as conducted at FCRC and elsewhere, are generally carried out in flasks incubated on shakers. Thus a wide range of aerobic microbial forms will grow in submerged habit under aeration varying in intensity depending upon many different factors affecting oxygen supply and transfer [11]. Oxygen supply and transfer as they are accomplished in shake flasks, are obviously different processes from those effected in tank-type fermentors.

The first steps in translation to the tank mode of fermentation will generally be undertaken in stirred jars of a few liters' capacity [11] which display operating characteristics translatable to those observed at the largest scale of operation. From the stirred jars, development may proceed progressively to larger and larger vessels.

Because of the many uncertainties in the comparison of one mode with another, common practice in translation from flask to tank or stirred jar is to select a set of conditions which are judged to be favorable based upon general observation of flask fermentation experience.

At FCRC, stirred-jar and tank fermentors range in operating volume or capacity from about 5–10,000 liters. In the translation from flask to fermentor however, the practice is to carry out first, tank fermentation experiments in operating volumes no greater than approximately 30 liters. Usual practice is to carry out aerobic fermentations in small fermentors at agitation rates of 100–300 revolutions per minute (rpm), air flow rates of about 0.2–1 volumes per volume per minute (vvm), or at such a rate as to maintain about 50% oxygen saturation in the medium under moderate back pressure of about 5 pounds per square inch (psi). From such a beginning, the effects of variations in operating conditions are examined to establish favorable conditions for reasonably good performance. It should be noted here that performance on transfer from one scale or one mode to another frequently shows baffling inconsistencies and therefore, translation from flask to tank fermentation does not usually respond to precise prediction.

With a definition of favorable operating conditions in the tank or stirred jar, we are prepared to move into our main pilot plant to undertake fermentation in one of the 30, 300, or 3000-gal fermentors (Figs. 2, 3). While the choice of fermentor size depends upon the immediate needs for a quantity of product, it also depends upon the degree of risk involved balanced against the costs of materials and labor. Obviously, the volume of fermentor operation must also depend upon the adequacy of processing equipment to handle the fermentor volume without undue delay since, as with most biologic materials, rapid handling is essential to preservation of the active product.

To attain, in large tanks, the most productive levels developed in small tanks, the formulae for scale-up as described by Humphrey, Aiba and Millis [7] may be used. With these formulae, aeration rates, agitation rates, and power input may be calculated for the large fermentor using the values found effective on the small scale. By controlling the services to the large fermentor at such calculated values, performance should approximate that observed under best conditions on the small scale.

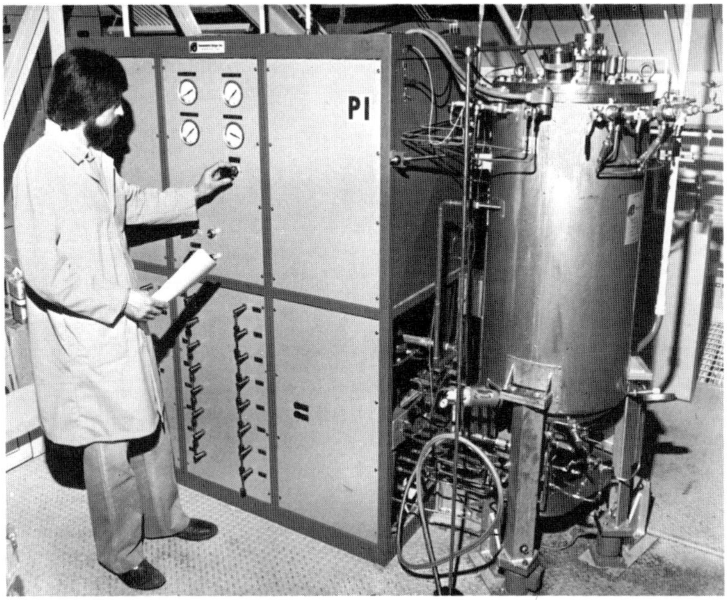

Fig. 2. 30 gal fermentor with operating console

The design of the five geometrically similar fermentors in the main FCRC pilot plant is illustrated in Fig. 4. The fermentors which are of conventional design are equipped with recording and controlling devices to permit careful control and replication of conditions from run to run. For each fermentor, automatic control of foam, pH, temperature and dissolved oxygen is provided. Sterile air is introduced through a perforated ring sparger while agitation is supplied by three impellors attached to a shaft which enters through the base and is anchored near the top by a stabilizer bearing. The seal on the shaft at the entrance to the fermentor is maintained with condensed steam which serves both to seal and to lubricate the drive shaft. All of the fermentors may be operated and controlled from a central control room (Fig. 5).

Control of charging of each fermentor is accomplished by means of load cells which record differences in the total weight of the fermentor and so measure weight of the fermentor contents.

Recovery Process

Obviously, the development of recovery and refining techniques is quite as important as fermentation development to satisfy the mission of the FCRC pilot plant. In the course of isolating and identifying new agents in the laboratory, chemical fractionation and recovery procedures are carried out, and, early in the scheme, these methods are carefully examined and adapted to provide recovery methods which are compatible with the equipment and facilities available in the pilot plant.

The unit operations which can be applied in the pilot plant to recover an active product, and important representative equipment installed to carry out these processes, as described in such a standard reference as PERRY'S Chemical Engineers Handbook [10], are as follows:

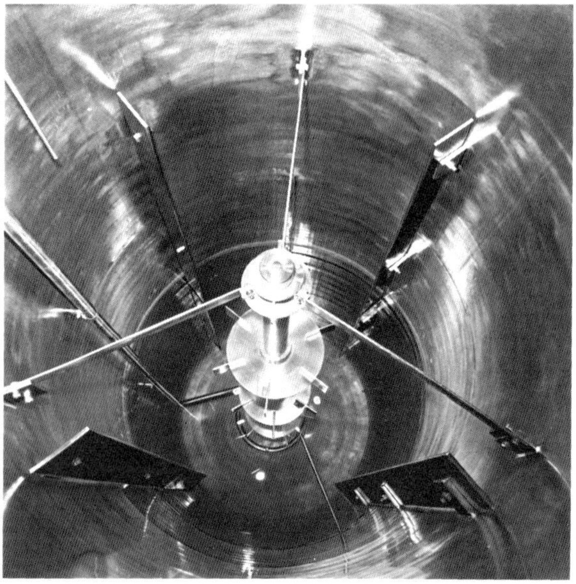

Fig. 3. View into interior of 3000 gal fermentor

1. Separation of mycelium or microbial cells and suspended solids by centrifugation:
   Two Sharples Model 16 centrifuges, tubular type, are capable of developing centrifugal force of about 6000 *g* at 10,000 rpm and at a flow rate of 20–25 gal per min (gpm).
   One CEPA Model Z-41 centrifuge, tubular type, is capable of about 17,000 *g* at 20,000 rpm and at a flow rate of about 5 gpm.
   One Fletcher basket centrifuge, 14 in., delivers about 2000 *g* at 3200 rpm and recovers about 0.3 ft^3 of cake per batch.
2. Separation of mycelium or microbial cells and suspended solids by filtration:
   One Shriver, ALP model, recessed plate filter press retains 1 ft^3 of filter cake per chamber employing 1–13 chambers at a nominal flow rate of 7.5 gpm per chamber (Fig. 6).
3. Clarification and product recovery by filtration:
   One Niagara Model 18-12-S horizontal plate filter has capacity for 12 plates, 22.40 ft^2 of filtration area and cake retention capacity of 1.62 ft^3. May be used for product recovery and for polish filtration.
   Three Knightware (ceramic) stoneware filters, 20–26 in. in diameter, provide product recovery by vacuum filtration. Capacity of funnel is 3–3.5 ft^3 (85–100 liters).
4. Disruption of cells for release of intracellular products:
   One Gaulin Model 15M homogenizer, effects disruption by shear obtained by directing a cell suspension under high pressure through a constricted passage and by flow reversal. Cell suspensions may be treated at 15 gph at pressures as great as 8500 psi.
5. Counter-current extraction:
   One Podbielniak Model B-10 extractor obtains multiple effect in a high speed centrifugal extractor by continuous counter-current contacting of two immiscible phases. At rotational speed of 3000 rpm, maximum flow of both phases combined is 60 gpm. Efficiency of extraction increases with reduction in flow rate.
6. Chromatography, gel filtration:
   One Pharmacia KS 370 sectional column provides effective column height by use of as

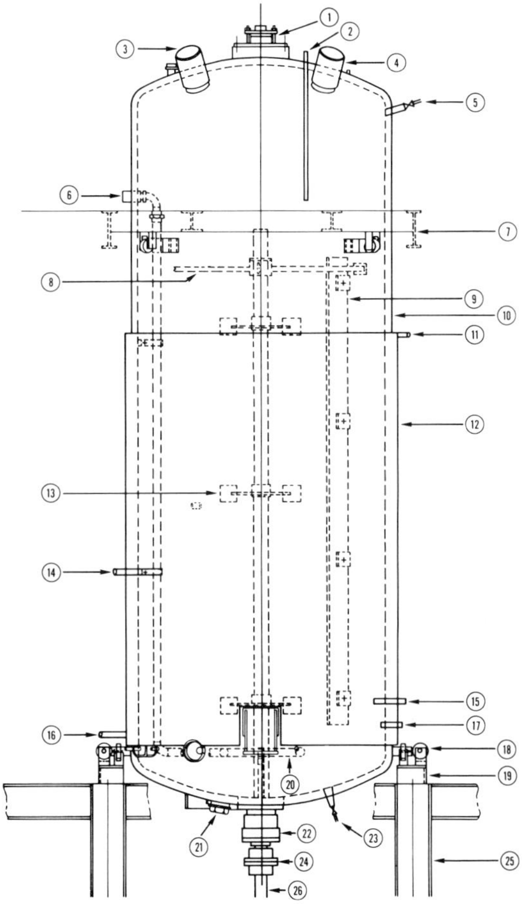

1. Pressure Relief System
2. Foam Probe
3. Light Source
4. Addition + View Port
5. Addition Port
6. Air Sparge Delivery
7. Support
8. Shaft Stabilizer and Guide Bushing
9. Baffle
10. Vessel Shell
11. Jacket Water to Heat Exchanger
12. Jacket for Cooling and Heating
13. Impeller
14. Dissolved Oxygen Probe
15. pH Probe
16. Cooling and Heating to Jacket
17. Temp. Sensor
18. Load Cell Alignment and Torque Relief System
19. Load Cells
20. Sparge Ring
21. Product Drop Valve
22. Seal
23. Sample Port
24. Drive Coupling
25. Support
26. Drive

Fig. 4. Plan of fermentor

many as six large diameter (37 cm), shallow (15 cm) cells connected in series. Volumetric flow rate is approximately proportional to cross section.

7. Evaporation:
   Two Pfaudler wiped film evaporators (Fig. 7) provide rapid evaporation under vacuum by moving the liquid being concentrated over the heating surface by means of rotating wiper blades. One unit provides 1.2 ft^2 of heating surface, while the second provides 13.3 ft^2. Heat transfer rate is approximately 25,000 BTU/h/ft^2 of heating surface.
8. Batch extraction:
   An assortment of processing tanks, some fixed and some portable. Of these, 11 are equipped with agitators and may be used for batch extraction under a variety of conditions. The processing tanks (Fig. 8) are also intended for use as feed and recovery tanks.
9. Size reduction:
   One Fitz Mill Model D comminutor for reduction of friable materials as well as tough plastic or fibrous woody materials to small particle size.

While the processes and equipment described above will permit effective recovery of most fermentation or natural products, there are obvious improvements that would contribute to

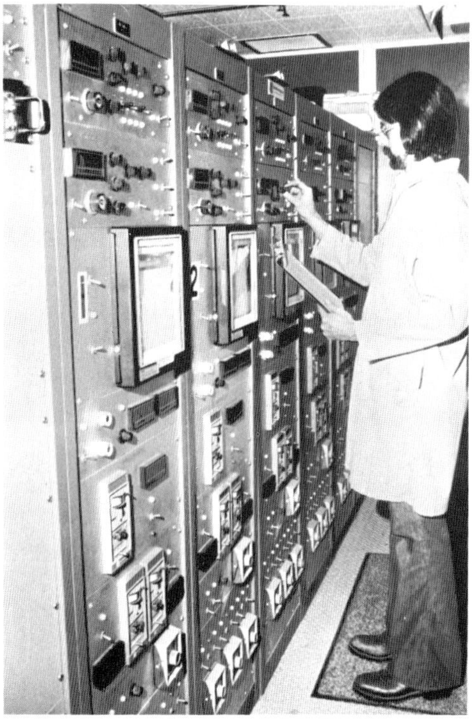

Fig. 5. Control panels for five fermentors in pilot plant control room

flexibility and to operation at high volume. To recover microbial cells in the volume generated at the 3000-gal fermentor level would require larger and more convenient capacity than is now available. To improve upon versatility, additional column capacity for chromatography and ion-exchange should be acquired. As operations develop and special needs are revealed, other modifications to the equipment will be made.

Two Representative Programs

In its first year, the FCRC pilot plant has conducted development and production studies on a number of fermentation or submerged culture products, including several crude enzyme preparations, two antitumor antibiotics, and one tissue culture product—interferon. So far, the pilot plant has been mainly concerned with fermentation and the microbial process and with recovery of crude products; operations have not yet extended to isolation, purification and refining.

Interferon

In the production of interferon which will be produced in large quantities, for and in cooperation with C. B. Anfinsen, of the National Institutes of Health, the objective is to

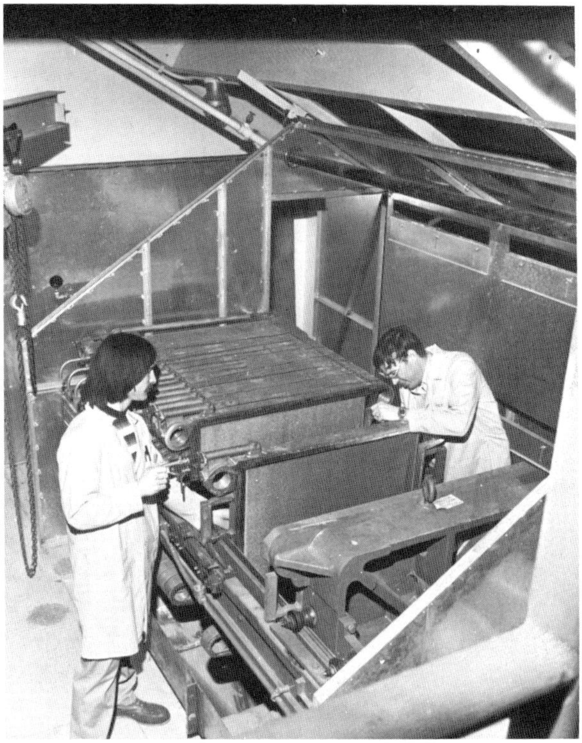

Fig. 6. Stainless steel Shriver filter press for filtration of fermentor product

produce about 10 mg or 10^{10} U for purposes of characterization. To this end, the plan is to produce approximately 10^{11} U in the culture liquor. The course to be followed at FCRC is shown schematically in the flow chart of Fig. 9.

For the past year, the pilot plant group has been engaged in development studies designed to improve yields, to reduce costs and to adapt the large scale fermentation equipment. Though many uncertainties persist, the results of the development program indicate that performance as outlined in the flow-chart can be attained in the production phase about to be undertaken. The process under development employs the Namalva cell line isolated from Burkitts lymphoma by workers at the Karolinska Institute in Stockholm as reported by KLEIN et. al. [8] In the projected process, when a viable cell count of at least 1.6×10^6 is obtained in the final tissue culture stage, the production of interferon is induced by inoculating the cell culture with Newcastle Disease Virus propagated in 10 day old embryonated eggs. After inoculation with the virus, the culture is diluted with the basic tissue culture medium supplemented with glutamine but without fetal calf serum [13].

We expect to attain interferon yields of 3000 U/ml in the interferon production liquor in a volume approximating 2800 liters per batch, or a fermentation yield in such a large volume batch of 8.4×10^9 U. Though efficiency of recovery is uncertain, we expect overall recovery to attain at least 10% or about 0.8 mg of interferon per batch (or per cell propagation run in the 300-gal fermentors).

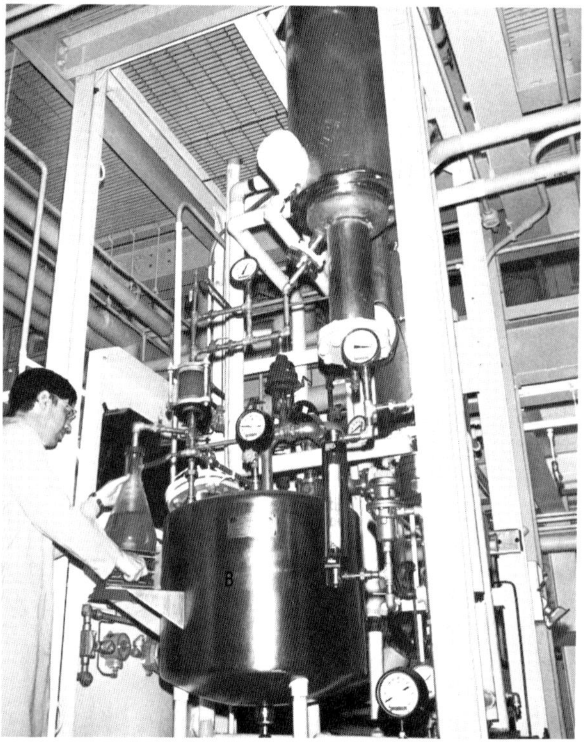

Fig. 7. Large wiped film evaporator at operating level

Carboxypeptidase G_1

A development program for the production of carboxypeptidase G_1 was begun, in cooperation with the New England Enzyme Center at Tufts University in Boston, to attempt production of carboxypeptidase G_1 equivalent to, or duplicating, that described by McCullough, Chabner and Bertino [9].

Applying the method of McCullough, et. al., by which they isolated *Pseudomonas stutzeri* and that of van Niel and Allen [12], described as highly specific for isolation of the species, ten cultures were obtained, all of which showed carboxypeptidase activity on methotrexate, but only two of which were pseudomonads. Evaluation of the isolates led to selection of a nonfermenting Gram-negative rod which was designated FCRC 252 and which gave good yields of the enzyme.

The flow chart shown in Figure 10, displays the procedure that has been developed for the production of pure carboxypeptidase G_1 derived from fermentation by culture FCRC 252. It presents a combination of pilot plant and laboratory activities and illustrates graphically how the large-scale equipment of the pilot plant in combination with the facilities, on a smaller scale, of the laboratory can be employed for the production of large quantities of fermentation products.

In the pilot plant, fermentors with working capacities of 200 gal have been used to produce cell material with yields ranging from 3–9 g of wet cells or cell paste per liter of fermentor

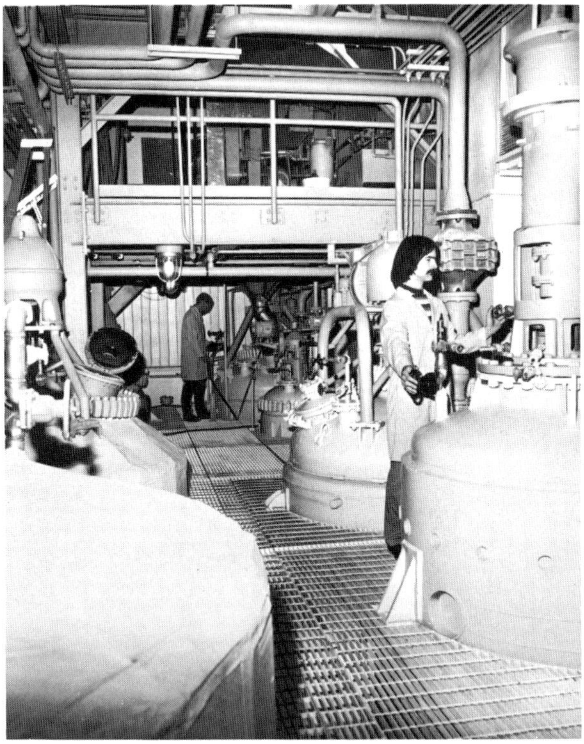

Fig. 8. Processing tanks in pilot plant recovery area

operating volume and with enzyme yields ranging from 14–154 U/g cells. The cycle in the fermentors was 16–20 h in duration.

From the fermentors, the fermentation product was run through a Sharples centrifuge to recover microbial cells. For good recovery very short exposure to the first processing steps is essential. Since the carboxypeptidase is contained within the cell, disruption of the cells was done on the large scale with the Gaulin homogenizer in which cell suspension could be treated at a rate of about 15 gph. The clear supernatant product of centrifugation contained a low concentration of enzyme accompanied by much protein impurity so that, at this stage, the enzyme preparation or solution had a specific activity of 0.2–1.0 U/mg protein.

At this stage, the supernate was submitted to laboratory treatment comprising protamine sulfate precipitation, ammonium sulfate precipitation, and heat denaturation with an overall yield varying from 55%–70%.

After initial purification steps in the laboratory, the material was returned to the pilot plant for larger scale handling on the Pharmacia sectional column in which gel filtration was carried out employing Sephadex G100 resin. This procedure, which results in three to six fold purification, is accomplished with about 50% yield.

The final purification of the large volume of enzyme is accomplished in laboratory equipment by affinity elution chromatography according to the method of H. E. Blair [4], resulting in pure enzyme with specific activity of 700 U/mg. The overall yield from production in the fermentor to recovery of the pure enzyme is about 10%.

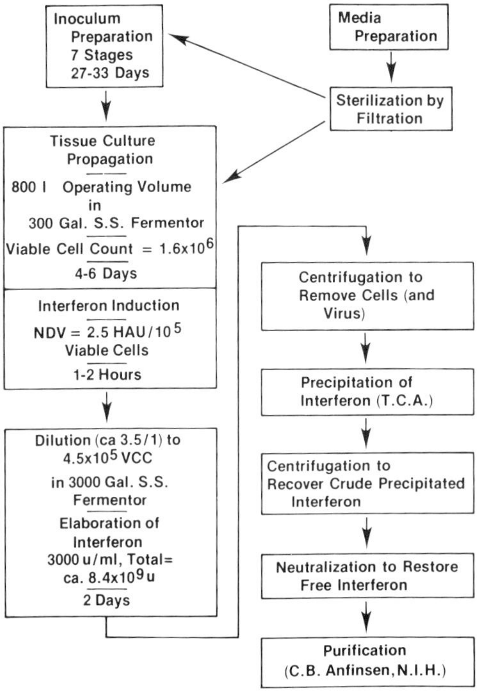

Fig. 9. Interferon production

Summary

In summary, operations in the FCRC pilot plant have included training an operating staff, operability trials, equipment modification and repair, and supplementation of the original equipment to gain greater versatility. In addition to effort spent on proving and improving the capacity of the pilot plant, development studies and production operations involving translation of laboratory operations to pilot plant level or volume have included:

1. Development of a production process for interferon as described above. As a by-product of the interferon program, samples of cell culture have been studied in the Basic Research Division of FCRC for the production of lymphokines.
2. Production of starting materials (cell paste) for carboxypeptidase G_1, using three different organisms, and production of refined material from the FCRC 252 organism as described herein.
3. Production of large quantities of crude phenylalanine ammonia lyase in the form of cell paste for Prof. Creed Abell at the University of Texas, Medical Branch, at Galveston.
4. Production of a crude staphylococcal nuclease for the program of Dr. David Sachs, National Cancer Institute, Bethesda, Maryland.
5. Developmental studies and limited production of a crude cysteine desulfhydrase according to the protocols of Dr. J. Uren, Sidney Farber Cancer Center, Boston, Massachusetts.

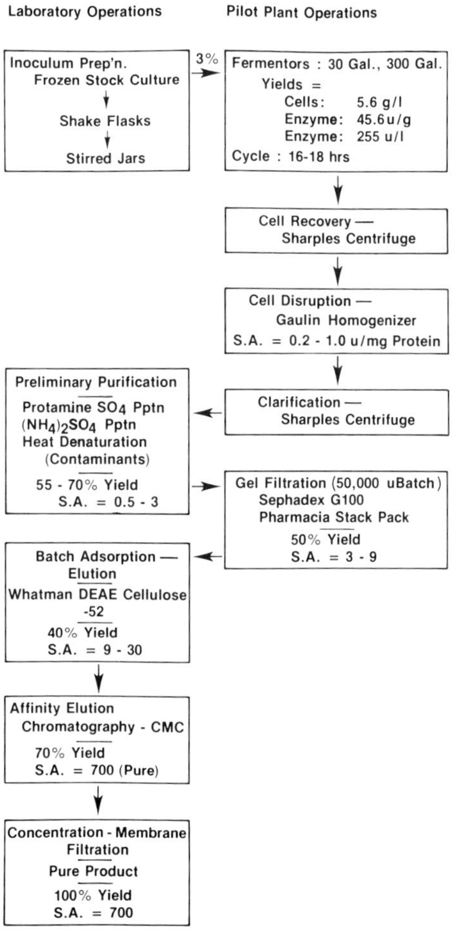

Fig. 10. Production of carboxypeptidase G_1 with FCRC 252

6. Preliminary production studies on the agent produced by Culture FCRC 14, discovered in the CFL search program.
7. Developmental fermentation studies on the antitumor antibiotic, piperazinedione 593A [6], in preparation for production of quantities of this antibiotic to support clinical studies under the auspices of the National Cancer Institute.

Acknowledgements

This work was supported by the National Cancer Institute under Contract No. NO1-CO-25423 to Litton Bionetics, Inc. The author wishes to recognize, with sincere thanks, the efforts of all of his colleagues at the Frederick Cancer Research Center in making this report possible. Special recognition is due to Dr. A. A. Aszalos for information on chemical aspects, Dr. A. L. Garretson for microbiologic assistance, Dr. B. K. Hamilton for advice on certain microbiologic features of the program and pilot plant operations, Mr. Frederick Klein for facts on interferon, Dr. Trent D. Buckman for information relating to carboxypeptidase and to Mr. I. T. Warder, formerly of the CFL staff, for plans and development of the pilot plant. It is impractical to list all of my other associates and colleagues to whom I am deeply indebted for their support in developing our program and our facility.

References

1. ARCAMONE, F., CASSINELLI, G., FANTINI, G., GREIN, A., OREZZI, P., POL, C., SPALLA, G.: Adriamycin, 14-hydroxydaunomycin, A new antitumor antibiotic from *S. peucetius* var. *caesius*. Biotechnol. Bioeng. **11**, 1101–1110 (1969).
2. ARCAMONE, F., CASSINELLI, G., diMARCO, A., GAETANI, M.: Adriamycin Derivatives. U.S. Pat. 3,590,028 (June 29, 1971).
3. ASZALOS, A. A., BACHUR, N. R., HAMILTON, B. K., LANGLYKKE, A. F., ROLLER, P. P., SHEIKH, M. Y., SUTPHIN, M. S.: THOMAS, M. C., WAREHEIM, D. A., WRIGHT, L. H.: Microbial reduction of the side-chain carbonyl of daunorubicin and N-acetyldaunorubicin. J. Antibiot. (Tokyo) **30**, 50–58 (1977).
4. BLAIR, H. E.: Personal communication (1977).
5. FUSKA, J., PROSKA, B.: Cytotoxic and antitumor antibiotics produced by microorganisms. Adv. Appl. Microbiol. **20**, 259–370 (1976).
6. GITTERMAN, C. O., RICKES, E. L., WOLF, D. E., MADAS, J., ZIMMERMAN, S. B., STOUDT, T. H., DEMNY, T. C.: The human tumor-egg host system IV. Discovery of a new antitumor agent, Compound 593A. J. Antibiot. (Tokyo) **23**, 305–310 (1970).
7. HUMPHREY, A. E., AIBA, S., MILLIS, N. F.: Biochemical Engineering, 2nd ed., New York-London: Academic Press 1973.
8. KLEIN, G., DOMBOS, L., GOTHOSKAR, B.: Sensitivity of Epstein-Barr virus (EBV) producer and non-producer human lymphoblastoid cell lines to superinfection with EB-virus. Int. J. Cancer **10**, 44–57 (1972).
9. MCCULLOUGH, J. L., CHABNER, B. A., BERTINO, J. R.: Purification and properties of carboxypeptidase G_1. J. Biol. Chem. **246**, 7207–7213 (1971).
10. PERRY, R. H., CHILTON, C. H., (Eds.): Chemical Engineers' Handbook, 5th ed., New York-St. Louis-San Francisco: McGraw-Hill Book Co. 1973.
11. SOLOMONS, G. L.: Materials and Methods in Fermentation, London-New York: Academic Press 1969.
12. VAN NIEL, C. B., ALLEN, M. B.: A note on *Pseudomonas stutzeri*. J. Bacteriol. **64**, 413–422 (1952).
13. ZOON, K. C., BUCKLER, C. E., BRIGDEN, P. J., ANFINSEN, C. B.: Production of human lymphoblastoid interferon by dilution of saturation density cultures with serum-free medium. Submitted to J. Clin. Microbiol. (1977).

Criteria for Selection of New Analogs of Antitumor Antibiotics

A. GOLDIN

A highly difficult area in the application of preclinical methodology involves the selection and development of new analogs of known antitumor agents for clinical trial. There are a considerable number of analogs of alkylating agents, purine and pyrimidine antagonists, folic acid antagonists, dimethane sulfonates, benzimidazols, antibiotics of a number of subcategories, and other classes of drugs which have demonstrable activity in antitumor test models but which have remained "dormant" with respect to development, pending any experimental observations that would provide a basis for further interest. The problems involved in the selection of new analogs of antitumor antibiotics are not dissimilar from those involved in the selection of new analogs in general. It is important to examine the preclinical criteria that may be employed in an attempt to identify analogs of antitumor antibiotics that are worthy of further development for the clinic. In general, standard preclinical testing methodologies may be employed to provide data as a guide for selection. Overall, if a new analog of a known antitumor antibiotic is to justify interest, the analog must be demonstrated to possess either quantitative or qualitative superiority over the parent compound in pharmacologic, toxicologic, immunologic, tumor cytotoxic, or other biologic properties that are therapeutically favourable. In such a determination, it is important to focus specific attention on the characteristics that are limiting for the parent antitumor antibiotic in clinical use. Various preclinical criteria for selection of new antitumor antibiotics for clinical use will be discussed below.

Preclinical Criteria for Selection of New Analogs I

An anolog of a parent antitumor antibiotic in clinical use may be deserving of further development if it has greater activity in an appropriate test system than the parent compound. This may be demonstrated in primary or secondary screening systems, in naturally refractory tumor systems, or in one or more tumors of a human tumor xenograft panel.

A basis for interest in the antitumor antibiotic adriamycin, stemmed from a demonstration that it was more effective than daunomycin, albeit only moderately so, in extending the survival time of animals with leukemia L1210 [24]. In animals inoculated with leukemia L1210, a single treatment with adriamycin one day following leukemic inoculation, or daily treatment from the first to the ninth day following leukemic inoculation, was more effective than daunomycin in increasing the survival time of the animals. The increase in response of adriamycin was not extensive but it was demonstrable over a series of dosage levels ranging from nontoxic to toxic doses.

In similar manner, adriamycin was more effective than daunomycin in the leukemia P388 system [24]. This was demonstrated on two treatment schedules, namely every six hours or every three hours administered on the first day following leukemic inoculation. On the six hourly schedule, the maximum increase in median survival time with adriamycin was greater than 445% and five out of eight animals were alive at sixty days. With daunomycin, the maximum increase in survival time was 95% and there was one out of eight animals alive at 60 days. On the three hourly schedule, the advantage of treatment with adriamycin was still evident but not as extensive. The percent increase in lifespan (ILS) was 154% for adriamycin as opposed to 104% for daunomycin.

Bleomycin is therapeutically active in the treatment of subcutaneously implanted B16 melanoma [31] in which site the tumor is generally somewhat naturally refractory. If an analog of bleomycin were more active than bleomycin itself in the treatment of s.c. inoculated B16 melanoma, it could provide a basis for further development of the analog.

Bleomycin is also active in inhibiting tumor growth and in increasing the survival time of animals with subcutaneously implanted Lewis lung carcinoma [31] which is another somewhat refractory tumor system. Again, an analog of bleomycin that was demonstrated to be more effective than bleomycin in the treatment of this tumor could warrant further investigation.

Umezawa and his colleagues [30] have prepared more than 200 bleomycin derivatives by fermentation and chemical synthesis. In one experimental model, the activity is determined on the basis of extent of inhibition of induction by methylcholanthrene of squamous cell carcinoma in mouse skin [30]. Bleomycin A5033 is a derivative of A_5 and contains succinylspermidine in the terminal amine moiety. At equal dosage, it showed approximately the same activity as the bleomycin mixture which is generally employed clinically in the inhibition of methylcholanthrene-induced mouse squamous cell carcinoma. Bleomycin A5196 (3.1 mg/kg/day) demonstrated activity similar to 12.5 mg/kg/day of the bleomycin mixture in inhibiting the number of mice developing 20-methylcholanthrene-induced squamous cell carcinoma. In addition, it produced significant, although modest (50% ILS), prolongation of survival time of animals with leukemia L1210. The latter observation is quite important since various bleomycins have demonstrated no effect in the leukemia L1210 system.

Bradner et al. [3] reported recently that a new bleomycin analog (BU-2231A), which differs from bleomycin in terminal amines and in the peptide chain, is highly active in the treatment of Walker 256 carcinosarcoma, moderately active in the treatment of P388 leukemia and B16 melanoma, and slightly active against Lewis lung carcinoma.

With the Ridgway osteogenic sarcoma system, it is possible on treatment with drugs to determine the extent of complete and partial regression of tumor, the duration of regression, and the incidence of regrowth and cures [19]. Actinomycin D has been demonstrated to produce a high incidence of complete and partial regressions in this tumor system and a high incidence of "cures." Adriamycin, daunomycin and bleomycin, although capable of producing regressions, do not generally result in an incidence of cures [19]. Attention could be focused on any anthracycline or bleomycin analog that would be capable of producing a high incidence of cures in this system.

In the Division of Cancer Treatment program at the NCI, a new antitumor screening panel has been instituted involving mouse colon, breast and lung tumor in syngeneic animals and human colon, breast and lung tumor growing as xenografts in athymic (nude) mice (Fig. 1).[1] Greater activity in any one of these systems as opposed to the parent analog could serve to focus attention on further development of a new analog.

It is of interest that hexamethylmelamine, which is essentially inactive in the primary murine screening systems, demonstrated definitive activity against colon, bronchus, ovary and kidney human tumor xeonografts growing in T-cell deprived mice (Table 1) [5]. This observation has created increased clinical interest in this compound.

---

[1] In Division of Cancer Treatment, NCI Treatment Linear Array, December 1976.

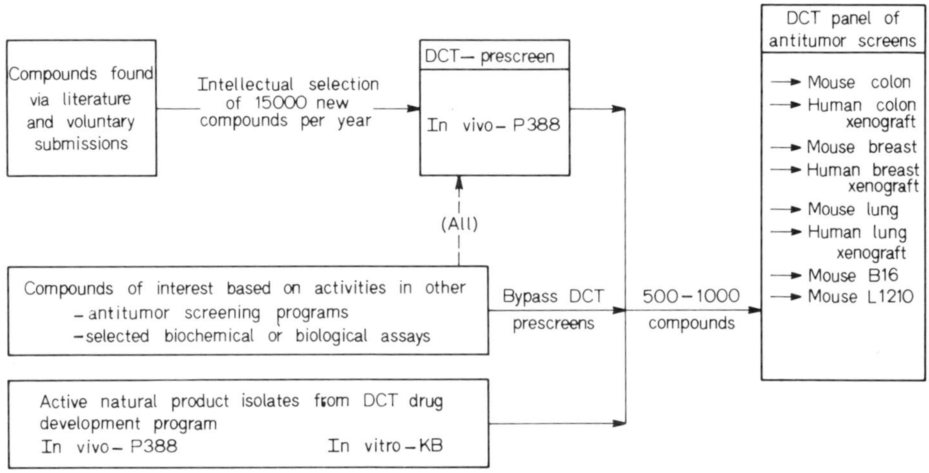

Fig. 1. Proposed flow of drugs through DCT screens

Table 1. Results of known anticancer agents against human tumors xenografted to T-cell deprived mice[a]

Drug	Colon 116	Colon 76	Human tumor xenografts Bronchus 246	Bronchus (mount)	Ovary 210	Kidney 381
Methotrexate	±	NR		±		
Cyclophosphamide			NR	NR	+	NR
Melphalan					+	
BCNU	+	+				
Cis-dichlorodiammineplatinum (II)					NR	
Adriamycin	±			NR		
Hexamethylmelamine	±		++	+	±	++
5-FU	+	NR		NR		

Definitions: [a] See reference 5
NR = no response; ± = slight response; + = tumor inhibition; + + = tumor regression.

Preclinical Criteria for Selection of New Analogs II

An additional criterion for selection of new analogs of antitumor antibiotics involves the demonstration of a broader spectrum of effectiveness against experimental tumors including transplantable, carcinogen-induced or spontaneous.

The activity of actinomycin D has been determined in a broad spectrum of experimental tumor systems [8]. It is curative for leukemia P388 and the Ridgway osteogenic sarcoma. It has produced marked inhibition of tumor growth, or increased life span in tumors such as B16 melanoma, leukemia L1210 and Gardner C3HED lymphosarcoma. It also has borderline activity against a number of tumors including lymphatic leukemia L5178Y, leukemia P355, lymphoma 8 and Walker carcinosarcoma 256. It has been inactive in a variety of tumor systems. Demonstration of a broader spectrum of activity of an actinomycin

Table 2. Summary of the antitumor efficacy of bleomycin in various animal models (US data)

Tumor systems	Evaluation of drug effect[a]
Leukemia L1210 (i.p.) (mice)	–
Leukemia P388 (i.p.) (mice)	+
B16 Melanoma (s.c.) (mice)	++
B16 Melanoma (i.p.) (mice)	–
Ependymoblastoma (i.c.) (mice)	+
Lewis lung (i.m., s.c., i.v.) (mice)	+
Madison lung carcinoma (i.m.) (mice)	+
Walker 256 carcinosarcoma (i.p.) (rat)	++
Walker 256 carcinosarcoma (i.m.) (rat)	++
Ridgway osteogenic sarcoma (s.c.) (mice)	++

[a] *Survival time*: ILS% 0–24—; 25–49+; ≥50 ++; *Solid tumors*: % Inhibition; 0–49—; 50–74+; ≥75 ++.

Table 3. Summary of the antitumor efficacy of bleomycin in various animal models. (Japanese data)

Tumor systems	Evaluation of drug effect[a]
SR—C57B1/6—2008-B (i.p.) (mice	+
MM_2 Mammary carcinoma (i.p.) (mice)	++
Friend Ascites SFAT-5 (i.p.) (mice)	–
MH, Hepatoma (i.p.) (mice)	++
Plasmacytoma X-5563 (i.p.) (mice)	+
SR-C3H/HeTH_{62} (i.p.) (mice)	++
SR—C3H/H_e TH_{62} (s.c.) (mice)	++
Ehrlich (s.c.) (mice)	++
Sarcoma-180 (s.c.) (mice)	++

[a] *Survival time*: ILS%; 0–24-; 25–49+; ≥ 50 ++; *Solid tumors*: % Inhibition; 0–49-; 50–74+; 75++.

derivative or activity in a system where actinomycin D is inactive, or improvement of activity in a system where actinomycin D has been demonstrated to show activity, would stimulate interest in a new analog.

The activity of bleomycin has been determined in a spectrum of tumor systems both in the United States (Table 2) and in Japan (Table 3).[2] It is inactive in certain systems such as leukemia L1210 and Friend ascites and has shown only moderate activity in other tumor systems. Adriamycin has demonstrated broad spectrum activity in animal tumor systems including lymphoma, leukemia, myeloma, sarcoma, carcinoma and melanoma [10]. With bleomycin or adriamycin analogs, as for analogs of actinomycin D, activity in a broader spectrum of tumor systems would identify new analogs as worthy of further development.

[2]Collected data of various U.S. and Japanese investigators.

Preclinical Criteria for Selection of New Analogs III

Schedule and route characterization may be taken into account in relation to selection of new analogs. Criteria could include greater effectiveness over a variety of schedules, significant difference in scheduling dependency characteristics and more latitude in choice of routes of administration.

A schedule dependency comparison has been made of adriamycin, rubidazone and daunomycin in the L1210 system. Over a series of schedules, adriamycin was demonstrated to be more effective than daunomycin. Adriamycin also appeared to be more effective than rubidazone, although on some schedules rubidazone appeared to be equally effective (Table 4) [11, 12].

Adriamycin, rubidazone and daunomycin were all highly effective in the treatment of i.p. inoculated B16 melanoma (Table 5) [11, 12]. Although, on some schedules, adriamycin appeared to be more effective than daunomycin, there were no clear cut differences in schedule dependency characteristics between adriamycin and rubidazone. All three drugs were essentially ineffective in the treatment of s.c. inoculated B16 melanoma. Although in the treatment of s.c. Lewis lung carcinoma the drugs produced some inhibition of tumor growth, possibly more extensive with rubidazone, they were essentially ineffective in increasing survival time [10, 11].

Over several schedules, adriamycin was more effective than carminomycin in the treatment of leukemia L1210 or leukemia P388 (Table 6) [11, 12]. Carminomycin and daunomycin appeared to be approximately equally effective in increasing survival time in these two leukemia systems.

On an intermittant schedule of treatment of leukemia L1210, adriamycin appeared to be more effective than daunomycin employing the i.p. or s.c. routes of drug administration [24]. Neither drug was effective on oral administration. Demonstration of activity on oral administration for an anthracycline derivative such as has been observed for carminomycin[3] and also 4-demethoxydaunorubicin [6], indicates some fundamental difference in biologic action.

Table 4. Comparison adriamycin, daunomycin and rubidazone leukemia L1210

		Adriamycin		Daunomycin		Rubidazone	
Expt.	Schedule	Opt. dose mg/kg/inj.	ILS %	Opt. dose mg/kg/inj.	ILS %	Opt. dose mg/kg/inj.	ILS %
1	Q4D 1, 5, 9			2	44	16	81
2	Q4D 1, 5, 9			4	61	16	105
3	Q4D 1, 5, 9	2.5	31	5	21	10	63
4	Q4D 1, 5, 9	3.9	33	2.6	6	8.9	11
5	Q4D 1, 5, 9	8	63	5	20	5	63
6	QD 1-9	1	31	0.25	26	1	16
7	QD 1-9	1.8	43	1.8	44	3	50
8	Day 1 only	5	26	10	21	20	58
9	Day 1 only	5.9	28	5.9	6	20	28
10	Day 1 only	13.3	121	3	56	8	53
11	Q3H day 1 only	1	36 (2/8)	0.5	41	4	53
12	Q3H day 1 only	1.8	67 (1/10)	1.2	22	1.8	39
13	Q8D 1, 9	10	47	5	11	10	47
14	Q3H, Q4D 1, 5, 9	0.25	58	0.5	21	2	47

[3]Gauze, G. F. et al Personal Communication; and Division of Cancer Treatment Screening Data.

Table 5. Comparison adriamycin, daunomycin and rubidazone B16 melanoma and Lewis lung carcinoma

		Adriamycin		Daunomycin		Rubidazone	
Expt.	Schedule	Opt. dose mg/kg/inj.	ILS %	Opt. dose mg/kg/inj.	ILS %	Opt. dose mg/kg/inj.	ILS %
			i.p. B16 melanoma				
1	QD 1-9	1	188 (4/10)	0.5	94	3	100 (1/10)
2	QD 1-9	0.5	>172 (6/10)	88	88	6	>172 (6/10)
3	QD 1-9	1	>160 (7/10)	0.5	>160 (5/10)	3	126 (4/10)
4	QD 1-9	1	>144 (9/10)	0.5	>144 (5/10)	3	>144 (8/10)
5	Q4D 1, 5, 9	2	88	2	47	6	61
6	Q4D 1, 5, 9	2	>172 (5/10)	1	56	12	115 (4/10)
7	Q4D 1, 5, 9	1	>160 (6/10)	1	>160 (6/10)	6	>160 (6/10)
			s.c. B16 melanoma				
8	QD 1-9	4	31	1	10	6	10
			s.c. Lewis lung carcinoma				
9	QD 1-9	2	9 (42% TW1)[a]	2	0 (22% TW1)	12	0 (70% TW1)

[a] TW1 = Tumor weight inhibition.

Table 6. Comparison adriamycin, daunomycin and carminomycin L1210 and P388 leukemias

		Adriamycin		Daunomycin		Carminomycin	
Expt.	Schedule	Opt. dose mg/kg/inj.	ILS %	Opt. dose mg/kg/inj.	ILS %	Opt. dose mg/kg/inj.	ILS %
			Leukemia L1210				
1	QD 1-9	1.8	43	1.8	44	0.14	32
2	Q4D 1, 5, 9	8	63 (1/10)	5	20	0.39	40
3	Day 1 only	13.3	121	3	56	0.65	53
			Leukemia P388				
4	QD 1-9	1.08	136	0.65	77	0.14	77
5	Q4D 1, 5, 9	5	118 (1/10)	3	72	0.65	72
6	Day 1 only	13.3	104 (3/10)	5	59	0.65	72

Preclinical Criteria for Selection of New Analogs IV

Additional criteria for the selection of new analogs include diminished, limiting or undesirable, acute, chronic or delayed host toxicity, e.g., myelosuppressive action, gastrointestinal toxicity, cardiac toxicity, lung toxicity.

The cardiomyopathy induced by anthracyclines has complicated their therapeutic application. Rabbit, rat and mouse models are being utilized to evaluate the cardiotoxicity of anthracycline analogs [16, 20, 21, 33, 34]. A comparison was made in rabbit of the occurrence of cardiac toxicity following adriamycin, daunomycin, rubidazone and the adriamycin-DNA complex (1/10 LD_{50} per injection for each drug) on a treatment schedule of three times weekly (Table 7) [17]. The estimated total cardiotoxic doses in mg/M^2 for adriamycin and daunomycin were not essentially different. The total cardiotoxic dose for the adriamycin-DNA complex was somewhat higher, but the estimated cardiotoxic dose for rubidazone was almost six times higher than that observed with adriamycin. However, the optimal therapeutic dose of rubidazone is also somewhat higher than that observed for adriamycin. If an anthracycline analog elicited more extensive therapeutic effect than the parent compound at an equivalent cardiotoxic dose in an experimental tumor system, this could provide an important therapeutic possibility.

Table 7. Rabbit model for cardiac toxicity

Drug	mg/kg	Schedule	Total weeks on test	Estimated cardiotoxic dose[a] total mg/M^2[b]
Adriamycin	0.8	3 × week	10	250
Daunomycin	0.7	3 × week	17	375
Rubidazone	2.3	3 × week	18	1400
Adriamycin—DNA complex	1.4[c]	3 × week	>10	550

[a] Cardiomyopathy.
[b] mg/kg × 11 = mg/M^2.
[c] Adriamycin equivalent; Adriamycin: DNA = 1:9; See reference [16].

It should be noted that an Anthracycline Coordinating Group[4] at the Division of Cancer Treatment is instituting a study to determine the feasibility of employing the mouse model for the evaluation of cardiotoxicity of anthracycline derivatives on acute and chronic treatment. The stated objectives of the study include: a) determination of the feasibility of using the mouse model for evaluation of the cardiotoxicity of anthracycline derivatives; b) to determine whether the findings in the mouse will correlate with those in other experimental animals, with special attention to the development of a histologically defined anthracycline induced cardiomyopathy; c) to determine whether the acute cardiotoxic effects of anthracyclines correlate with chronic cardiotoxicity which in the rat, rabbit and monkey corresponds closely to the human toxicity. The parameters that may be of value in assessing cardiotoxicity include: heart weight, heart weight/body weight ratio, thin section light microscopy, electron microscopy, routine histopathologic evaluation, clinical evidence of congestive heart failure, and survival after chronic antibiotic treatment. The protocols include a) toxicity determination b) acute cardiotoxicity c) chronic cardiotoxicity for adriamycin, daunomycin and related analogs. If the mouse model proves feasible it will permit testing of a greater number of anthracycline analogs for cardiac toxicity in relation to potential clinical interest.

Bleomycin A5033 and bleomycin A5196 were demonstrated by Umezawa and colleagues [30] to elicit lower toxicity to the lung of aged mice than the bleomycin mixture. This reduction in toxicity for the lung, which constitutes an important factor in the limiting toxicity of the bleomycin mixture, provides a positive feature for these analogs.

[4] N. Bachur, Coordinator. The study has been devised by R. K. Johnson and D. M. Young.

Preclinical Criteria for Selection of New Analogs V

Criteria for selection of new analogs include the phenomenon of tumor cell resistance. There may be a delay in the origin of tumor cell resistance, or increased activity against tumors that are naturally resistant to the parent drug (as has been discussed above), or against tumors with acquired resistance to the parent drug. There have not been too many demonstrations of the ability of drugs to delay the origin of tumor cell resistance. One example involved combination treatment of leukemia L1210 with cytosine arabinoside plus cyclophosphamide over a series of transplant generations [9]. Treatment with this drug combination resulted in a two generation delay in the origin of tumor cell resistance to cytosine arabinoside as compared with the origin of resistance to cytosine arabinoside following treatment with the drug alone.

A subline of leukemia P-388 that acquired resistance to the parent drug adriamycin has been well characterized [13, 18]. It is cross resistant to noncovalent DNA binders including other anthracyclines, actinomycins, mithramycin, ellipticine, and other intercalators. It also is cross resistant to mitotic spindle poisons including vinca alkaloids, maytansine and podophyllotoxins. It is cross-resistant to the protein synthesis inhibitors, emetine, pactamycin, homoharringtonine, T2 toxin and streptoviticin A, and to miscellaneous compounds such as ICRF 159 and the terephthalanilides. Any anthracycline derivative that is active against this adriamycin-resistant P-388 leukemia subline would be a proper subject for further development. It may be noted that this subline of P388, resistant to adriamycin, is sensitive to covalent DNA binders including mitomycin C and anthramycin, antimetabolites including methotrexate, 5-fluorouracil, arabinosyl cytosine and glutamine antagonists, to alkylating agents including cyclophosphamide, nitrosoureas, cis platinum, piperazinedione and other mustards, to the protein synthesis inhibitors, anguidine and bruceantin, and to miscellaneous drugs such as neocarzinostatin, camptothecin and indicine N-oxide. This type of detailed study may be of interest in the development of patterns of resistance to analogs and antitumor agents in general.

An important problem pertains to the therapy that may be employed following the origin of tumor-cell resistance. In such a case it is possible to employ a second, unrelated drug, or an analog with a different mechanism of action which does not show cross-resistance to the original drug. For this purpose, a reference chart has been compiled by Skipper et. al. [29] listing the cross-resistance characteristics of antitumor agents. With the employment of a comprehensive chart of this nature it may be possible to determine what drugs or analogs may be utilized in treatment following the origin of tumor-cell resistance to the terapy that is being employed.

Taking these cross-resistance characteristics into account, it is of interest to consider, from the animal data, what drugs might be useful following the origin of resistance to the combination chemotherapy cyclophosphamide-methotrexate-5-flourouracil (CMF) that is being employed in the treatment of breast tumor by Bonadonna et. al. [1]. It could, for example, be possible to treat with adriamycin following the origin of resistance (Fig. 2). Adriamycin, employed alone, is an effective agent in the treatment of advanced breast cancer in the clinic. Also, in accordance with the animal test data, there is no cross resistance between adriamycin and cyclophosphamide, methotrexate or 5-flurouracil. On the other hand, following the origin of resistance to CMF, treatment with L-phenylalanine mustard (melphalan) would be questionable since there is cross resistance between cyclophosphamide and L-phenylalanine mustard [29]. However, this is still uncertain since more recently, Schabel reported sensitivity to melphalan following the origin of cyclophosphamide resistance [26]. This kind of information may also be useful in the determination of interest in analogs. Thus, if an analog did not show cross resistance to the parent drug, alone or in

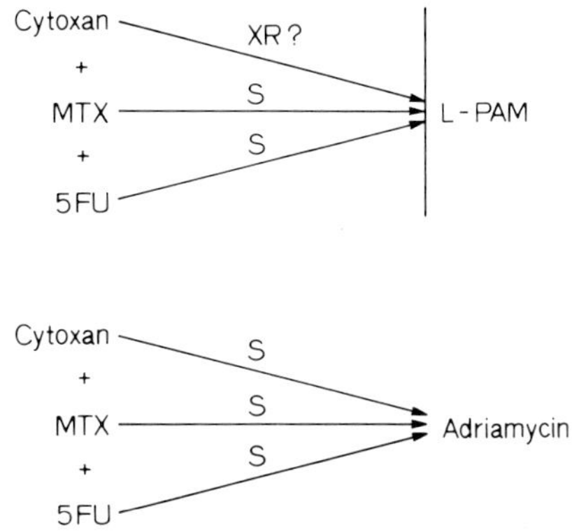

Fig. 2. CMF combination treatment to be followed by L-PAM or Adriamycin

combination in an appropriate animal model, the analog could be used in the clinic following the origin of resistance.

Preclinical Criteria for Selection of New Analogs VI

The demonstration of therapeutic synergism of an analog when employed in combination with a parent drug would imply that there was a difference in pharmacologic or biochemical action of the analog. More extensive therapeutic synergism with the analog than with the parent compound, in combination with a structurally unrelated agent, would also suggest interest in the analog. There has been a paucity of studies in this area. In one example, the combination of ftorafur plus 5-fluorouracil was investigated in the treatment of leukemia L1210 [7]. It was determined that at optimal dosage, the combination was not more effective in increasing survival time than 5-fluouracil alone, thereby failing to support the suggestion of a significant difference in pharmacologic or biochemical action of the ftorafur analog. In another study, a comparison was made of adriamycin plus vinblastine or adriamycin plus vincristine in the treatment of leukemia L1210 against the drugs employed individually [9, 11]. The extent of therapeutic effect appeared to be greater with the combination of adriamycin plus vincristine than that observed with adriamycin plus vinblastine. If vincristine had been an unknown analog this data would suggest a strong interest in it.

Preclinical Criteria for Selection of New Analogs VII

Additional criteria for selection of new analogs are greater penetration to intracranial or other sequestered sites, and specific organ localization which could result in the elicitation of more extensive antitumor effectiveness. In one study, BCNU was highly effective against an intracranially inoculated subline of leukemia L1210 that had high dihydrofolate reductase levels [14]. On parenteral administration of BCNU there was a marked increase in life span

of these mice and a marked reduction in the dihydrofolate reductase levels in the brain, indicative of tumor cell destruction. More extensive action against intracranial tumor than the parent compound would be an important feature for an analog.
Following injection of ^{3}H-bleomycin into mice, 50%–64% and 46%–49% of the active form of the drug remained in lung and skin respectively [30]. More extensive localization of the active form of a bleomycin analog in tumor, which might result in increased antitumor effect, would suggest that a bleomycin analog could be of value. It should be noted that bleomycin A5196 showed high concentrations in lung, liver, spleen and tumor of mice bearing the solid form of Ehrlich tumor [30].

Preclinical Criteria for Selection of New Analogs VIII

Another criterion for selection involves the demonstration of greater effectiveness in preventing metastasis or in the effective treatment of metastatic tumor. In one example employing advanced Lewis lung tumor in which the disease had metastasized to the lungs, treatment was more effective with methyl-CCNU as compared with CCNU or BCNU in inhibiting local tumor growth and in increasing the survival time of the animals. The latter result is indicative of greater inhibition of lung metastasis and thereby created interest in this compound [25].

Preclinical Criteria for Selection of New Analogs IX

Further on the question of criteria for selection of new analogs, greater action against oncogenic virus, viral transformation or viral induced tumor or reinduction of tumor would create an interest in an analog. Evidence has been provided that with the virus induced AKR lymphoma it is possible on treatment with various drug combinations to essentially eradicate the disease [27, 28]. However there may be reinduction of the disease and any analog that would prevent this reinduction would have an important property of interest. Also, any analog that might be more effective than the parent compound in the treatment of viral-induced tumors such as Moloney or Rauchser leukemia, or prevent tumor induction following inoculation of the Moloney sarcoma virus would be an important candidate for further study.

Preclinical Criteria for Selection of New Analogs X

Further criteria for selection of new analogs includes the possession of more desirable pharmacologic or biochemical characteristics. This may encompass: a) diminished detoxification or excretion; greater maintenance of blood and tissue levels; depot form with steady release; b) more satisfactory dosage form including greater solubility or greater stability; c) the drug could be more active on oral administration; d) there could be increased entry into tumor cells; increased or prolonged binding to active sites and so forth. Any analog demonstrating such characteristics would be of great interest.

Preclinical Criteria for Selection of New Analogs XI

Further, with respect to characteristics that would create an interest in analogs, there could be different action in relation to tumor and/or vital host cell kinetics. This could encompass an effect of the analog at a different phase of the cell cycle than the parent compound, more extensive selective tumor-cell kill, greater retention of activity at various stages of the tumor growth curve or more extensive action against nondividing Go cells. Alternatively if Go cells could be recruited successfully they could be rendered more sensitive to therapy with a second agent.

Preclinical Criteria for Selection of New Analogs XII

Where a parent compound exerts carcinogenic activity, an analog that is not carcinogenic could be of considerable importance.

Preclinical Criteria for Selection of New Analogs XIII

Criteria of selection of new analogs may include action on the immune status of the host. If the analog had less immunosuppressive action, if it demonstrated more extensive immunostimulation, or if it were more effective in altering antigenicity of tumor cells, this could create interest in a compound. Belomycin has been reported to not elicit any immunosuppressive effect [23, 30, 32], but this is somewhat exceptional since most antitumor agents are immunosuppressive to a greater or lesser degree and this may interfere with antitumor effectiveness. Any congener of a known antibiotic that has diminished immunosuppressive or increased immunostimulatory action could be of potential value.

Two examples of immunosuppression in animal tumor systems may be cited. In one study, employing the L1210 system, in which animals were pretreated prior to leukemic inoculation, melphalan and cyclophosphamide were more immunosuppressive than 6-mercaptopurine or methotrexate [15]. In another study involving the Moloney-sarcoma-virus-induced tumor both adriamycin and daunomycin treatment resulted in progressive growth of the tumor overcoming the immunity of the host which following an initial period of growth-caused regression of the tumor [4].

It has been demonstrated that a number of antitumor drugs such as DTIC may alter tumor antigenicity [2, 22] and any antibiotic analog that could alter antigenicity more extensively than the parent compound would provide a useful tool for investigation.

Preclinical Criteria for Selection of New Analogs XIV

In view of the great clinical interest, criteria for selection of new analogs should include superiority of an analog over the parent compound in combined modalities with surgery, radiation or immunotherapy. If an analog of an antitumor antibiotic did show a more extensive therapeutic effect than the parent compound on a combined modality regimen, it could indeed arouse profound interest. This area has been largely unexploited in animal tumor systems.

In summary, there are a variety of factors that may be employed in determining further clinical interest for analogs of known antitumor antibiotics. It is important to delineate the limiting characteristics in the clinical application of the parent antitumor antibiotic and to then choose the appropriate systems to identify and characterize new analogs. The analogs should then be investigated in depth in order to determine whether they may provide some advantage either in antitumor selectivity or in the diminution of host toxicity with retention of antitumor effectiveness.

Summary

If a new analog of a known antitumor antibiotic is to justify interest, it must be demonstrated to possess either quantitative or qualitative superiority over the parent compound in pharmacologic, toxicologic, immunologic, tumor cytotoxic, or other biologic properties that are therapeutically favorable. The most commonly used criterion is in vivo activity in experimental tumor systems. This may be demonstrated in primary screening systems or in secondary screening systems, or in refractory tumor systems, or in one or more tumors of a human xenograft panel. Data on adriamycin and bleomycin analogs give evidence of some of these approaches. An additional criterion for selection of analogs involves the demonstration of a broader spectrum of effectiveness against a panel of experimental systems. Actinomycin D is used as an example.

There are a variety of factors that may be employed in determining further clinical interest for analogs of known antitumor antibiotics. It is important to delineate the limiting characteristics in the clinical application of the parent antitumor antibiotic and to then choose the appropriate systems to identify and characterize new analogs and investigate them in depth in order to determine whether they may provide some advantage either in antitumor selectivity or in the diminution of host toxicity with retention of antitumor effectiveness.

References

1. BONADONNA: G., BRUSAMOLINO, E., VALAGUSSA, P., ROSSI, A., BRUGNATELLI, L., BRAMBILLA, C., DE LENA, M., TANCINI, G., BAJETTA, E., MUSUMECI, R., VERONESI, U.: Combination chemotherapy as an adjuvant treatment in operable breast cancer. N. Engl. J. Med. **294**; 405–410 (1976).
2. BONMASSER, E., BONMASSAR, A., VADLAMUDI, S., GOLDIN, A.: Immunological alteration of leukemic cells in vivo after treatment with an antitumor drug. Proc. Natl. Acad. Sci. USA **66**, 1089–1095 (1970).

3. BRADNER: W. T., IMANISHI, H., HIRTH, R. S., WODINSKY, I.: Antitumor activity and toxicity of BU-2231-A, a new bleomycin analogue. Proc. Am. Assoc. Cancer Res. **18**, 35 (1977).
4. CASAZZA, A. M., ISETTA, A. M., GIULIANI, F., DI MARCO, A.: Immunodepressive activity of daunomycin and adriamycin. In: Adriamycin Review. Staquet, M. et al (eds.) Ghent, Belgium: European Press Medikon 1975, pp. 123–131.
5. DETRE, S. I., DAVIES, A. J. S., CONNORS, T. A.: New models for cancer chemotherapy. Cancer Chemother. Rep. Pt. II, **5** (1), 133–145 (1975).
6. DI MARCO, A., CASAZZA, A. M. PRATESI, G.: Antitumor activity of 4-demethoxydaunorubicin (NSC 256,439) administered Orally. Cancer Treat. Rep. **61**, (5), 893–894 (1977).
7. GARIBJANIAN, B. T., JOHNSON, R. K., KLINE, I., VADLAMUDI, S., GANG, M., VENDITTI, J. M., GOLDIN, A.: Comparison of 5-fluorouracil and ftorafur. II. Therapeutic Response and Development of Resistance in Murine Tumors. Cancer Treat. Rep. **60** (9), 1347–1361 (1976).
8. GOLDIN, A., JOHNSON, R. K.: Evaluation of actinomycins in experimental systems. Cancer Chemother. Rep. Pt. I, **58**, (1), 63–77 (1974).
9. GOLDIN, A., JOHNSON, R. K.: Experimental Grounds for Combination Chemotherapy. Excerpta Medica International Congress Series No. 353, Proc. XI Int. Cancer Cong. Florence 1974, Vol. V, pp. 308–313.
10. GOLDIN, A., JOHNSON, R. K.: Experimental tumor activity of adriamycin (NSC 123127). Cancer Chemother. Rep. Pt. III, **6**, 137–145 (1975).
11. GOLDIN, A., JOHNSON, R. K.: Antitumor effect of adriamycin in comparison with related drugs, and in combination chemotherapy. In: Adriamycin Review. STAQUET, M. et al (eds.) Ghent, Belgium: European Press Medikon 1975 pp. 37–54.
12. GOLDIN, A., JOHNSON, R. K.: Adriamycin activity in experimental tumors. In: Ergebnisse der Adriamycin—Therapie. GHIONE, M., FETZER, J., MAIER, H. (eds.): Berlin: Springer-Verlag 1975, pp. 3–13.
13. GOLDIN, A., JOHNSON, R. K.: Resistance to antitumor agents. EORTC Monograph Series (In Press) (1977).
14. HUMPHREYS, S. R., THOMAS, L. B., CHIRIGOS, M. A., GOLDIN, A., CRAWFORD, E. J., FRIEDKIN, M.: Use of dihydrofolate reductase as a biochemical index of chemotherapy. Nature **195**, 453–455 (1962).
15. HUMPHREYS, S. R., GLYNN, J. P., GOLDIN, A.: Suppression of the homograft response by pretreatment with antitumor agents. Transplantation **1**, 65–69 (1963).
16. JAENKE, R. S.: An anthracycline antibiotic-induced cardiomyopathy in rabbits. Lab. Invest. **30**, 292–304 (1974).
17. JAENKE, R. S., Colo., St. U.: personal communication.
18. JOHNSON, R. K., OVEJERA, A. A., GOLDIN, A.: Activity of anthracyclines against an adriamycin (NSC-123127)—resistant subline of P-388 leukemia with special emphasis on cinerubin A (NSC-18334). Cancer Treat. Rep. **60** (1), 99–102 (1976).
19. LASTER, W. R., Jr.: Ridgway osteogenic sarcoma—A promising laboratory model for special therapeutic trials against an advanced—staged, drug-sensitive animal tumor system. Cancer Chemother. Rep. Pt. II, **5** (1), 151–168 (1975).
20. LENAZ, L., PAGE, J. A.: Cardiotoxicity of adriamycin and related anthracyclines. Cancer Treat. Rev. **3** (3), 111–120 (1976).
21. MYERS, C. E., MCGUIRE, W., YOUNG, R.: Adriamycin: amelioration of toxicity by α-tocopherol. Cancer Treat. Rep. **60** (7), 961–962 (1976).
22. NICOLIN, A., VADLAMUDI, S., GOLDIN, A.: Antigenicity of L1210 leukemic sublines induced by drugs. Cancer Res. **32**, 653–657 (1972).
23. OHNO, R., NISHIKAWA, H., KAWASHIMA, K., UETANI, T., HIRANO, M., MIURA, M., YAMADA, K.: Lack of immunosuppressive effect of bleomycin on the primary response of mice to sheep red blood cells. Gann **62**, 267 (1971).
24. SANDBERG, J. S., HOWSDEN, F. L., DI MARCO, A., GOLDIN, A.: Comparison of the antileukemic effect in mice of adriamycin (NSC-123127) with daunomycin (NSC-82151). Cancer Chemother. Rep. Pt. 1, **54** (1), 1–7 (1970).
25. SCHABEL, F. M., Jr.: Nitrosoureas: A review of experimental antitumor activity. Cancer Chemother. Rep. **60** (6), 665–698 (1976).
26. SCHABEL, F. M., Jr., LASTER, W. R., Jr., TRADER, M. W., WITT, M. H.: Combination chemotherapy with cyclophosphamide plus melphalan against leukemia L1210. Proc. Am. Assoc. Cancer Res. **16**, 24 (1975).
27. SKIPPER, H. E., SCHABEL, F. M., Jr.: Quantitative and Cytokinetic Studies in Experimental Tumor Models. Cancer Medicine. HOLLAND, J. F., FREI, E. (eds.): Phila.: Lea & Febiger 1973, Vol. III, pp. 629–650.
28. SKIPPER, H. E., SCHABEL, F. M., Jr., TRADER, M. W., LASTER, W. R., Jr.: Response to therapy of spontaneous, first passage, and long passage lines of AK leukemia. Cancer Chemother. Rep. **55**, 345–366 (1969).

29. SKIPPER, H. E., HUTCHISON, D. J., SCHABEL, F. M., Jr., SCHMIDT, L. H., GOLDIN, A., BROCKMAN, R. W., VENDITTI, J. M., WODINSKY, I.: A quick reference chart on cross resistance between anticancer agents. Cancer Chemother. Rep. Pt. I, **56** (4), 493–498 (1972).
30. UMEZAWA, H.: Development and mechanism of action of bleomycin. In: New Drug Seminar on Bleomycin. SOPER, W. GOTT, A.: Natl. Cancer Inst. 1974.
31. VENDITTI, J. M.: Relevance of transplantable animal tumor systems to the selection of new agents for clinical trial. In: Pharmacological Basis of Cancer Chemotherapy. Univ. of Texas System Cancer Center, Baltimore: The Williams & Wilkins Co. 1975, pp. 245–270.
32. YAMAKI, H., TANAKA, N., UMEZAWA, H.: Effects of several tumor-inhibitory antibiotics on immunological response. J. Antibiot. (Tokyo) **22**, 315 (1969).
33. YOUNG, D. M.: Pathologic effects of adriamycin (NSC-123127) in experimental systems. Cancer Chemother. Rep. Pt. III, **6** (2), 159–175 (1975).
34. ZBINDEN, G., BRANDLE, E.: Toxicologic screening of daunorubicin (NSC-82151) adriamycin (NSC-123127), and their derivatives in rats. Cancer Chemother. Rep. Pt. I, **59** (4), 707–715 (1975).

Preclinical Status of Macromomycin at the National Cancer Institute

V. H. Bono Jr. and D. Abraham

Macromomycin (MCR) is an antitumor antibiotic protein isolated from the culture filtrate of *Streptomyces* macromomyceticus by Chimura et. al. [1]. It was found to have antibacterial activity against Gram-positive organisms and to have antitumor activity against L1210 leukemia. It was also found by Kunimoto et. al. [2] that its effects on DNA synthesis and cell division of HeLa cells are reversed by incubation with trypsin. This suggests an action of the drug at the surface of the cell membrane.

The NCI has received and tested MCR from both Bristol Laboratories, USA and Kanegafuchi Laboratories, Japan (Table 1).

This material was received over a period of 2½ years. Crude MCR was at most 30% MCR and the purified material was more than 95% MCR.

Antitumor Activity

The antitumor activity of MCR was determined by the screening laboratories of the Drug Evaluation Branch, DCT, NCI and has been reported by Lippman et. al. [3]. It was reported as active against L1210 leukemia, P388 leukemia and B16 melanoma. The results of treating i.p. L1210 leukemia with i.p. administered MCR are shown in Table 2.

The ratio T/C represents the median survival time (MST) of treated groups of mice divided by the MST of untreated groups, expressed as a percentage. The optimal T/C values were all about the same for several dose schedules.

The activity of i.p. MCR against i.p. P388 leukemia is shown in Table 3.

Three different lots were tested. The optimal doses required reflect the differences in purity of the lots. The optimal activities were all comparable for the different lots and different dose schedules.

The results of treating i.p. B16 melanoma with i.p. MCR are shown in Table 4.

Four lots have been tested with optimal T/C values ranging from 139–160. Here also, the optimal dose required for each lot reflects its purity. The activity of MCR was independent of lot or dose schedule.

Stability of Antitumor Activity of MCR

MCR is unstable in solid form, even when stored at −20°C. It is reported to be even more unstable in light and to be stabilized by maltose. We have found that MCR loses its therapeutic activity against L1210 leukemia, P388 leukemia and B16 melanoma on prolonged storage. Table 5 shows the loss of activity of lot NF, purified MCR from Kanigafuchi Laboratories, against L1210 leukemia.

The relative age is the time in months after the first assay. For three-dose schedules, initial T/C values in the 145 range, fell to inactive levels over a 7 month period.
A similar loss of activity was found in the treatment of P388 leukemia (Table 6) and for B16 melanoma (Table 7).
The loss of activity against B16 melanoma occurred with both a Bristol Laboratories lot NB and the purified lot NF.

Studies on Lewis Lung Carcinoma

Intraperitoneally administered MCR is inactive against subcutaneous (s.c.) implanted Lewis lung carcinoma. However, when MCR is injected directly into the tumor site, it prolongs the life span of the mice. The experiments to be described were conducted for the NCI by Dr. W. R. Laster at Southern Research Institute, in collaboration with Dr. M. M. Lippman at the N.C.I.
Groups of 10 mice with s.c. Lewis lung carcinoma were treated daily for 20 days with intratumor injections of MCR. The results are shown in Table 8.
The dose administered and day of death of the various groups of mice is tabulated. The untreated mice died with a MST of 28 days, with no tumor-free survivors on day 146. At increasing doses of MCR, the animals lived longer and there were increasing numbers of tumor-free survivors.
The 7 survivors treated with 1 mg MCR/kg and the 2 survivors treated with 0.25 mg MCR/kg were reinoculated with Lewis lung carcinoma to determine whether they had developed a resistance to the tumor as part of the mechanism of their survival (Table 9).
Previously untumored and untreated mice died with a MST of 20 days after Lewis lung carcinoma implant. Both survivors of the 0.25 mg/kg dose died on day 22 and the survivors of the 1 mg/kg dose died with a MST of 24 days after reinoculation. Thus it appeared that these animals had not developed a demonstrable resistance to Lewis lung cells and that their survival was not due primarily to an immune effect.
The effect of intratumor injection of MCR on the development of pulmonary metastases was also studied. Groups of mice were treated with MCR for 12 days, and on day 12 the lungs were minced and aliquots injected s.c. into a new group of mice to assay for the presence of Lewis lung cells in the lung tissue. The results are shown in Table 10.
All the test animals receiving lung tissue from untreated Lewis-lung-bearing mice died between day 24 and 41, indicating the presence of pulmonary metastases. Of the animals treated with 0.125 mg/kg, 1/6 had no pulmonary metastases. At higher doses most of the animals were free of metastases. The absence of metastases on day 12 was at a time when the primary tumor was still in active growth. This result suggests that either there is a decrease in the release of cells from the primary tumor or an increased sensitivity of metastatic cells to death from MCR.

Effects of MCR in Cell Culture

MCR inhibits the growth of L1210, P388 and KB cells in cell culture. Table 11 shows the ED_{50} values for several lots of MCR.
These figures represent the concentrations which inhibit growth by 50% over a standard time

period. The difference in values for each lot reflects the relative purity of the three lots. For lot MB and lot NF, P388 cells were more sensitive than L1210 cells. This difference in potency was not seen in the optimal doses for the treatment of P388 and L1210 leukemia in vivo, and it probably reflects some characteristic related to growing the cells in culture.

The time-course of inhibition of the growth of L1210 cells is shown in Table 12.

Untreated L1210 cells have a doubling time of 12 h. At a dose of 0.5 μg/ml, the growth rate was slowed to a doubling time of 24 h. At 0.5 μg/ml and above, cell division essentially ceases.

The effects of MCR on cell cycle progression were evaluated by flow microfluorometry (FMF). In this technique, cells are stained for DNA content with a fluorescent dye and the DNA content of each cell is measured in a flow system using a laser light activating source. In this way the DNA content of 100,000 cells can be measured in 1 min. The results are displayed as a curve of the number of cells plotted against increasing DNA content.

A computed DNA-content distribution (DCD) curve of a model of cells in log-phase growth is shown in Fig. 1. It can be seen that the shape of this curve is due to a population of G1-phase cells, with a relative DNA content of 1.0, a smaller population of G2-phase cells, with a relative DNA content of 2.0, and a population of S-phase cells with intermediate DNA values.

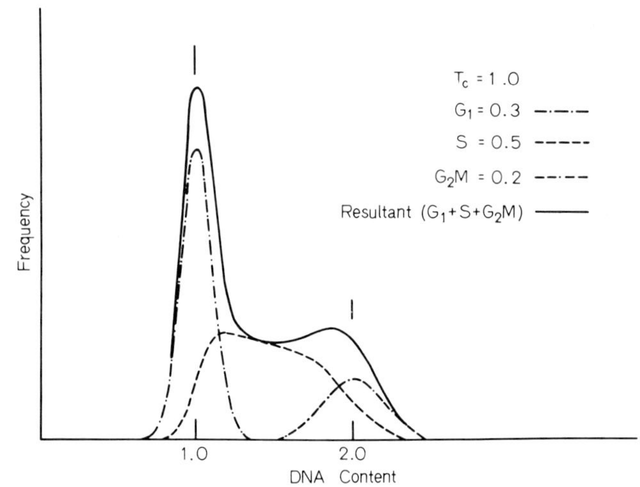

Fig. 1. Computed log-phase DCD curve. A model of an exponentially growing population with a relative cycle cycle time, Tc = 1.0, was used. The relative duration of G1-phase was 0.3 (-.-.-.), of S-phase was 0.5 (----), and of G2 + M phase was 0.2 (--.--.). The resultant DCD curve (____) is the sum of these contents

The effects of MCR on cell cycle progression of L1210 cells after 6 h of exposure are shown in Figure 2. The first large peak of the control curve marks the position of G1-phase cells and the second smaller peak marks the position of the G2-phase cells. At a 0.5 μg/ml, MCR produces an increase in the number of G2-phase cells and also an increase in the number of cells in late S-phase. There is a marked decrease in G1-phase cells. This suggests that cells can progress at a normal rate from G1 to S-phase and through early S-phase but that their progression is slowed in late S-phase and G2-phase. At 5 μg/ml the results are similar but the increase in number of S-phase cells occurs throughout S-phase. This suggests that at a high concentration progression through early S-phase is also slowed. MCR has no effect on progression through the mitotic process since it does not cause a rise in mitotic index.

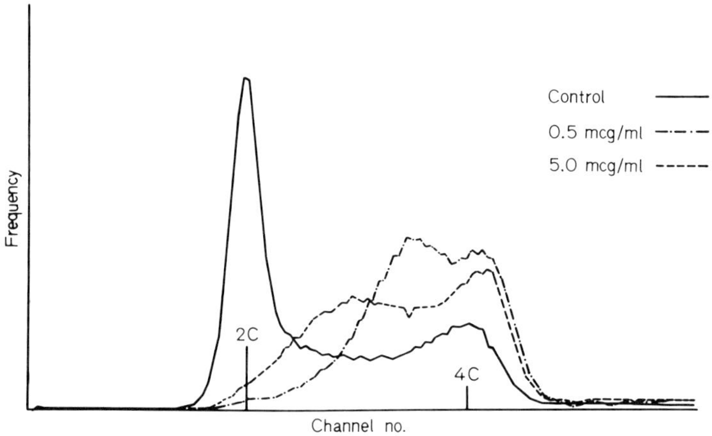

Fig. 2. Effect of 6 h exposure to macromomycin. L1210 cells were exposed to the following concentrations: 5 μg/ml (----), 0.5 μg/ml (-.-.), and control (______). After 6 h, samples were taken for FMF analysis. The 2C and 4C marks along the x-axis represent the positions of diploid and tetraploid cell DNA contents

Conclusion

MCR is an antitumor protein with activity against P388 leukemia, our primary screen and against L1210 leukemia and B16 melanoma two of the tumors in the new NCI tumor panel. It has yet to be tested against the murine or human xenograft colon and breast tumors of the new panel.

Its further development, at NCI, has been hindered by the instability of the bulk drug. Kanigafuchi Laboratories is currently preparing a stabilized formulation of the bulk drug containing maltose. We are awaiting a supply for further testing and drug development.

Tables

Table 1. Source and lot numbers of macromomycin (NSC 170105)

Lot	Source	Date	Purity
MA	Bristol Lab.	Feb. 1973	Crude
MB	Bristol Lab.	May 1973	Crude
NB	Bristol Lab.	Nov. 1974	Crude
NF	Kanegafuchi	Sept. 1975	Purified

Table 2. Response of L1210 leukemia to macromomycin therapy

Lot	Schedule	Optimal dose (mg/kg)	Optimal T/C
NF	Day 1 only	2.0	145
NF	Day 1-9	1.0	148
NF	Day 1, 5, 9	2.0	145

Table 3. Response of P388 leukemia to macromomycin therapy

Lot	Schedule	Optimal dose (mg/kg)	Optimal T/C
MA	Day 1-9	16	159
NB	Day 1-9	8	160
NB	Day 1, 5, 9	15.6	152
NF	Day 1-9	0.5	148
NF	Day 1, 5, 9	2.0	153

Table 4. Response of B16 melanoma to macromomycin therapy

Lot	Schedule	Optimal dose (mg/kg)	Optimal T/C
MA	Day 1-9	40	160
MB	Day 1-9	270	170
NB	Day 1-9	8	146
	Day 1, 5, 9	7.8	153
NF	Day 1-9	0.12	139
	Day 1-20	0.25	145
	Day 1, 5, 9	0.5	151

Table 5. Loss of activity of macromomycin against L1210 leukemia

Lot	Relative age (months)	Schedule	Optimal dose (mg/kg)	Optimal T/C
NF	0	Day 1 only	2.0	145
	6	Day 1 only	4.0	132
	7	Day 1 only	2.0	124
NF	0	Day 1-9	1.0	148
	7	Day 1-9	1.0	93
NF	0	Day 1, 5, 9	2.0	145
	6	Day 1, 5, 9	2.0	133
	7	Day 1, 5, 9	2.0	117
	12	Day 1, 5, 9	2.0	120

Table 6. Loss of activity of macromomycin against P388 leukemia

Lot	Relative age (months)	Schedule	Optimal dose (mg/kg)	Optimal T/C
NF	0	Day 1, 5, 9	1.0	132
	1	Day 1, 5, 9	2.0	153
	6	Day 1, 5, 9	4.0	117

Table 7. Loss of activity of macromomycin against B16 melanoma

Lot	Relative age (months)	Schedule	Optimal dose (mg/kg)	Optimal T/C
NB	0	Day 1–9	8.0	146
	3	Day 1–9	7.8	138
	9	Day 1–9	8.0	98
NF	0	Day 1, 5, 9	0.5	151
	2	Day 1, 5, 9	0.5	144
	6	Day 1, 5, 9	1.0	122

Table 8. Response of Lewis lung carcinoma to macromomycin therapy

(Intratumor injections: daily, day 1–20)

Dose (mg/kg)	Day of death (Postimplant) 13	20	22	24	25	26	27	28	29	31	32	33	34	36	37	39	40	43	48	Survivors[a]
1.0		1		1												1				7
0.5								1		1			1	1					1	5
0.25									1			3					1	2	1	2
0.125						1	1		1		1	1				1	1			3
0	1	1	1		1			1	1	3					1					0

[a] Tumor-free survivors on day 146.

Table 9. Reinoculation[a] of Lewis lung survivors after treatment with macromomycin

Prior dose (mg/kg)	Survivors	Day of death (Post-reinoculation) 14	17	18	19	20	21	22	23	24	25	27	29	30	Survivors[b]
1.0	7					1			1	2	1	2			0
0.25	2							2							0
0	NA	1	4	4	4	4	4	1	7	3	4	2	1	1	0

[a] Reinoculated 117 days after last dosage of drug.
[b] Tumor-free survivors on day 30.

Table 10. Pulmonary metastases after treatment with macromomycin (Intratumor injections: daily, day 1-12)

Whole lung bioassay of treated mice

Dose of prior treatment (mg/kg)	Day of death (Post-bioassay)											Survivors[a]
	24	31	33	34	35	36	38	41	42	49	181	
1.0		1										5/6
0.5											1	5/6
0.25		1										5/6
0.125					1	1	1		1	1		1/6
0	1		1	1		1	1	1				0/6

[a] Tumor-free survivors on day 182.

Table 11. Activity of macromomycin in cell culture

		ED_{50} (µg/ml)	
Cell line	Lot-MB	Lot-MB	Lot-NF
KB	16	4.5	0.01
P388	18	0.22	0.002
L1210	30	2.1	0.038

Table 12. Effect of macromomycin on the growth of L1210 cells in culture

Conc.	Cell density (cells × 10^5/ml)			
(µg/ml)	0 h	3 h	6 h	24 h
0	3.0	3.7	4.5	13.9
0.5	3.0	3.4	3.6	5.7
5	3.0	3.3	3.3	3.7
50	3.0	3.3	3.3	3.3

References

1. Chimura, H., Ishizuka, M., Hamada, M., Hori, S., Kimura, K., Iwanga, J., Takeuchi, T., Umezawa, H.: A new antibiotic, macromomycin, exhibiting antitumor activity and antimicrobial activity. J. Antibiot. (Tokyo) **21**, 44-49 (1968).
2. Kunimoto, T., Hori, M., Umezawa, H: Macromomycin, an inhibitor of membrane function of tumor cells. Cancer Res. **32**, 1251-1256 (1972).
3. Lippman, M. M., Laster, W. R., Abbott, B. J., Venditti, J., Baratta, M.: Antitumor activity of macromomycin B (NSC-170105) against murine leukemias, melanoma and lung carcinoma. Cancer Res. **35**, 939-945 (1975).

New Microbial Secondary Metabolites Under Preclinical Development for Cancer Treatment

H. UMEZAWA

Numerous antitumor antibiotics have been discovered since the author initiated the screening study and reported the isolation of three antitumor antibiotics in 1953. During the last 15 years, there has been great progress in studies of the mechanisms of cytotoxic actions of antitumor compounds. These studies have shown that antitumor compounds bind or react with DNA, inhibit DNA or RNA synthesis, inhibit protein synthesis, interfere with membrane function, or interact with microtubules. The mechanisms of cytotoxic action and of therapeutic action have been studied for some antitumor antibiotics which have exhibited therapeutic effects on certain types of human tumors. It is possible that even those antitumor compounds which inhibit a life function common to normal and malignant cells can exhibit therapeutic action against certain types of human tumors. This therapeutic effect may occur if a tumor has a special characteristic, in a biochemical process or in its structure, in relation to the action of the antitumor compound: e.g., a tumor may lack a system to repair the damage caused by an antitumor compound; the antitumor compound may be distributed in a higher concentration in the tumor than in other tissues; the tumor may have a stronger activity to activate (or a weaker activity to inactivate) an antitumor compound than other tissues. Therefore, antitumor antibiotics which showed unique actions have been selected for clinical studies.

Besides development of new types of antitumor antibiotics for cancer treatment, a great effort is being spent in development of more useful derivatives or analogs of effective antitumor drugs.

The microbial products which have no obvious function in the growth of microbial cells are called "microbial secondary metabolites." Studies on antibiotics and enzyme inhibitors of small molecular size have revealed a great ability of microorganisms to produce various bioactive compounds which have widely varying structures. At present, experimental data which indicate the involvement of plasmids in biosyntheses of many microbial secondary metabolites are increasing. It is suggested that mutations occur in a natural environment and that various genetic units thus produced, cause production of compounds of various structures. Evolution and transfer of genetic materials involved in production of secondary metabolites generally do not cause cell death but cause production of different compounds. Therefore, if a proper and exact screening method is devised, then there is a great possibility of finding a compound which has the purposed activity. In fact, the author has found products which enhance cellular immune response and which seem to be useful in the treatment of cancer.

In this paper, the author will report on his studies of effective antitumor antibiotics and their derivatives or analogs, and the microbial products enhancing immune response under preclinical development.

Selection of Antitumor Antibiotics with Potential Utility

Establishing the selection procedure for antitumor antibiotics worth clinical study is an urgent problem for the development of effective cancer chemotherapeutic agents. Among 30 antitumor antibiotics found by the author, phleomycin was selected for preclinical study because of its unusually high therapeutic index against Ehrlich carcinoma. In the study of antibiotics of a similar type, bleomycin (which had much lower renal toxicity than phleomycin) was found. The therapeutic effect of bleomycin on a squamous cell carcinoma of the penis and its distribution at a high concentration in skin promoted further clinical studies [2].

The chemical structure and the behavior of bleomycin in vivo are shown in Fig. 1 and 2 [16]. Bleomycin binds with cupric ion and forms an equimolar bleomycin-copper complex. The amino group of the α-aminocarboxamide moiety, the pyrimidine chromophore, the imidazole group and the carbamoyl group are copper ligands of bleomycin molecule. The α-aminocarboxamide group and the carbamoyl group have been shown to be involved in binding or reaction with DNA. The DNA strand scission caused by bleomycin is inhibited by cupric ions but the bleomycin-copper complex does not cause DNA strand scission. Bleomycin-copper complex is resistant to bleomycin hydrolase, which hydrolyzes the carboxamide group of copper-free bleomycin. Part or all of injected bleomycin binds with the cupric ion in blood. After penetration into cells, the cupric ion of the bleomycin-copper complex is reduced by a sulfhydryl compound in cells and transferred to a cellular protein which has an ability to bind with cuprous ion. Copper-free bleomycin, thus formed in cells, is acted upon by bleomycin hydrolase. Copper-free bleomycin, which was not inactivated by bleomycin hydrolase, reaches the nucleus and inhibits growth of cells by causing strand scission of DNA, inhibiting DNA ligase, causing DNA-membrane breakage, inhibiting cell division etc. Free-radical producing or reducing agents (sulfhydryl compounds, ascorbic acid, hydrogen peroxide etc.) enhance the action of bleomycin on DNA in the presence of ferrous ion or oxygen, or enhance the inactivation of bleomycin by ferrous ion and oxygen. It is not certain whether these free-radical producing or reducing agents actually enhance bleomycin action in cells or inactivate bleomycin in cells. The behavior of bleomycin in vivo indicates that the cells which contain only small amounts of bleomycin hydrolase should be more sensitive to bleomycin than other cells. The therapeutic effect of bleomycin on squamous cell carcinoma has been shown to be due to a low content of this enzyme and a high distribution of the antibiotic in this tumor. It suggests that a characteristic distribution in various organs or tissues and knowledge of the metabolism of an antitumor antibiotic may be useful information to predict a type of tumor sensitive to treatment with this antibiotic. Bleomycin is effective on squamous cell carcinoma induced by methylcholanthrene, but not on sarcoma induced by the same agent in mouse skin. It conforms with the therapeutic effect of bleomycin on human squamous cell carcinoma.

Antitumor compounds worth clinical study may be selected on the basis of their characteristic actions or action mechanisms. Macromomycin [3] was found to bind to animal cells and inhibit their growth [6]. Its cytotoxic effect was eliminated by treatment of cells with trypsin, after exposure to macromomycin. Moreover, treatment of Ehrlich carcinoma or L1210 leukemia with this macromolecular antibiotic produced resistance to the second inoculation of the same tumor cells. Based on these interesting actions, macromomycin was selected for preclinical study. The properties and antitumor actions of macromomycin are described by Watanabe in this book in detail.

In a screening study, we found a new benzodiazepine antibiotic named neothramycin [15] (Fig. 3). Compared with other known benzodiazepine antibiotics (e.g., anthramycin, tomaymycin, sibiromycin and dextrocrysin), neothramycin has much lower toxicity: LD_{50};

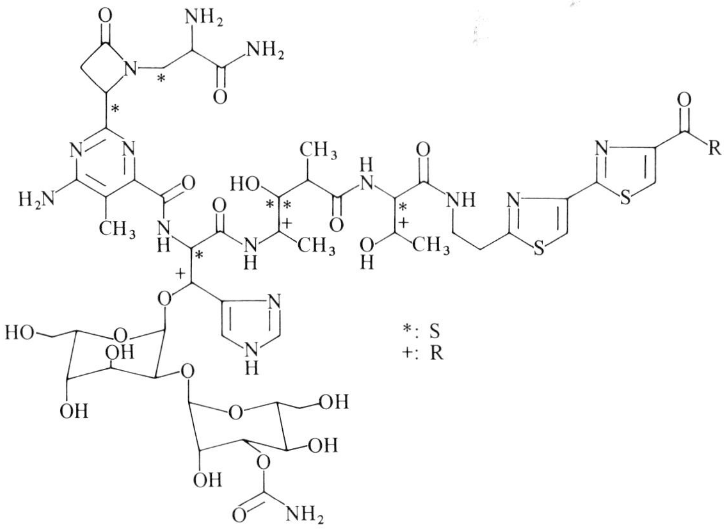

A1: R=NH–$(CH_2)_3$–SO–CH_3

Demethyl–A2: R=NH–$(CH_2)_3$–S–CH_3

A2: R=NH–$(CH_2)_3$–$S^{+}(CH_3)_2$

A2′–a: R=NH–$(CH_2)_4$–NH_2

A2′–b: R=NH–$(CH_2)_3$–NH_2

A2′–c: R=NH–$(CH_2)_2$–

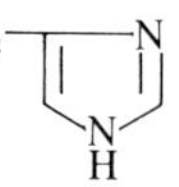

A5: R=NH–$(CH_2)_3$–NH–$(CH_2)_4$–NH_2

A6: R=NH–$(CH_2)_3$–NH–$(CH_2)_4$–NH–$(CH_2)_3$–NH_2

B1′: R=NH_2

B2: R=NH–$(CH_2)_4$–NH–C(=NH)–NH_2

B4: R=NH–$(CH_2)_4$–NH–C(=NH)–NH–$(CH_2)_4$–NH–C(=NH)–NH_2

Bleomycinic acid: R=OH

Fig. 1. Structures of bleomycins produced in media containing natural nitrogen sources

mice, 18–20 mg/kg (male), 20–30 mg/kg (female) i.v. and i.p., 33 mg/kg (male) s.c.; rats, 15.5 mg/kg i.v., 14.0 mg/kg i.p., 118 mg/kg oral. The other new benzodiazepine antibiotic, N-methylanthramycin, in which the amino group of the carboxamide moiety of anthramycin is methylated, showed a much stronger toxicity than neothramycin: 1 mg/kg caused death of mice. Neothramycin inhibited L1210 moderately, Yoshida rat sarcoma strongly, and sarcoma 180 weakly. It showed almost no inhibition of Ehrlich carcinoma. Moreover, a

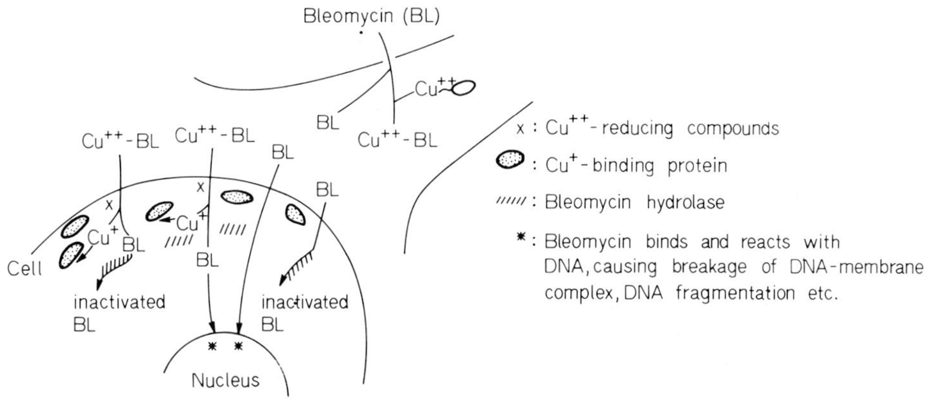

Fig. 2. Behavior of bleomycin in vivo

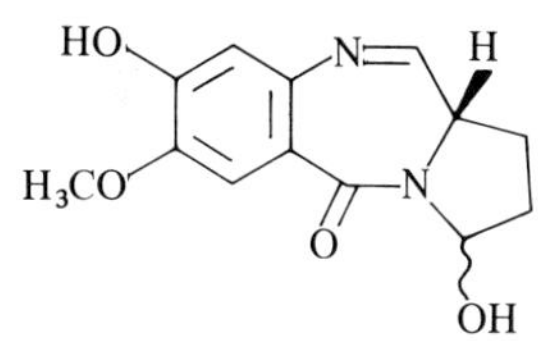

Fig. 3. Structure of neothramycin

relatively strong effect was found by Sato (Sasaki Institute, Tokyo) on various rat hepatomas. This antitumor spectrum was different from other antitumor antibiotics found by the author. Therefore, on the basis of this spectrum and its strong effect on rat hepatomas, neothramycin was thought to be worth clinical study.

A high therapeutic index against some experimental tumors, a strong action against experimental animal tumors which are resistant to treatment with most antitumor compounds, an unusual antitumor spectrum, a characteristic unusual action, and a characteristic distribution among various organs have been utilized to select antitumor antibiotics worth clinical examination. An antitumor compound which shows therapeutic effect with a high therapeutic index on a certain type of chemically induced tumor or a human tumor in nude mice may exhibit therapeutic effect on a similar type of human tumors.

Development of More Useful Derivatives and Analogs of Effective Antitumor Antibiotic Drugs

The study of analogs or derivatives of antitumor antibiotics which have shown a strong therapeutic effect in cancer treatment will provide more effective and more useful therapeutic agents. As described in this book in detail by Matsuda et al., various bleomycins, different from one another in the terminal amine moiety, have been prepared by fermentation or by chemical derivation of bleomycinic acid [16]. They are different from one another in the degree of pulmonary and renal toxicity, and those which have lower pulmonary toxicity have been selected for the clinical study. The terminal amine moiety (Fig. 1) is not involved in DNA strand scission, but it might be involved in the mechanism of penetration into cells. Therefore, it may also be possible to find new bleomycins which have a wider antitumor spectrum. Modification of the α-aminocarboxamide moiety may give other derivatives which are resistant to bleomycin hydrolase and which have different antitumor spectra.

Adriamycin, discovered by Arcamone et al., has been shown to exhibit a strong therapeutic effect on various types of cancer. The study of its analogs and derivatives will determine the compounds which have lower cardiac toxicity and are more useful in cancer treatment. Therefore, with my colleagues, I undertook the isolation of anthracycline pigments from the strains which had been found in the screening study of antitumor antibiotics in my laboratories. In this study, one of them, aclacinomycin A [8], was selected for clinical study on the basis of its low cardiac toxicity and its high distribution in lung and spleen of mice.

Aclacinomycin A showed lower activity than adriamycin in inhibition of L1210 leukemia and P388 mouse leukemia. It inhibited a mouse mammary carcinoma. In a test using hamsters, it showed about 16 times lower cardiac toxicity than adriamycin. As shown in Fig. 4, after i.v. injection, aclacinomycin was found to be distributed at high concentrations in lung and spleen. Moreover, in lung and spleen, aclacinomycin A was not converted into its inactive metabolites, i.e., in these organs aclacinomycin A remained as itself or as glycosidic metabolites.

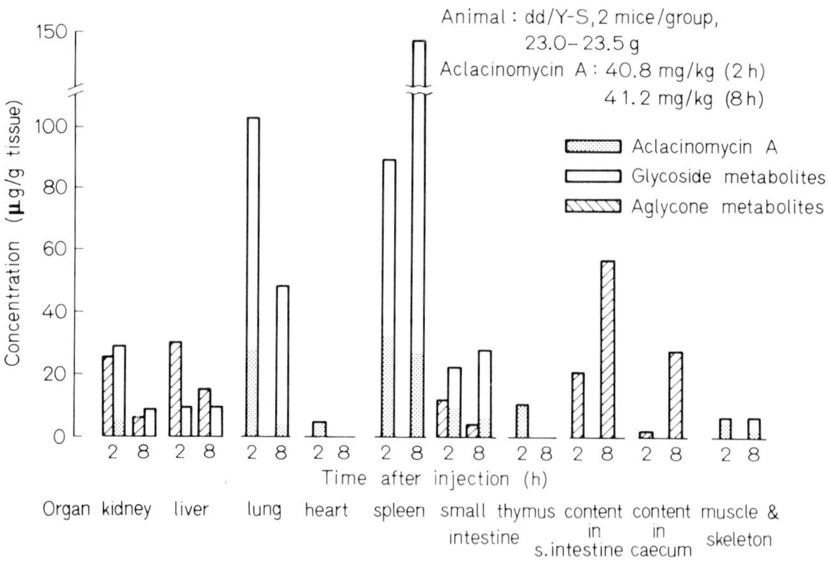

Fig. 4. Concentrations of [³H]-aclacinomycin A and its metabolites in various organs of mice 2–8 h after i.v. injection

As shown in Fig. 5, aclacinomycin A undergoes various metabolic reactions in vivo: The L-cinerulose moiety is reduced to L-amicetose or L-rhodinose to give MA144M1 or MA144N1; α-L-cinerulosyl-2-deoxy-L-fucose moiety splits to give 1-deoxypyrromycin; the sugar part is removed by hydrolysis to give aklavinone, or removed by reductive deglycosidation to give 7-deoxyaklavinone or 7,7'-bis(7-deoxyaklavinone), designated MA144E1; aklavinone is further dehydrated to bisanhydroaklavinone. The enzyme which catalyzes the reductive

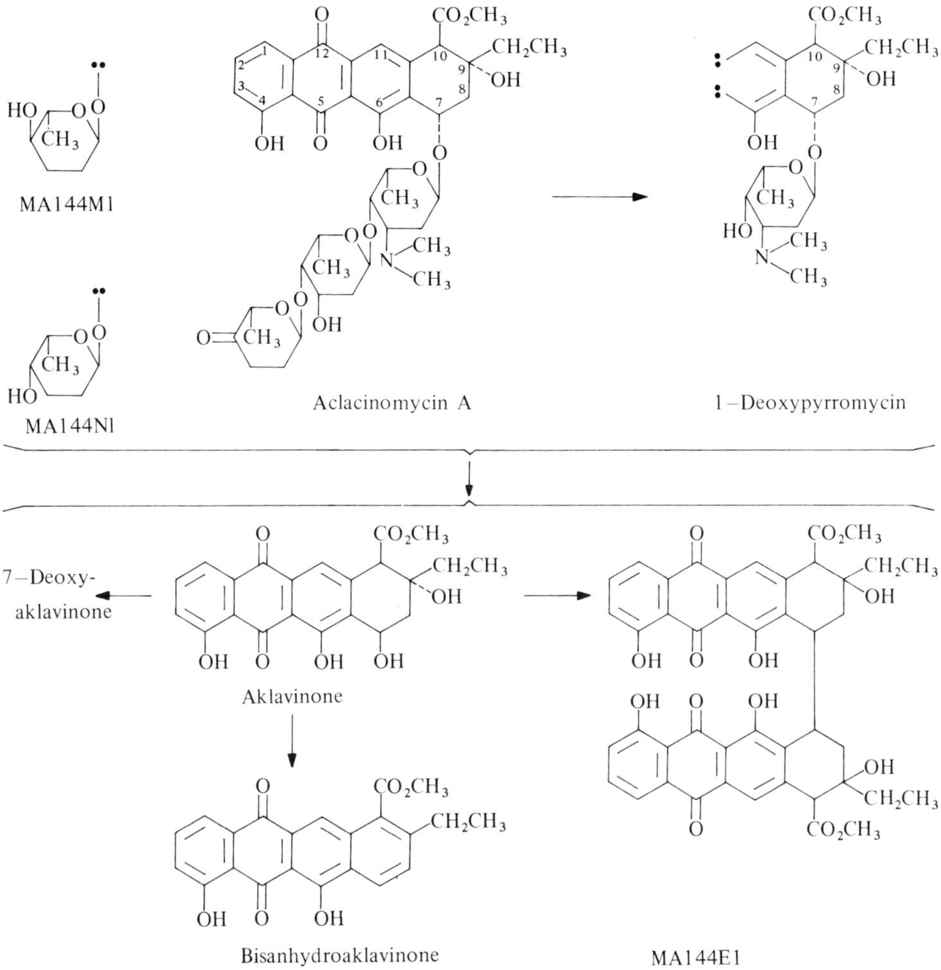

Fig. 5. Metabolism of aclacinomycin A

deglycosidation has been confirmed by Oki et. al. [9] to be identical with microsomal NADPH-cytochrome C reductase. Among these metabolites, those which lack the sugar moiety show neither antitumor nor cytotoxic action. The metabolites containing sugar moeties have the antitumor activity.

After i.v. injection of 10 mg/kg, aclacinomycin A was excreted into urine in both sugar-containing and sugar-lacking forms, as shown in Fig. 6. The results suggest that active glycosidic forms, especially MA144N1, remain for a fairly long period in the body. The metabolite MA144N1 may be worth further examination. The distribution of radioactivity after i.v. or oral administration of [^{14}C]-aclacinomycin A (prepared by fermentation in a medium containing $^{14}CH_3$-methionine and 1-[^{14}C]-propionic acid) indicated that aclacinomycin A is orally well absorbed and that the distribution pattern among various organs is similar after i.v. and oral administration. After i.v. injection or oral administration, high concentrations of aclacinomycin and glycosidic metabolites are observed in lung and spleen.

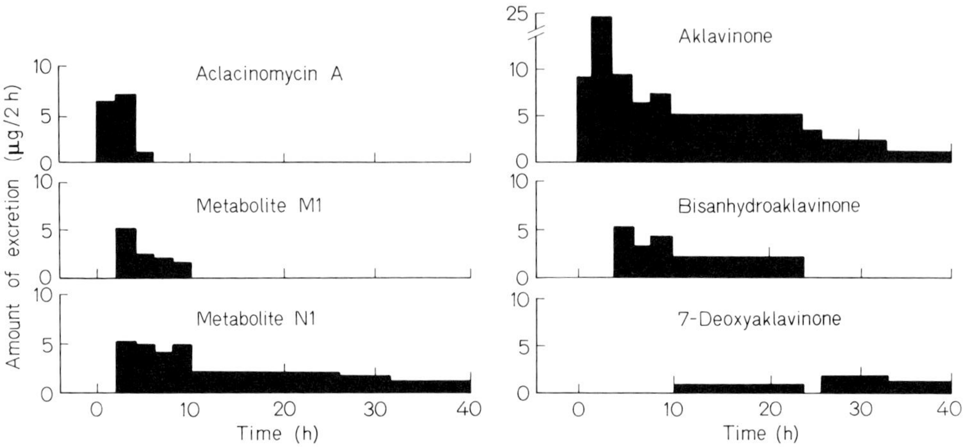

Fig. 6. Excretion of aclacinomycin A and metabolites in urine after i.v. injection of 10 mg aclacinomycin A/kg rabbit

Aclacinomycins A and B are yellow colored pigments. Both yellow and red pigments were produced by the strain producing aclacinomycins. Therefore, we undertook a detailed study of yellow and red pigments produced by this strain (Table 1).

Red pigments contained the 1-hydroxyl group and (probably due to the two copper ligands (1-OH and 12=0; 4-OH and 5=0) in the molecule) were precipitated by addition of cupric ion and thus separated from yellow pigments. Thereafter, each pigment was purified by silica gel chromatography. Thus, the strain producing aclacinomycins was found to produce more than 19 anthracycline compounds [10]. As shown in Table 1, all yellow anthracycline glycosides contained the same chromophore as aclacinomycin A. There were different in the sugar moiety: the sugar moiety of aclacinomycin A was 4-[4-(α-L-cinerulosyl)-α-2-deoxy-L-fucosyl]-rhodosamine; that of MA144G1 was 4-[4-(α-D-cinerulosyl)-α-2-deoxy-L-fucosyl]-rhodosamine; that of MA144M1 was 4-[4-(α-L-amicetosyl)-α-2-deoxy-L-fucosyl]-rhodosamine; that of MA144N1 was 4-[4-(α-L-rhodinosyl)-α-2-deoxy-L-fucosyl]-rhodosamine; that of MA144S1 was 4-(α-2-deoxy-L-fucosyl)-rhodosàmine; that of 1-deoxypyrromycin was rhodosamine. Among these yellow pigments containing sugar moieties, MA144M1, MA144N1 and 1-deoxypyrromycin have been found in metabolites of aclacinomycin A. Therefore, these anthracycline glycosides may be produced by reduction or hydrolysis of the sugar moiety of aclacinomycin A. In aclacinomycin B, L-cinerulose is linked to 2-deoxy-L-fucose through two bridges. N-Monodemethyl aclacinomycin A was also isolated. Aklavinone, 7-deoxyaklavinone, bisanhydroaklavinone and 7,7'-bis (7-deoxy-aklavinone) (MA144E1) which have been found as metabolites of aclacinomycin A (Fig. 5) were also found in cultured broths. These anthracycline compounds lack a sugar moiety and therefore, may be produced during fermentation by hydrolysis or by reductive deglycosidation of anthracycline glycosides.

All red pigments containing sugar moieties contained the same aglycone as cinerubin. The following glycosidic pigments have been isolated: cinerubin A (1-hydroxyaclacinomycin A), cinerubin B (1-hydroxyaclacinomycin B), 1-hydroxy-MA144M1, 1-hydroxy-MA144S1 and pyrromycin. Also, anthracycline compounds lacking a sugar moiety, i.e., 7-deoxy-ε-pyrromycinone and ε-pyrromycinone have been isolated from cultured broths (Table 2).

As shown in Table 2, the following anthracycline glycosides, containing the same aglycone as aclacinomycin A, have been isolated from cultured broths of mutants of the aclacinomycin-producing strain: the sugar moiety of MA144U1 was (2-deoxy-L-fucosyl-2-deoxy-L-fucosyl)-

Table 1. Anthracycline compounds produced by the aclacinomycin-producing strain MA144M1 (*Streptomyces galilaeus*)

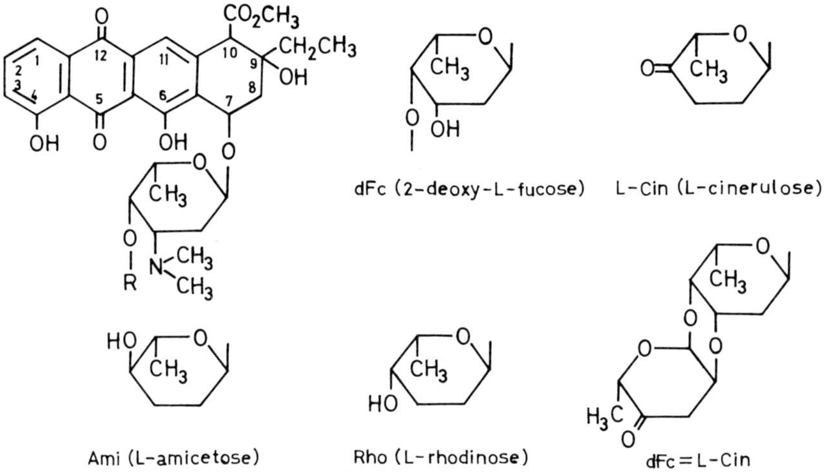

Components	Structure	Rf value[a]
A1	Aclacinomycin A: R = dFc-L-Cin	0.50
B1	Aclacinomycin B: R = dFc-L-Cin	0.77
L1	N-monodemethylaclacinomycin A	0.31
G1	MA144G1: R = dFc-D-Cin	0.38
M1	MA144M1: R = dFc-Ami	0.25
N1	MA144N1: R = dFc-Rho	0.21
S1	MA144S1: R = dFc	0.14
T1	1-Deoxypyrromycin: R = H	0.03
F	Bisanhydroaklavinone (7=8, 9=10)	0.95
D1	Aklavinone (7-OH)	0.86
C1	7-Deoxyaklavinone	0.90
E1	MA144E1[b]	0.82
A2	1-Hydroxyaclacinomycin A[c]	0.50
B2	1-Hydroxyaclacinomycin B[d]	0.77
M2	1-Hydroxy-MA144M1	0.25
S2	1-Hydroxy-MA144S1	0.14
T2	Pyrromycin	0.03
C2	7-Deoxypyrromycinone[e]	0.90
D2	ε-Pyrromycinone	0.86

[a] Rf value: Thin-layer chromatography on silica gel using chloroform-methanol (20:1 v/v).
[b] 7,7'-*bis* (7-deoxyaklavinone).
[c] Cinerubin A.
[d] Cinerubin B.
[e] ζ-Pyrromycinone (1-hydroxy-7-deoxyaklavinone).

rhodosamine; that of MA144U5 was (L-cinerulosyl-2-deoxy-L-fucosyl)-2-deoxy-L-fucose; that of MA144U6 was (L-rhodinosyl-L-rhodinosyl)-2-deoxyfucose; that of MA144U8 was L-rhodinosyl-2-deoxy-L-fucose.

Activities of anthracycline glycosides, containing the same aglycone as aclacinomycin A, to inhibit L1210 leukemia are shown in Table 2. N-Monodemethyl aclacinomycin A had almost no activity and those (U5, U6, U8) which had no dimethylamino group showed no activity. All anthracycline glycosides containing rhodosamine showed the activity.

Table 2. Antitumor activities of anthracycline glycosides, produced by the strain MA144M1 and its mutants, against L1210 leukemia

Compounds	Sugar moiety	ILS (%)					
		16[a]	8[a]	4[a]	2[a]	1[a]	0.5[a]
Aclacinomycin A	RA-DF-LCin	Toxic	−2	103	97	56	22
Aclacinomycin B	RA-DF-LCin	Toxic	−50	−15	75	86	42
N-monodemethyl-aclacinomycin A	mdRA-DF-LCin	—	10	14	−10	0	—
MA144G1	RA-DF-DCin	—	—	70	20	−4	−7
MA144M1	RA-DF-Ami	Toxic	−35	85	62	35	4
MA144S1	RA-DF	Toxic	84	113	33	14	0
1-Deoxypyrromycin	RA	48	33	13	−2	0	0
MA144U1[b]	RA-DF-DF	Toxic	82	48	52	39	20
MA144U5[b]	DF-DF-LCin				No effect		
MA144U6[b]	DF-Rho-Rho				No effect		
MA144U8[b]	DF-Rho				No effect		
1-Hydroxy MA144M1	Ra-DF-Ami	—	Toxic	Toxic	73	55	45
1-Hydroxy MA144N1	RA-DF-Rho	—	Toxic	Toxic	62	71	40

[a] mg/kg/da. [b] products of mutants.
L1210: 10^5 cells/mouse, ip-ip, CDF_1 mice (2-4 mice/group), treatment on day 0-9.
RA: Rhodosamine DF: 2-Deoxy-L-focose Cin: Cinerulose Ami: Amicetose
Rho: Rhodinose mdRA: monodemethyl rhosamine

We also studied orange-red pigments produced by a daunomycin-producing strain which had been isolated by us and designated as the strain ME130-A4. In this study, we isolated 14 anthracycline pigments and the structures of 12 pigments were determined. Five of them were identified to be known compounds i.e., daunomycin, dihydrodaunomycin, N-acetyldaunomycin, 7-deoxydihydro-daunomycinone and ε-rhodomycinone. The other one was suggested to be the 7-epimer of 7-deoxydihydrodaunomycinone. The other six were new daunomycin analogues [5]. Among them, two were determined to be N-formyldaunomycin and N-formyldihydrodaunomycin [5]. The other four were named baumycins A1, A2, B1 and B2 [5] and their structures were determined as shown in Fig. 7 [14]. A1 and A2, and also B1 and B2, were stereoisomers to each other, respectively. Among them, baumycin A1 showed a stronger activity than daunomycin in inhibiting L1210 leukemia. Baumycins A1 and A2 may be interesting daunomycin analogs. We are also studying these types of derivatives of adriamycin and daunomycin.

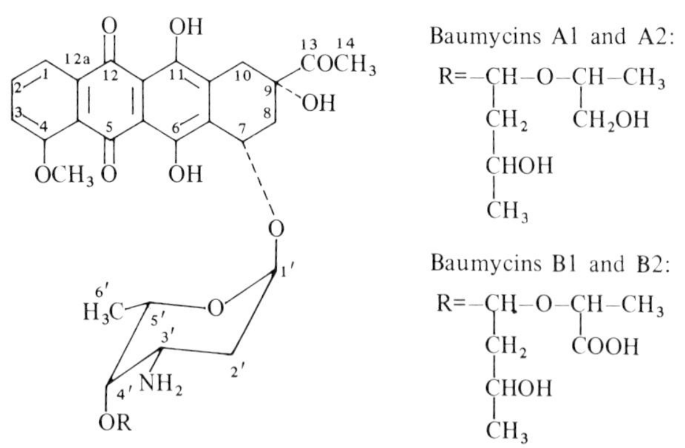

Fig. 7. Structures of baumycins A1, A2, B1, B2 (A1 and A2 as well as B1 and B2 are stereoisomers in R)

Microbial Products Enhancing Immune Response

As described, production of various compounds by microorganisms is due to the presence of a great variety of genetic structures in plasmids and chromosomes of microorganisms. Therefore, it is rational to search not only for antitumor compounds but also for compounds which enhance immune resistance to cancer.

We found that administration of very low doses of coriolin group antibiotics and their derivatives increased the number of antibody-forming cells [4]. Coriolins A and C, produced by a mushroom, and diketocoriolin B (a derivative of coriolin B [13]) (Fig. 8) prolonged the survival period of mice inoculated with L1210 mouse leukemia. The latter was confirmed to inhibit Na-K-ATPase [7]. The i.p. injection of 0.01–31.2 μg diketocoriolin B per mouse significantly increased the number of antibody-forming cells. Inhibition of Na-K-ATPase suggests that this compound might bind with the enzyme on the surface of cells involved in immunity.

Aoyagi and the author [1] found that, as shown in Fig. 9, intact animal cells liberated N-terminal amino acids (dipeptide or tripeptide) from synthetic peptides but the enzymes involved in these hydrolyses were not released into the medium. This indicates that these aminopeptidases appear on the cell surface and hydrolyze the substrates in the medium.

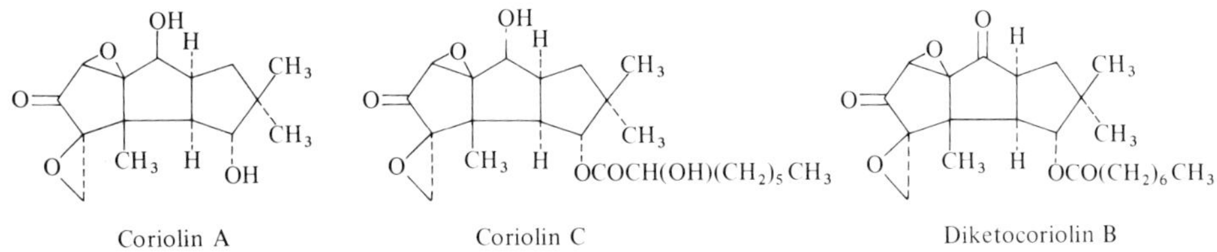

Fig. 8. Structures of coriolins

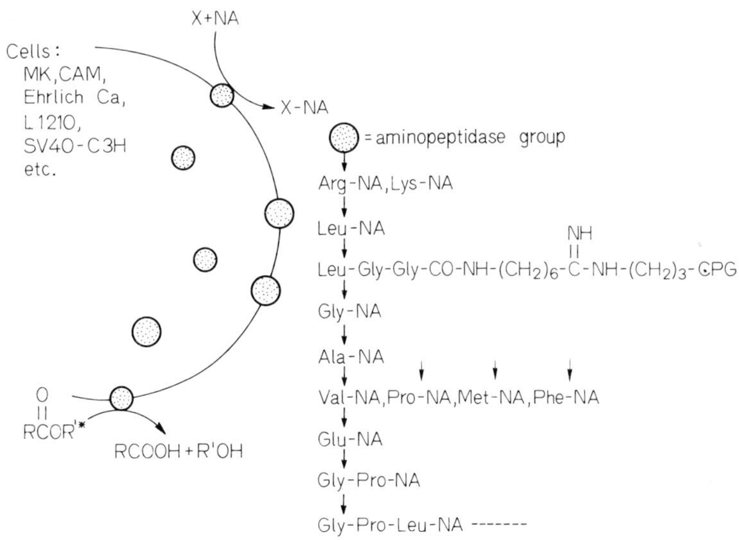

Fig. 9. Hydrolysis of N-terminal amino acids, dipeptides or tripeptides by aminopeptidases on surface of animal cells

*p-nitrophenylacetate.

Therefore, the author proposed that inhibitors of such enzymes might bind to the surface of cells involved in immunity and increase or decrease the activity of such cells. In fact bestatin (Fig. 10), which inhibited aminopeptidase B and leucine aminopeptidase, increased delayed-type hypersensitivity [18]. The i.p. injection of 1.0–100 μg/mouse at the time of immunization, that is, at the time of injection of sheep red-blood cells into the footpad, enhanced the reaction elicited by a second injection of cells into the footpad of the other side (Table 3). The strongest effect was shown by 0.1–100 μg/mouse. The i.p. injection of bestatin at the time of eliciting the reaction did not show any influence. A large dose such as 1000 μg bestatin per mouse at the time of immunization, or 24 h before or after immunization, increased the number of antibody-forming cells, but the low doses which exhibited great activity in enhancing delayed-type hypersensitivity did not increase the number of antibody-forming cells. Delayed-type hypersensitivity, enhanced by bestatin, is specific to the antigen. Bestatin produced no effect when mice were immunized by sheep red blood cells and human red blood cells were injected or vice versa.

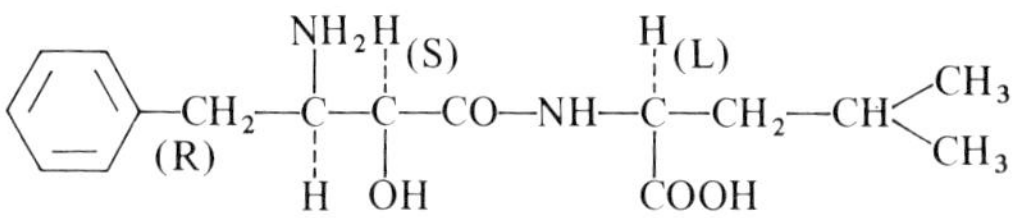

Fig. 10. Structure of bestatin

Table 3. Enhancement of delayed-type hypersensitivity by bestatin

Immunized with	Increased thickness of footpad (× 0.1 mm)
10^8 SRBC, s.c.	4.5 ± 0.6 (± S.E.)
10^8 SRBC bestatin, 1mg, i.p.	6.0 ± 1.0
10^8 SRBC bestatin, 100μg, i.p.	9.2 ± 1.2
10^8 SRBC bestatin, 10μg, i.p.	10.5 ± 1.9
10^8 SRBC bestatin, 1μg, i.p.	7.4 ± 1.3

Sheep red blood cells (10^8) were s.c. injected into the right footpad of CDF_1 mice (male, 8 weeks old), and the indicated doses of bestatin were i.p. injected 4 days after, 10^8 cells were subcutaneously injected to the left footpad and the reaction was elicited; 24 h after, the width of left leg was measured.

Bestatin, (2S,3R)-3-amino-2-hydroxy-4-phenylbutanoyl-L-leucine [17, 12], which is produced by *Streptomyces olivoreticuli*, strongly inhibits aminopeptidase B (K_i = 6.0 x 10^{-8} *M*) and leucine aminopeptidase (K_i = 2.0 x 10^{-8} *M*). The type of inhibition is competitive with substrates such as L-arginine β-naphthylamide, for the former, and L-leucine β-naphthylamide for the latter. It does not inhibit aminopeptidase A and endopeptidases. The 2S-configuration of the 3-amino-2-hydroxy-3-phenylbutanoyl moiety in bestatin is the absolute structural requirement for activity and all stereoisomers with the 2R-configuration have little or no activity [11]. The stereoisomers of the 2S-configuration inhibited aminopeptidase B or leucine aminopeptidase and the i.p. injection of 0.1 μg enhanced delayed-type hypersensitivity. However, isomers of 2R-configuration only slighly inhibited the enzymes, and doeses of 100 μg or more were required to enhance delayed-type hypersensitivity. This suggests that enhancement of delayed-type hypersensitivity is due to binding of bestatin with aminopeptidases on the cellular surface of immune cells.

As found by Ishizuka and Takeuchi in my institute, if Ehrlich carcinoma cells are inoculated into the footpad of mice, tumor growth in this location is resistant to treatment with antitumor compounds such as bleomycin, mitomycin C, adriamycin etc. Using this experimental system, the effects of bestatin on cancer immunity have been studied. When 10^6 Erhlich carcinoma cells were mixed with 2 μg bestatin and inoculated subcutaneously into the footpad, tumor growth occurred at the site of inoculation but the resistance was produced to a second inoculation of the same tumor cells into the opposite footpad.

10^6 Ehrlich carcinoma cells were inoculated into the footpad and treatment with bleomycin alone, bestatin alone or the combination was started 24 h later and continued for 6 days. Tumor size was measured 30 days after the inoculation. Treatment with 100 μg bleomycin alone per mouse or 1–1000 μg bestatin alone per mouse showed no inhibition of tumor growth, but combination treatment of bleomycin with 1–100 μg bestatin showed strong inhibition (Table 4). A large dose of bestatin such as 1000 μg/mouse daily did not enhance the bleomycin effect. In the other experiment, 10^6 cells were inoculated into the right footpad and treatment was started 24 h later and continued for 6 days. On the day after the last treatment, 10^6 cells were inoculated into the left footpad. Tumors produced by the first inoculation were measured on the 14th day after the first inoculation and tumors produced by the second inoculation were measured on the 14th day after the second inoculation. It was shown that bestatin (10 μg/mouse) along produced resistance to the second inoculation and the combination treatment of bleomycin (100 μg/mouse) with bestatin (10 μg/mouse) produced complete resistance to the second inoculation.

Table 4. Effect of bestatin on bleomycin treatment of Ehrlich carcinoma inoculated into footpad

	Bestatin with			
	None		BLM (100 μg/mouse)	
Bestatin (μg/mouse)	Tumor size (× 0.1 mm)	Inh.%	Tumor size (× 0.1 mm)	Inh. %
0	48.9	0	44.9	8
1000	59.3	0	46.1	6
100	73.5	0	0	100
10	49.6	0	0	100
1	49.4	0	22.6	78

10^6 Ehrlich carcinoma cells were inoculated s.c. into footpad of dd/Y mice and 1 day after treatment with bleomycin alone, bestatin alone or with both was started. 100 μg bleomycin/mouse or indicated doses of bestatin were injected i.p. daily for 6 days. The size of tumor was measured 30 days after the inoculation.

Bestatin increases also effects of other antitumor agents. When 10^6 Ehrlich carcinoma cells were inoculated into the footpad, i.p. injection of 20 μg adriamycin per mouse on day 1, 3 and 5 of the inoculation did not show a significant inhibition, but addition of bestatin treatment (10 μg or 100 μg orally, daily for 10 days) showed strong inhibition. The tumor growth was suppressed and there was almost no increase of the size of the tumor after day 14 of the inoculation. When 10^6 L1210 cells were inoculated into the footpad and 20 μg adriamycin per mouse was injected i.p. on day 1, 2, and 3 of the inoculation, all mice died and the mean survival was 15.2 days. Addition of bestatin, 10 μg orally for 10 days, to the adriamycin treatment prolonged the survival period. The mean survival was longer than 20.7 days and two out of six rats survived.

The data indicate that destruction of cells by an anticancer agent may provide antigen, and that bestatin may promote production of immune resistance.

Treatment with bestatin alone exhibited a strong inhibition against Gardner lymphosarcoma and IMC-carcinoma. As shown in Table 5, 10^5 cells of Gardner lymphosarcoma, obtained from the ascites form, were s.c. inoculated into C3H/He mice and the weight of each tumor

Table 5. Effect of bestatin on Gardner lymphosarcoma

Bestatin µg/mouse/day	Tumor weight on day 30, mg, mean (range)	% inhibition
0	1375.3 (570–2174)	—
10	303.3 (105–561)	77.9
100	551.8 (93–947)	59.9

Cells were collected from the ascites form, and washed with physiologic saline and 10^5 cells were s.c. inoculated into the inguinal area of C3H/He mice. 8 mice for each dose. Bestatin was orally administered daily on day 1–5.

was measured on day 30. Oral administration of 10 µg or 100 µg bestatin/mouse/day (eight mice for each dose group), for 5 days on day 1–5, showed a strong inhibition: 77.9% inhibition by 10 µg/mouse/day; 59.9% inhibition by 100 µg/mouse/day, although, as shown in Table 5, the degree of inhibition fluctuated in each mouse of each dose group: 52%–92% inhibition in the 10 µg/mouse/day group; 31%–93% inhibition in the 100 µg/mouse/day group.

IMC-Carcinoma is the carcinoma which appeared spontaneously in CDF_1 mice in my laboratories. Intraperitoneal inoculation of 10^6 cells of this ascites tumor cells caused death of mice after 8–10 days. When the cells are subcutaneously inoculated, the subcutaneous tumor continues growing and the weight of tumor increases to more than 10 g. As shown in Table 6, treatment with 1, 10 or 100 µg bestatin/mouse/day orally for 5 days on day 1–5, on day 8–12, or on day 14–18, showed strong inhibition. The size of tumor in the control on day 30 of the inoculation was relatively even (13.3–7.0 g in eight mice), but as shown in Table 6, the size of tumor of treated groups fluctuated more. It should be emphasized that even when the treatment was started from day 8 or day 14 of the inoculation, a marked inhibition occurred. A stronger inhibition was observed in the treatment on day 8–14 than in the treatment on day 1–5. This suggests that the tumor on day 8–12 might provide more useful antigens than the tumor on day 1–5 of the inoculation. Although bestatin alone was effective on IMC-carcinoma, the effect was suppression of the rate of growth of tumors. We thought that bestatin treatment combined with tumor antigens might cause shrinking of existing tumors.

Table 6. Effect of bestatin on IMC-carcinoma

Bestatin µg/mouse/day	Treatment, days and % mean inhibition (range)			
	-7–-1	1–5	8–12	14–18
1	—	43.1 (52–27)	48.7 (89–0)	55.0 (76–3)
10	—	41.7 (75–26)	82.0 (89–76)	71.0 (84–58)
100	42.3 (91–0)	36.3 (63–0)	71.6 (82–61)	71.3 (81–62)

Bestatin was orally administered: −7 means daily for 7 days before inoculation of the tumor cells; 1–5 means daily for 5 days on day 1–5 of the inoculation. 10^6 tumor cells collected from the ascites form were washed with saline and inoculated on day 0. Tumors were weighed on day 30.

Mean weight of tumors in untreated mice was 10.31 ± 0.74 g (13.3–7.0 g).

As reviewed by Watanabe et al. in this book in detail, treatment with macromomycin produces the resistance to a second inoculation of the same tumor cells. However, we confirmed that macromomycin neither enhanced delayed-type hypersensitivity nor increased the number of antibody-forming cells. It seems that macromomycin does not affect the immune system but may affect tumor cells and provide tumor antigens to the immune system. Therefore, we examined the effect of bestatin in combination on the inoculation of macromomycin-treated IMC-carcinoma cells. 10^6 cells of IMC-carcinoma were inoculated s.c. into the inguinal area of CDF_1 mice. On day 21, 10^7 cells, mixed with 10 μg macromomycin, were injected s.c. into the opposite inguinal area and, at the same time, bestatin treatment (10 μg/mouse/day) was started and continued daily up to day 40 of the first cell inoculation. Tumors, which had been found by other experimenters to have grown up to about 6 g on day 21, increased their size up to about day 25–30 and thereafter shrunk gradually with slight necrosis. On day 40, the mice gained the weight and looked completely healthy except for a small tumor in the inoculated place. Without bestatin treatment, after inoculation of the mixture of the tumor cells with macromomycin, severe necrosis and bleeding occurred in the tumor and on day 40 mice were in a state of severe cachexia. In the control, the tumor continued to grow and mice with severe cachexia died 35–40 days after the inoculation.

The results suggest that combination of a cell immunity-enhancing agent with tumor antigens may be useful in treatment of cancer.

As already shown (Fig. 9), aminopeptidase A appears on the cell surface. Esterase also appears on the cell surface. An inhibitor of aminopeptidase A increased the number of antibody-forming cells. An inhibitor of esterase suppressed delayed-type hypersensitivity and decreased the number of antibody-forming cells. Experimental data have indicated that compounds which bind to enzymes on the surface of animal cells increase or decrease immune response. We have also found that an inhibitor of the other cellular surface enzyme also enhances cancer immunity.

Summary

Limitless numbers of various genetic structures have been formed in chromosomes and plasmids and numerous bioactive compounds are produced by microorganisms. Therefore, it may be said that compounds useful in treatment of cancer will be found more and more in microbial secondary metabolites and more effective antitumor antibiotics and their derivatives, or more effective products producing immune resistance to cancer, will be discovered. In these studies, as discussed in this paper, the most urgent problem is to establish a rational screening principle or system to select compounds worth clinical examination. This is particularly important in the analog area. Bleomycin is an analog of phleomycin chosen because of lower renal toxicity. It has become an antitumor agent of significant value. Macromomycin is a new structure which has been found to bind with animal cells and inhibit growth. Neothramycin is a new benzodiazepine antibiotic which has lower toxicity than other structures studied in this class and is active against L1210, Yoshida sarcoma, and Sarcoma 180. Aclacinomycin A is an analog of adriamycin chosen for clinical study based on its low cardiac toxicity and high distribution in mouse lung and spleen. Coriolins are another new structural class. Diketocoriolin B has activity in L1210 leukemia and has been shown to inhibit Na-K-ATPase. Bestatin is a compound which inhibits aminopeptidase B and leucine aminopeptidase has been shown to increase delayed hypersensitivity. Bestatin also increases the effects of other antitumor agents such as adriamycin, and bleomycin.

References

1. Aoyagi, T., Suda, H., Nagai, M., Ogawa, K., Suzuki, J., Takeuchi, T., Umezawa, H.: Aminopeptidase activities on the surface of mammalian cells. Biochim. Biophys. Acta **452** 131-143 (1976).
2. Carter, S. K., Ichikawa, T., Mathe, J., Umezawa, H. (eds.): Fundamental and Clinical Studies of Bleomycin. Monograph on Cancer Research No. 19 by Japanese Cancer Association. Tokyo: University of Tokyo Press 1976.
3. Chimura, H., Ishizuka, M., Hamada, M., Hori, S., Kimura, K., Iwanaga, J., Takeuchi, T., Umezawa, H.: A new antibiotic, macromomycin exhibiting antitumor and antimicrobial activity. J. Antibiot. (Tokyo) **21**, 44-49 (1968).
4. Ishizuka, M., Iinuma, H., Takeuchi, T., Umezawa, H.: Effect of diketocoriolin B on antibody formation. J. Antibiot. (Tokyo) **25**, 320-321 (1972).
5. Komiyama, T., Matsuzawa, Y., Oki, T., Inui, T., Takahashi, Y., Naganawa, H., Takeuchi, T., Umezawa, H.: Baumycins, new antitumor antibiotics related to daunomycin. J. Antibiot. (Tokyo) **30**, 619-621 (1977).
6. Kunimoto, T., Hori, M., Umezawa, H.: Reversible binding of macromomycin, a macromolecular peptide antibiotic to cell membrane. J. Antibiot. (Tokyo) **24**, 203-205 (1971).
7. Kunimoto, T., Umezawa, H.: Mechanism of action of diketocoriolin B. Biochim. Biophys. Acta **298**, 513-525 (1973).
8. Oki, T., Matsuzawa, Y., Yoshimoto, A., Numata, K., Kitamura, I., Hori, S., Takamatsu, A., Umezawa, H., Ishizuka, M., Naganawa, H., Suda, H., Hamada, M., Takeuchi, T.: New antitumor antibiotics, aclacinomycins A and B. J. Antibiot. (Tokyo) **28**, 830-834 (1975).
9. Oki, T., Komiyama, T., Tone, H., Inui, T., Takeuchi, T., Umezawa, H.: Reductive cleavage of anthracycline glycosides by microsomal NADPH-cytochrome C reductase. J. Antibiot. (Tokyo) **30**, 613-615 (1977).
10. Oki, T., Shibamoto, N., Matsuzawa, Y., Ogasawara, T., Yoshimoto, A., Kitamura, I., Inui, T., Naganawa, H., Takeuchi, T., Umezawa, H.: Production of nineteen anthracyclic compounds by *Streptomyces gallilaeus* MA-144-M1. J. Antibiot. (Tokyo) **30**, 683-687 (1977).
11. Suda, H., Aoyagi, T., Takeuchi, T., Umezawa, H.: Inhibition of aminopeptidase B and leucine aminopeptidase by bestatin and its stereoisomer. Arch. Biochem. Biophys. **177**, 196-200 (1976).
12. Suda, H., Takita, T., Aoyagi, T., Umezawa, H.: The structure of bestatin. J. Antibiot. (Tokyo) **29**, 100-101 (1976).
13. Takahashi,- S., Naganawa, H., Iinuma, H., Takita, T., Maeda, K., Umezawa, H.: Revised structures and stereochemistry of coriolins. Tetrahedron Lett., No. 22, 1955-1958 (1971).
14. Takahashi, Y., Naganawa, H., Takeuchi, T., Umezawa, H., Komiyama, T., Oki, T., Inui, T.: The structures of baumycins A1, A2, B1, B2, C1 and C2. J. Antibiot. (Tokyo) **30**, 622-624 (1977).
15. Takeuchi, T., Miyamoto, M., Ishizuka, M., Naganawa, H., Kondo, S., Hamada, M., Umezawa, H.: Neothramycins A and B, new antitumor antibiotics. J. Antibiot. (Tokyo) **29**, 93-96 (1976).
16. Umezawa, H.: Bleomycin: Discovery, Chemistry and Action. Fundamental and Clinical Studies of Bleomycin. Gann Monograph on Cancer Research No. 19. Tokyo: University of Tokyo Press 1976, pp. 3-36.
17. Umezawa, H., Aoyagi, T., Suda, H., Hamada, M., Takeuchi, T.: Bestatin, an inhibitor of aminopeptidase B produced by actinomycetes. J. Antibiot. (Tokyo) **29**, 97-99 (1976).
18. Umezawa, H., Ishizuka, M., Aoyagi, T., Takeuchi, T.: Enhancement of delayed-type hypersensitivity by bestatin, an inhibitor of aminopeptidase. J. Antibiot. (Tokyo) **29**, 857-859 (1976).

The Current Status of Chemotherapy for Gastric Cancer in Japan with Special Emphasis on Mitomycin C

Y. Koyama

The current status of the chemotherapy of gastric cancer in our country is divided into three parts. First is the chemotherapy in advanced cases; second, an adjuvant chemotherapy to surgery; and third, an adjuvant chemotherapy to radiotherapy. Adjuvant chemotherapy to radiotherapy has only been started very recently; radiotherapy is performed under laparotomy followed by chemotherapy. Sometimes, chemotherapy is performed before laparotomy and irradiation. Since the current clinical data on adjuvant chemotherapy to radiotherapy is limited, it will not be presented here.

Chemotherapy of Advanced Cases

Clinical data on the single use of antibiotics in gastric cancer are:
27% with MMC
36% with CHRM
19% with NCS
15% with ADM
very low with BLM
The schedule of the combination chemotherapy is attached (Table 1). The letter "A" or "E" in Table 1 denotes cyclophosphamide. In Table 2, Ps means prednisolone and Ts means chromomycin hemisuccinate and the dosage of this drug is 1.5-2 times more than that of chromomycin.

Table 1. Dosage (mg/kg) of drugs in combined chemotherapy

Type of chemotherapy	MMC	CQ	CHRM	CA	CPA	5FU	FT	TSPA	BLM	VCR	CC	Admin.
MF	0.16-0.2					7.5						
MFT	0.04		0.02			10						1-2×/wk
MFCT	0.08		0.02	0.4		10						2×/wk
MFC	0.08			0.8		10						1-2×/wk
FAMT	0.04		0.01		4	10						1-2×/wk
FAM	0.08				4	10						1-2×/wk
METT	0.04		0.01		2			0.2				q 4 ds
FCQ		0.04-0.08		0.8		10						1-2×/wk
FOBEM	0.08				8	5			0.3	0.02		1×/wk
NeoMFC	0.08-0.12						16-24				12	po 1×/wk
MFtC	0.08			0.8			8-16					1-2×/wk

Table 2. Clinical data of combined chemotherapy in stomach cancer

Type of chemotherapy	No. of cases	Effective	
		cases	%
MF	92	23	25.0
MFT	142	32	22.6
MFC	259	100	38.6
MFCT	46	9	19.6
FAMT	122	50	41.2
FAM	24	4	16.7
METT	26	4	15.4
FCQ	32	9	28.1
NeoMFC	21	10	47.6
MFtC	27	7	25.9
MTPs	18	4	22.0
FTPs	40	17	42.5
FtTPs	47	11	23.4
FTs	28	9	32.1
FTsPs	24	13	54.1
FOBEM	12	2	17.0

Data on combination chemotherapy (Table 2) are:

56% with FTsPs	25% with MFtC
47% with Neo MFC	23% with FtTPs
42% with FTPs	22% with MFT
41% with FAMT	22% with MTPs
38% with MFC	19% with MFCT
32% with FTs	17% with FOBEM
28% with FCQ	16% with FAM
25% with MF	15% with METT

As can be concluded from these data, better results are obtained with MFC, FAMT, NeoMFC and FTPs. Since the combination with ADM has just been started, results are not yet available.

Adjuvant Chemotherapy to Surgery

There are three study groups in the controlled trials of adjuvant chemotherapy to surgery in gastric cancer in Japan. In this paper, the data of the National Hospitals group will be presented. The gastric cancer study group of the Cancer Chemotherapy Cooperating Research Committee of National Hospitals under the Ministry of Health and Welfare, started co-operative studies on adjuvant chemotherapy to curable surgery on July 1, 1959, and seven consecutive studies were carried out up to this year. Each study lasted from 2-2½ years. Twenty national hospitals participated in these studies which were carried out on a nationwide scale (Fig. 1).

Patients participating in these programs have never undergone chemotherapy and were histologically diagnosed as carcinoma. The controls without chemotherapy were set up in each study, and for randomization, the Fisher-Yates' table and the envelope method were used. Chemotherapies tried were as follows (Table 3): In the first study, daily dosage of 0.2 mg/kg thio-TEPA (TSPA) or 0.08 mg/kg mitomycin C (MMC) was administered i.v.

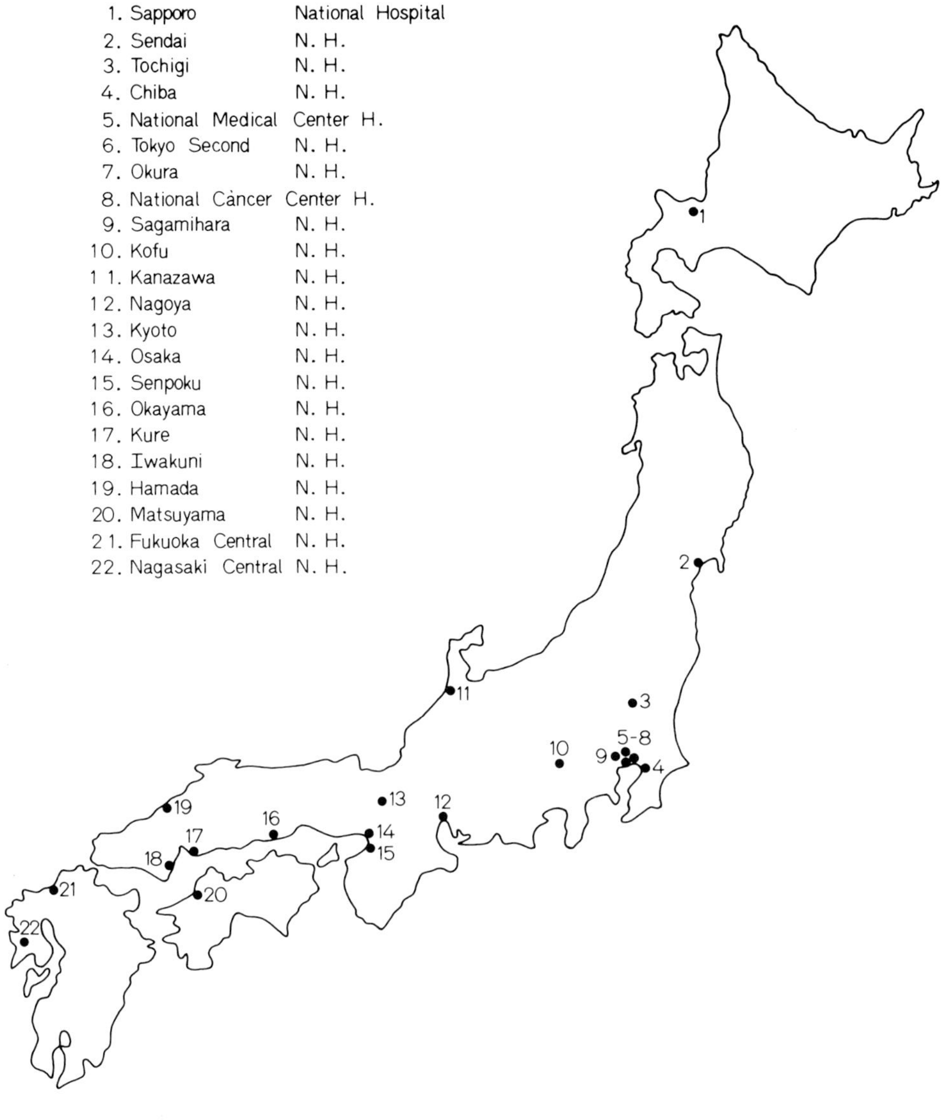

Fig. 1. Location of 22 National Hospitals on the map of Japan

and the total dosage of TSPA was more than 1.0 mg/kg or 0.8 mg/kg for MMC. During the operation, 5 mg TSPA or 4 mg MMC were administered i.p. This was a moderate dosage protocol of MMC.

In the second study, the chemotherapeutic procedure was the same, except that the daily dosage of MMC and TSPA was reduced to half that used in the first study, and the total dosage of MMC was 0.8 mg/kg and that of TSPA, 2.0 mg/kg. This was a small dosage protocol of MMC.

In the third study, 0.2 mg/kg MMC was given i.v. by the one shot method twice a week (totaling 0.8 mg/kg); or a daily dosage of 2.0 mg/kg cyclophosphamide (CPA) mixed with 0.01 mg/kg of chromomycin A3 (CHRM) was given i.v. (totaling 60 mg/kg CPA and

Table 3. Method of chemotherapy in gastric carcinoma

Study	Drug	Dosage		
		During the operation (i.p.)	During and after surgery (i.v.)	
			Daily dosage	Total dosage
First	MMc TSPA Control	4 mg 5 mg —	0.08 mg/kg daily 0.2 mg/kg daily —	over 40 mg over 50 mg —
Second	MMC TSPA Control	4 mg 5 mg —	0.04 mg/kg daily 0.1 mg/kg daily —	0.8 mg/kg 2.0 mg/kg —
Third	MMC CPA-CHRM Control	4 mg CPA 200 mg —	0.2 mg/kg 2×/wk CPA 2.0 mg/kg daily CHRM 0.01 mg/kg daily —	0.8 mg/kg 60 mg/kg —
Fourth	MMC Control	4 mg —	0.4 mg/kg on the day of surgery 0.2 mg/kg on the following day —	0.6 mg/kg —
Fifth	MMC-CPA 5FU Control	MMC 8 mg — —	MMC 0.2 mg/kg on the day of surgery CPA 4 mg/kg daily 5 mg/kg daily, and 10 mg/kg every other day —	0.2 mg/kg 60 mg/kg 150 mg/kg —
Sixth	MMC-5FU (Simultaneous) perop. MMC-postop. 5FU Control	MMC 4 mg — —	MMC 0.12 mg/kg 5 FU 10 mg/kg 2×/wk simultaneously MMC 0.2 mg/kg on the day of surgery 5FU 10 mg/kg every other day —	0.72 mg/kg 60 mg/kg 0.2 mg/kg 90 mg/kg —

0.3 mg/kg CHRM). During the operation, 4 mg MMC or 200 mg CPA were administered i.p. This was a large dosage protocol of MMC.

In the fourth study, 0.4 mg/kg MMC was administered i.v. on the day of surgery and 0.2 mg/kg MMC on the following day (totaling 0.6 mg/kg). During the operation, 4 mg MMC was given i.p. This was a push therapy protocol of MMC.

In the fifth study, 0.2 mg/kg MMC was given i.v. and 8 mg MMC was administered i.p. during the operation and then 4 mg/kg CPA was given i.v. daily for the ensuing 15 days (totaling 60 mg/kg CPA). This was a combination therapy of MMC. Alternatively 5 mg/kg 5FU was injected i.v. on the day of surgery and the ensuing 5 days, and then 10 mg/kg 5FU was given every other day for 4 weeks (totaling 150 mg/kg 5FU).

In the sixth study, 0.12 mg/kg MMC and 10 mg/kg 5FU was given i.v. and 4 mg MMC was administered i.p. during the operation. Then, simultaneously, 0.12 mg/kg MMC and 10 mg/kg 5FU was given i.v. twice a week (totaling 0.72 mg/kg MMC and 60 mg/kg 5FU).

This was a MMC-5FU simultaneous administration therapy. Alternatively 0.2 mg/kg MMC was injected i.v. on the day of surgery and then 10 mg/kg 5FU was given every other day for the ensuing 3 weeks (totaling 0.2 mg/kg MMC and 90 mg/kg 5FU). (This was peroperative MMC and postoperative 5FU therapy).

In the seventh study, 4 mg MMC was given i.p. during the operation, 0.2 mg/kg MMC was administered i.v. on the day of operation and the ensuing 3 days after the operation, and then 10 mg/kg 5FU was given three times a week for the ensuing 3 weeks (totaling 0.4 mg/kg MMC and 90 mg/kg 5FU). Alternatively 0.04 mg/kg carbazilquinone (CQ) and 5 mg/kg 5FU were administered simultaneously twice a week for 5 weeks (totaling 0.4 mg/kg CQ and 50 mg/kg 5FU).

In these studies, chemotherapy started on the day of the operation.

In the first study, 149 cases used MMC, 142 cases used TSPA, and 131 cases of the control; total 422 cases. In the second, 101 cases used MMC, 98 cases used TSPA, and 101 cases of the control; total 300 cases. In the third, 148 cases used MMC, 162 cases used CPA with CHRM, and 142 cases of the control; total 452 cases. In the fourth study, there were 187 cases using MMC, and 187 cases of the control; total 374 cases. In the fifth study, there were 146 cases using MMC-CPA, 161 cases using 5FU, and 159 cases of the control; total 466 cases. In the sixth study, there were 146 cases of MMC-5FU simultaneous administration group, 149 cases of peroperative MMC and postoperative 5FU therapy groups, and 172 cases of the control; total 467 cases.

The age distribution of patients in each treatment group was approximately the same in each study (Fig. 2).

All cases were divided into two groups according to the histologic classification of the Japanese Research Society for Gastric Cancer: the adenocarcinoma and carcinoma simplex. They were further divided into four subgroups, classified by the same society according to the stages of the disease. The relative survival rate was calculated and statistically significant difference was presented only where there was 95% confidence. A 5 year follow-up study has been completed for the first four studies but not on the fifth and sixth studies.

Results of the first study (Fig. 3):

The survival rate of the MMC group was slightly higher than that of the control after 1 and 2 years. In adenocarcinoma, there was no difference, and in carcinoma simplex, the MMC group showed a high survival rate in the course of the 5 year follow-up.

In the second study, no differences were found (Fig. 4).

In the third study, no differences were found in the total cases and in adenocarcinoma. In carcinoma simplex, the control was slightly higher than that of the MMC-group only after 2 years (Fig. 5).

In the fourth study, the survival rate of the MMC group was higher than that of the control after 5 years. In adenocarcinoma, the survival rate of the MMC group was higher than that of the control after 5 years. In carcinoma simplex, the rate for the MMC group was high after 2–5 years (Fig. 6).

In the fifth study, no differences were found in the total cases and in adenocarcinoma. In carcinoma simplex, the rate for 5FU was high after 3 years (Fig. 7).

From the stage classification, in Stage I and Stage II, there were no significant differences between the control and the treated groups. In Stage III, a high survival rate with MMC was obtained after 1 and 2 years in the first study, after 2–5 years in the fourth study, and the 5FU group was high after 3 and 4 years in the fifth study (Fig. 8).

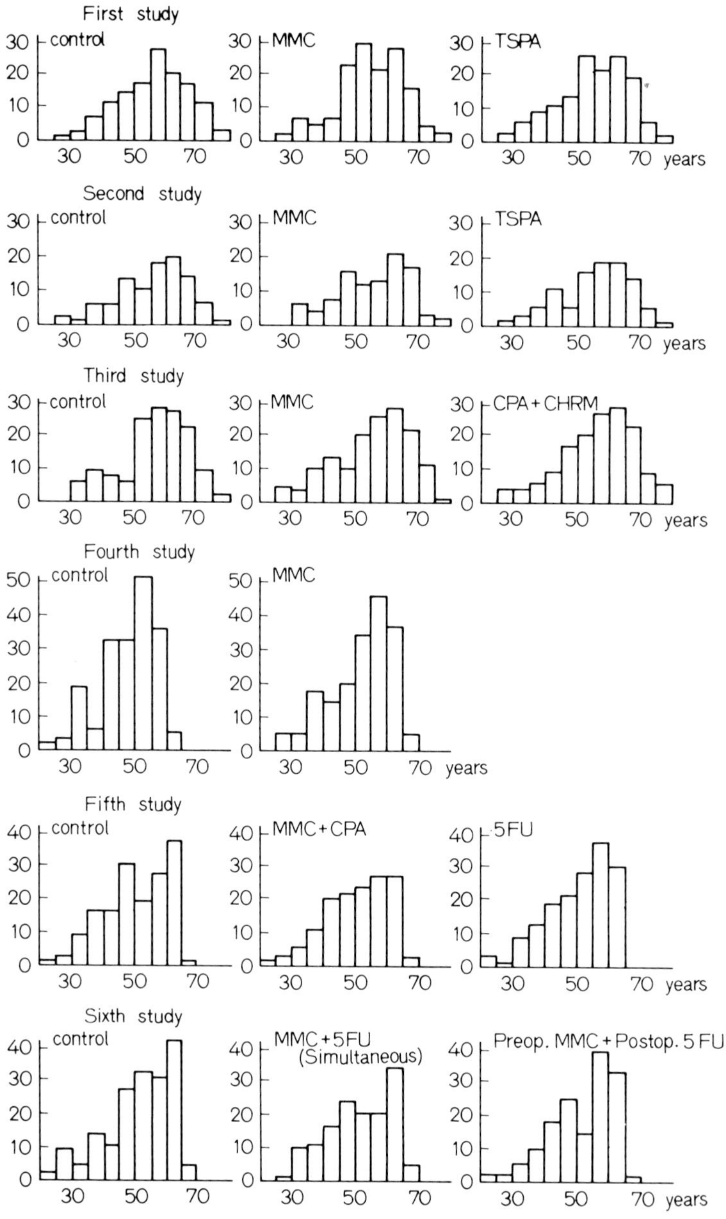

Fig. 2. Age distribution of gastric cancer patients

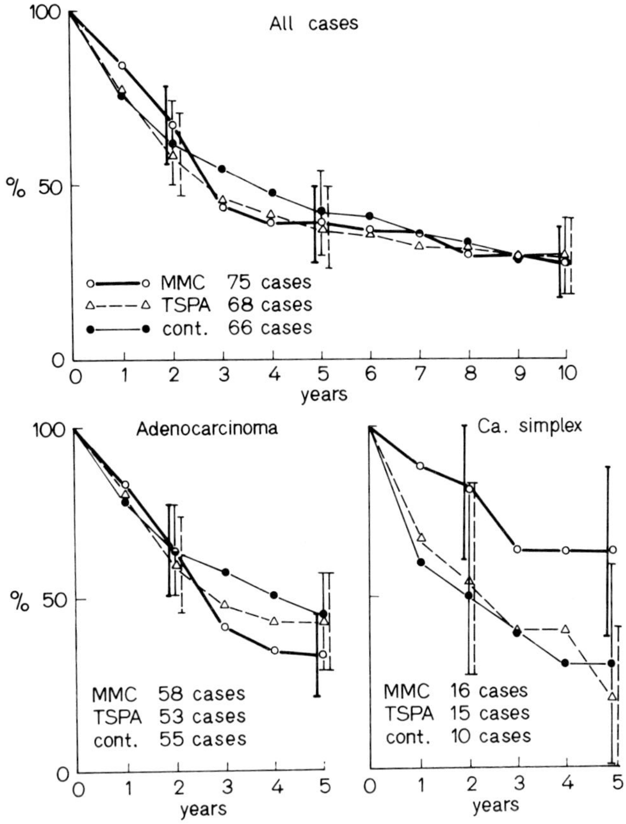

Fig. 3. Survival rate of gastric carcinoma (the First study)

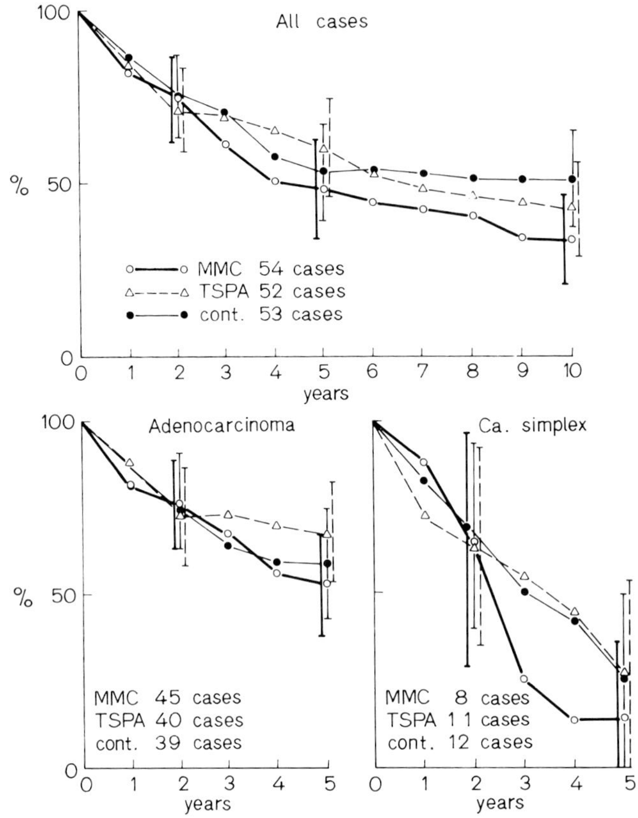

Fig. 4. Survival rate of gastric carcinoma (the Second study)

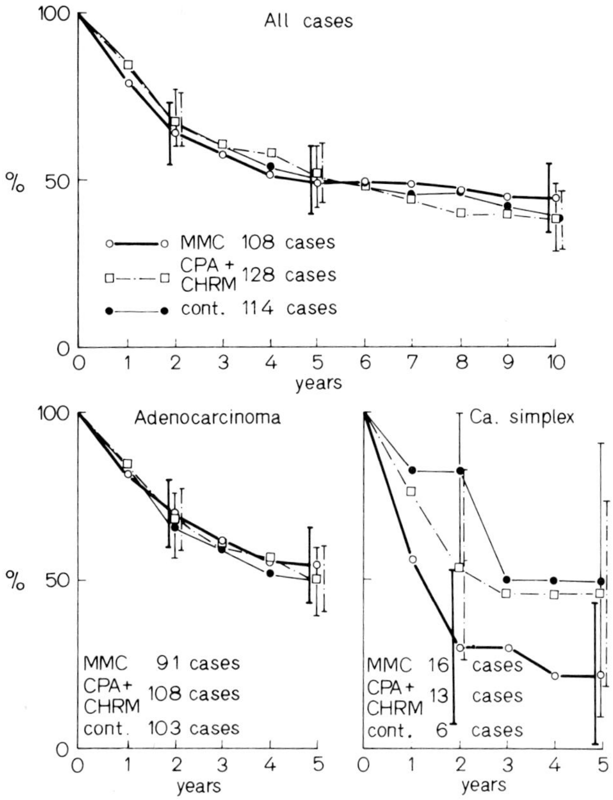

Fig. 5. Survival rate of gastric carcinoma (the Third study)

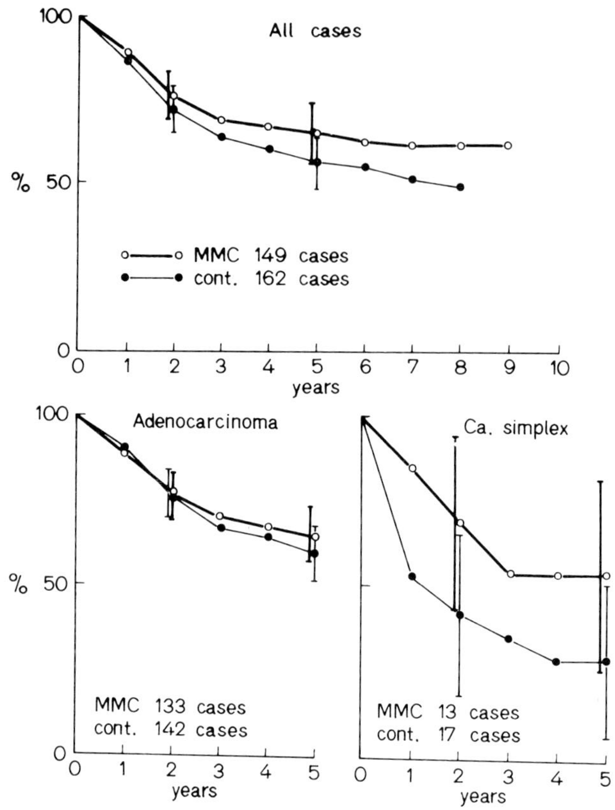

Fig. 6. Survival rate of gastric carcinoma (the Fourth study)

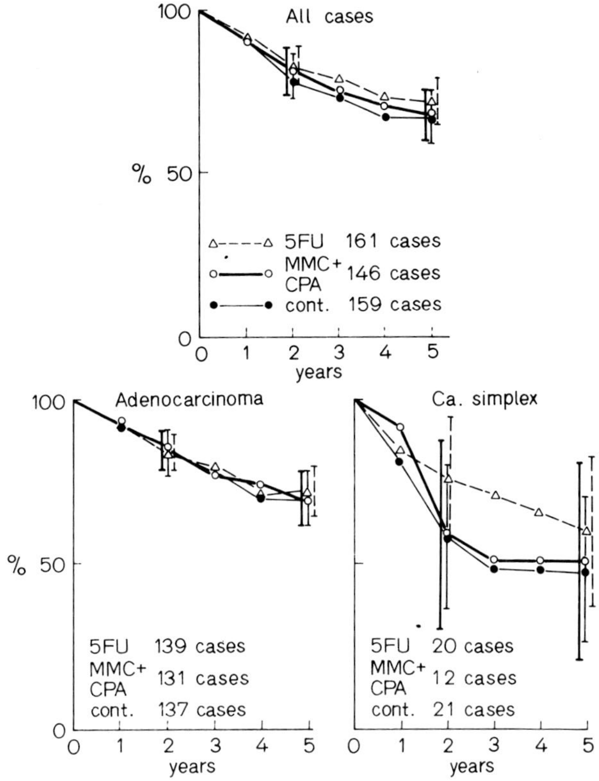

Fig. 7. Survival rate of gastric carcinoma (the Fifth study)

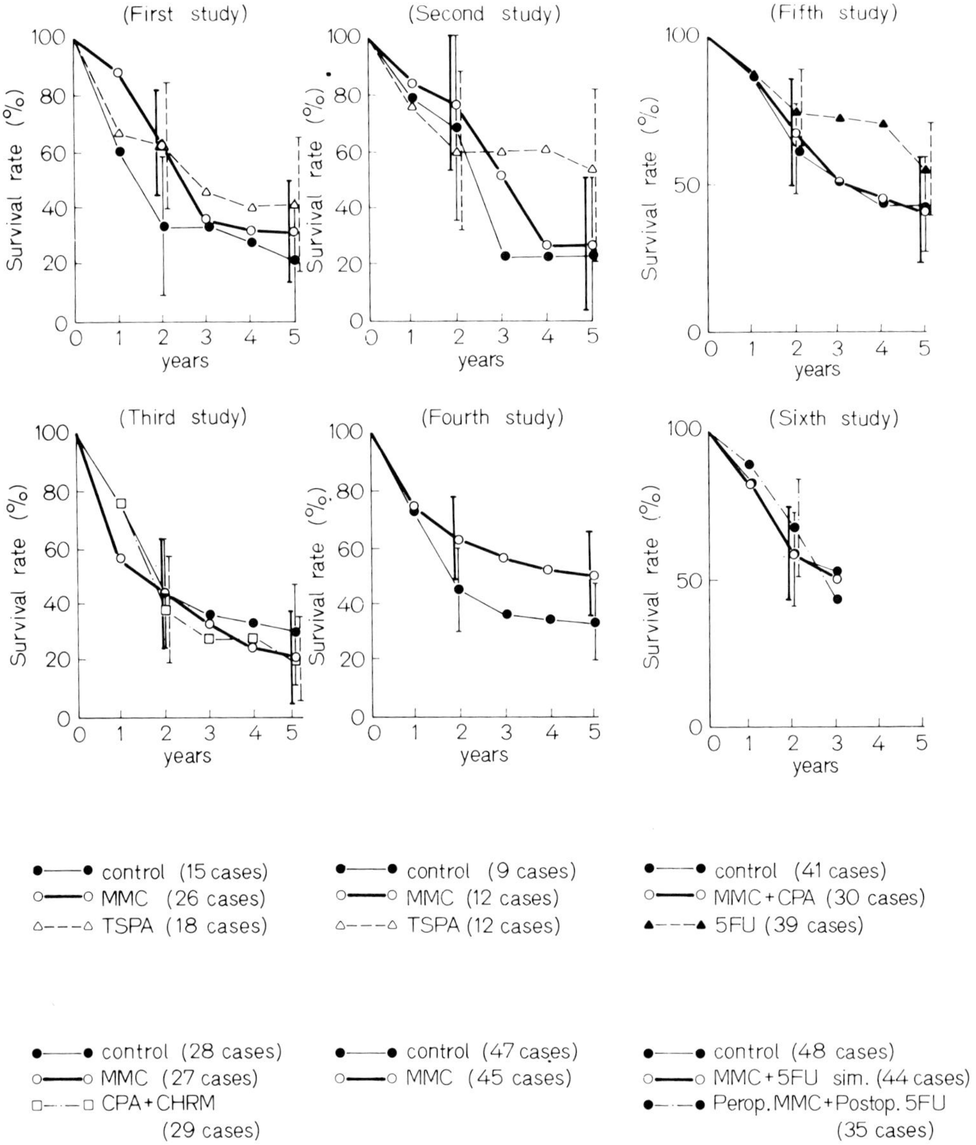

Fig. 8. Survival rate of gastric carcinoma (Stage III)

Summary

1. Significant differences in the survival rate between the control and MMC groups were observed for carcinoma simplex, in Stage III in the first and fourth studies, and also for 5FU group in the fifth study for carcinoma simplex and Stage III.
2. For Stage I patients, chemotherapy as an adjuvant to surgery may not be necessary because it decreased the survival rates in the second, third and fourth studies.
3. Total dosage of more than 0.6 mg/kg MMC is necessary to obtain a significant difference in the survival rate between the control and the treated groups.

Further controlled clinical studies are necessary to determine the effects of a long-term and multiple combined chemotherapy as an adjuvant to surgery in gastric cancer. These problems are under consideration in the following studies.

References

1. FURUE, H., NAKAO, I., KANKO, T., YOKOYAMA, T., FURUKAWA, K.: Chemotherapy of gastric cancer. GANN-TO-KAGAKURYOHO (Cancer & Chemother.) **2**, 351–359 (1975).
2. HARA, Y., TOBITA, Y.: Chemotherapy in cancer of the digestive organ. NIPPON-RINSHO (Jap. J. Clin. Med.) **33**, 1825–1832 (1975).
3. KIMURA, T.: Chemotherapy as an adjuvant to surgery in gastric carcinoma. GANN-TO-KAGAKURYOHO (Cancer & Chemother.) **2**, 391–405 (1975).
4. KOYAMA, Y.: Clinical evaluation of chemotherapy in gastric, lung, breast, liver and cervix cancers and hematopoietic organ tumors. Annual report of the co-operative research committee on cancer chemotherapy in National Hospitals. Tokyo, (1976) (in press).
5. KOYAMA, Y.: Summary of the clinical data on antitumor antibiotics in Japan. (1977) (in this book).
6. KOYAMA, Y., KIMURA, T., TAKEMASA, Y.: Chemotherapy as an adjuvant to surgery in stomach cancer. In: Progress in Antimicrobial and Anticancer Chemotherapy. Tokyo: University of Tokyo Press 1970, Vol. II, p. 242–249.
7. KURIHARA, M., IZUMI, T., SHIRAKABE, H., NAMIHISA, T., HAYAKAWA, H.: Cancer chemotherapy of gastrointestinal tract. GANN-TO-KAGAKURYOHO (Cancer & Chemother.) **1**, 443–455 (1974).
8. MURAKAMI, T.: The general rules for the gastric cancer study in surgery. Jap. J. Surg. **3**, 61–71 (1973).
9. NAKAJIMA, T., KAJITANI, T., FUKAMI, A., OHASHI, I.: Effect of adjuvant chemotherapy with Mitomycin C on the recurrence of gastric cancer after radical surgery. GANN-NO-RINSHO (Jap. J. Cancer Clin.) **21**, 897–904 (1975).
10. NAKAJIMA, T., KAJITANI, T., FUKAMI, A., OHASHI, I.: Prognostic study of adjuvant chemotherapy with Mitomycin C for the gastric cancer after surgery. GANN-NO-RINSHO (Jap. J. Cancer Clin.) **22**, 21–27 (1976).
11. NAKAO, I., FURUKAWA, K., KANKO, T., YOKOYAMA, T., HARASHIMA, S., FUNADA, A., MASUDA, Y., FURUE, H., KUBO, A.: Combination Chemotherapy in gastric cancer. GANN-TO-KAGAKURYOHO (Cancer & Chemother.) **2**, 377–384 (1975).
12. NAKAZATO, H.: Evaluation of adjuvant chemotherapy to surgery. NIPPON-RINSHO (Jap. J. Clin. Med.) **33**, 1818–1824 (1975).
13. SAITO, T., YOKOYAMA, M.: Treatment of solid tumors, mainly cancer of the digestive organ. NAIKA (Internal Medicine) **38**, 922–929 (1976).
14. SUGA, S., HIROTA, Y., SHIMACHI, T., KOIDE, A., IWATA, T., NAKANE, M., KODAMA, M., MASUDA, T., YAMAMOTO, T., MIYAGI, Y., YOSHIDA, T., AIZAWA, N.: Chemotherapy of advanced gastric cancer, especially with Mitomycin C. 5-Fluorouracil, and Cytosine arabinoside. GANN-NO-RINSHO (Jap. J. Cancer Clin.) **18**, 209–213 (1972).
15. YOKOYAMA, M., SAITO, T.: Evaluation of cancer chemotherapy from viewpoint of survival of patients with gastric cancer. GANN-TO-KAGAKURYOHO (Cancer & Chemother.) **2**, 367–375 (1975).

Mitomycin C: Experience in the United States, with Emphasis on Gastric Cancer

P. S. Schein, J. S. MacDonald, D. Hoth and P. V. Woolley

Mitomycin C is an antibiotic alkylating agent isolated from the fermentation of *Streptomyces caespitosus* in 1958. Clinical trials were initiated in Japan soon after the demonstration of antitumor activity against a broad spectrum of transplanted animal tumours [2]. Mitomycin C was reported to have a high degree of efficacy for human cancer, which prompted a cooperative multiinstitution evaluation of this agent in the United States. A preliminary summary of the results of the initial experience was reported in 1959 by Jones [11]. Of 120 patients treated, objective responses were observed in 21 (18.5%) including breast cancer, Hodgkin's disease, lymphocytic lymphoma and chronic granulocytic leukemia. Treatment was discontinued in 87% of patients because of severe hematologic toxicity. It was concluded that mitomycin C had an extremely narrow therapeutic index, while demonstrating only limited efficacy. The result was a sharply reduced interest for mitomycin C as an anticancer agent in the United States.

Because of the variance in results from Japanese and American investigators, Frank and Osterberg in 1960 undertook an analysis of 14 clinical trials conducted in Japan [7]. A total of 351 individual case records were reviewed using the following criteria as evidence of an objective response: reduction in tumor size, decreased pleural or ascitic fluid, marked reduction in jaundice, or a significant improvement in peripheral blood or bone-marrow findings in patients with leukemia. The overall tumor response was found to be 37%. Responses were recorded in gastric cancer (35%), breast cancer (42%), and lung cancer (37%). In addition, higher levels of activity were recorded in a smaller number of patients with chronic myelogenous leukemia, reticulum cell sarcoma, and seminoma. It was found that both toxicity and anti-tumor effect were a function of the total dose administered; hematologic toxicity was an accompaniment of tumor response in 68% of cases and was severe in cases which had received a cumulative dose of 40–50 mg.

In the same year, Ferguson and Humphrey introduced a dose schedule of 50 ug/kg for 6 consecutive days followed by alternate day treatment until toxicity [6]. This regimen was to remain a standard method of administration of mitomycin C in the United States and was employed in many of the major trials carried in this country. An alternative dose schedule of 150 ug/kg for 5 days was developed by Moertel and coworkers [15]. While the toxicity of these regimens were considered adequately tolerated, it was repeatedly noted that platelet and white blood cell depressions were delayed in onset, with nadirs occurring 3–6 weeks after the initiation of therapy. This pattern of delayed and cumulative bone marrow toxicity is remarkably similar to that observed with the chloroethyl nitrosoureas, BCNU and CCNU. In recognition of this phenomenon, the dosage schedules of these latter two agents had been adjusted to allow for prolonged periods of recovery in order to prevent serious cumulative toxicity. However, in the case of mitomycin C, it was not until 1974 that a similar prolonged intermittent schedule of administration was reported. Baker and coworkers described an overall 37% objective response rate for patients with solid tumor who received a single 20 mg/m^2 dose every 6–8 weeks [1]. This included responses in 8 out of 20 cases with upper gastrointestinal cancer. The hematologic toxicity associated with this regimen was considered acceptable. In view of the delayed nature of the toxicity, it is quite possible that our past method of daily mitomycin C administration has been inappropriate. The intermittent schedule is now being actively employed in the design of combination chemotherapy regimens employing this agent.

Recently, the use of oral mitomycin C has undergone a Phase I study [4]. The drug was administered in gelatin capsules, at doses of 10–15 mg/m^2; all patients were fasted prior to treatment. There was considerable variability in both peak serum concentration and disappearance curves after oral absorption. The toxic effects of mitomycin C were similar to those observed with parenteral treatment and could be correlated with the peak serum concentrations. The oral route was not recommended for further clinical investigation.

Aside from the treatment limiting bone marrow depression, several additional clinical toxicities have been described for mitomycin C. These have included a severe inflammatory reaction at injection sites if the drug is extravasated, and acute but mild gastrointestinal disturbance consisting of anorexia, nausea, vomiting and diarrhea.

A less frequent problem has been renal toxicity, manifested by an increased serum BUN and creatinine concentration and histologic evidence of glomerular sclerosis [12]. This complication of treatment is usually delayed in onset, occurring several months after initiation of therapy in patients who have received large total doses. Renal toxicity appears to be less important with the intermittent schedule and doses of 10–20 mg/m^2 [18].

The therapeutic activity of mitomycin C, administered as a single agent for selected tumors, has been defined in seven major trials conducted in the United States. The overall response rate for gastric cancer is 24%. Activity has also been reported for pancreatic (18%), colorectal (18%), and breast cancer (31%), in addition to head and neck and pulmonary malignancies. The principal limitation has been the duration of responses, which have lasted only an average of three months [15].

Mitomycin C has been incorporated into several drug combinations for solid tumors. The initial programs employed the daily loading method of administration. Horton et al. have reported the use of a combination of mitomycin C, thio-TEPA, 5-fluorouracil, and fluoxymesterone administered daily to 56 patients with solid tumors [9]. Responses were observed in four out of 22 patients with colonic carcinoma, and three out of 12 cases with breast cancer. At the Mayo Clinic, combinations of mitomycin C, 5-fluorouracil, and BCNU, and mitomycin plus 5-FU were compared to 5-fluorouracil used alone in a controlled randomized trial [19]. For colorectal cancer, neither combination was demonstrated to produce objective response rates superior to that achieved using 5-fluorouracil as a single agent. In contrast, two out of five patients with gastric cancer evidenced an objective response after treatment with 5-FU (9 mg/kg/day × 5) plus mitomycin C (0.11 mg/kg/day × 5) and two out of four responded to a mitomycin C plus BCNU combination.

The combination of mitomycin C, 5-fluorouracil and cytosine arabinoside was reported by Hoshino et al. [10] to have a marked synergistic activity for the murine leukemia L-1210. Subsequent clinical studies conducted by Ota et al. [17] in Japan demonstrated a response rate of 55% in patients with gastric cancer and 60% in patients with colonic cancer. DeJager and coworkers at Memorial Hospital initiated a clinical trial with the same regimen in an attempt to confirm the activity of the combination [5]. Mitomycin C (0.04–0.08 mg/kg), 5-FU (7.5–10 mg/kg) and cytosine arabinoside (0.6 or 2.0 mg/kg), MFC, were given i.v. twice a week until the development of treatment-limiting hematologic toxicity. For 32 patients with gastric cancer there was 31% response, whereas negligible activity was demonstrated for colonic and pancreatic cancer. The role of cytosine arabinoside in the MFC combination is not known and it is possible that the activity for gastric cancer is mediated solely by 5-FU and mitomycin C.

Macdonald et al. have recently described a new combination chemotherapy program for gastric cancer, FAM, in which mitomycin C is administered by the single dose intermittent schedule [13]. The FAM regimen is administered in 9-week courses: 5-FU (600 mg/m^2) is given i.v. on days 1, 8, 28, and 35 of each cycle; adriamycin (30 mg/m^2) is administered on days 1 and 28; and mitomycin C is given as a single dose of 10 mg/m^2 on day 1 only, of each treatment course. 29 patients with advanced measurable gastric cancer have been treated and 16 (55%) have evidenced an objective response. The median duration of response is 10 months with a range of 2+–17+ months. The median survival of the responding patients is in excess of 13 months, with 25% still alive as long as 24 months after initiation of therapy. In contrast, the median survival of nonresponders was 2.5 months and all patients had died within 6 months. The regimen was well tolerated, with myelosuppression as the principal treatment-limiting toxicity. The median nadir white blood cell and platelet counts were 2500/mm^3 and 100,000/mm^3 respectively. There was little evidence of cumulative bone marrow depression, with 75% of initial doses being administered after one year of treatment. The FAM regimen is now being evaluated for activity in primary adenocarcinoma of lung, with preliminary report demonstrating an objective response rate of 33%.

Wiggans et al. have utilized a combination similar to the FAM regimen for advanced pancreatic cancer; in this study, streptozotocin (1.0 gm/m^2) was administered on day 1, 8, 28 and 35 in substitution for adriamycin [20]. 10 out of 23 patients (43%) achieved a partial or complete (one patient) response. The median duration of response is in excess of 6 months, with four patients alive and still in a remission state. The median survival of all patients in this series is 6 months. Patients demonstrating an objective response have a median survival in excess of 7.5 months, with a range of 3–23+ months, compared to 3 months for the non-responding group.

In summary, mitomycin C appears to have an established role in the treatment of gastric cancer and other solid tumors. The use of a single dose intermittent schedule has allowed for the safe and effective use of this agent in recently developed combination chemotherapy regimens.

References

1. Baker, L. H., Caoili, E. M., Izbicki, R. M., Opipari, M. I., Vaitkevicius, V. K.: A comparative study of mitomycin C and porfiromycin. Proc. Am. Soc. Clin. Oncol. **15**, 182 (1974).
2. Carter, S. K.: Mitomycin C (NSC-26980) clinical brochure. Cancer Chemother. Rep., part 3 **1**, 99–114 (1968).
3. Comis, R. L., Carter, S. K.: Integration of chemotherapy into combined modality treatment of solid tumors III. Gastric cancer. Cancer Treat. Rev. **1**, 221–238 (1974).
4. Crooke, S. T., Bradner, W. T.: Mitomycin C: A review. Cancer Treat. Rev. **3**, 121–139, 1976.
5. DeJager, R. L., Magill, G. B., Golbey, R. B., Krakoff, I. H.: Combination chemotherapy with mitomycin C, 5-fluorouracil, and cytosine arabinoside in gastrointestinal cancer. Cancer Treat. Rep. **60**, 1373–1375 (1976).
6. Ferguson, D., Humphrey, E.: Mitomycin C. Cancer Chemother. Rep. **8**, 154 (1960).
7. Frank, W., Osterberg, A. E.: Mitomycin C (NSC-26980), an evaluation of Japanese reports. Cancer Chemother. Rep. **9**, 114–119 (1960).
8. Godfrey, T. E., Wilbur, D. W.: Clinical experience with mitomycin C in large infrequent doses. Cancer **29**, 1647–1652 (1972).
9. Horton, J., Olson, K. B., Gehrt, P., Spear, M.: Combination therapy with 5-fluorouracil (NSC-19893), mitomycin (NSC-26980), vincristine (NSC-67574), and thioTEPA (NSC-6396) for advanced cancer. Cancer Chemother. Rep. **49**, 59–61 (1965).
10. Hoshino, A., Kato, T., Amo, H., et al.: Combination chemotherapy of mitomycin C, 5-fluorouracil and cytosine arabinoside in L-1210 mouse leukemia. In: Proceedings of the 10th International Cancer Congress, Houston, Texas. Houston: Medical Arts Publishing Co. 1970, pp 409–410.
11. Jones, R., Jr.: Mitomycin C. A preliminary report of studies of human pharmacology and initial therapeutic trial. Cancer Chemother. Rep. **2**, 3–7 (1959).
12. Liu, K., Mittleman, A., Sproul, E. E., Elias, E. G.: Renal toxicity in man treated with mitomycin-C. Cancer **28**, 1314–1320 (1971).

13. MACDONALD, J., SCHEIN, P., UENO, W., WOOLLEY, P.: 5-Fluorouracil, mitomycin C, and adriamycin—FAM: A new combination chemotherapy program for advanced gastric carcinoma. Proc. Am. Soc. Clin. Onc. **17**, 264 (1976).
14. MANHEINER, L. H., VITAL, J.: Mitomycin-C in the therapy of far-advanced malignant tumors. Cancer **19**, 207–212 (1966).
15. MOERTEL, C. G., REITEMEIER, R. J., HAHN, R. G.: Mitomycin C therapy in advanced gastrointestinal cancer. J. Am. Med. Assoc. **204**, 1045–1048 (1968).
16. MOORE, G. E., BOSS, I. D. J., AUSMAN, R., NADLER, S., JONES, R., Jr., SLACK, N., RIMM, A. A.: Effects of mitomycin C. (NSC-26980) in 346 patients with advanced cancer. Eastern clinical drug evaluation program. Cancer Chemother. Rep. **52**, 657–684 (1968).
17. OTA, K., KURITA, S., NISHIMURA, M., et al.: Combination therapy with mitomycin-C (NSC-26980), 5-fluorouracil (NSC-19883), and cytosine arabinoside (NSC-63878) for advanced cancer in man. Cancer Chemotherap. Rep. **56**, 373–385 (1972).
18. RATANATHARATHORN, V., CADNAPAPHORNDAI, P., ROSENBERG, B., BAKER, L. H., TABER, S., RUFFER, B. W., MCDONALD, F. D., VAITKEVICIUS, V. K.: Clinical and pathologic study of mitomycin-C nephrotoxicity: A retrospective analysis. Proc. Am. Soc. Clin. Oncology **18**, 293 (1977).
19. REITEMEIER, R. J., MOERTEL, C. G., HAHN, R. G.: Combination chemotherapy in gastrointestinal cancer. Cancer Chemother. Rep. **30**, 1425–1428 (1970).
20. WIGGANS, G., SMYTHE, T., UENO, W., MACDONALD, J., SCHEIN, P., FLANNERY, E.: Streptozotocin, mitomycin, and 5-fluorouracil, SMF, chemotherapy for advanced pancreatic carcinoma: Phase II trial. Cancer (In Press).

A Review of the Bleomycin Experience in the United States

M. A. FRIEDMAN

Since the original identification of bleomycin (BLM) as a promising anticancer agent by the Japanese investigators and its subsequent introduction into the United States, active world wide efforts have been made to evaluate this drug clinically. In the United States, these efforts were initially unfocused, with many institutions of oncology and cooperative groups pursuing broad Phase II trials looking for promising single agent activity. After this preliminary exploration of dosage, schedule, and method of administration, the antitumor activity of BLM was confirmed for squamous tumors of the head and neck, squamous tumors of the cervix, for testicular tumors, and for lymphoproliferative disorders [5]. Coincident with these investigations, it became clear that BLM had not only unique antitumor potential but also unique toxic properties. Unlike most other antineoplastics, BLM demonstrated little myelotoxicity. Its acute toxicities proved to be dermatitis and allergy, and its major dose-limiting chronic toxicity, pulmonary fibrosis.

However, it rapidly became apparent that BLM, used as a single agent, effected only transient objective remissions. Therefore, explorations of this drug in combination with other drugs or modalities were initiated [11]. This review will update the status of combined BLM trials in the United States, with emphasis on ongoing, currently uncompleted, or proposed investigations. Since the number of trials and active investigators is large, an encyclopedic cataloging would be impossible. I have, therefore, restricted this review to the most comprehensive studies reported.

In compiling this broad experience, several consistent strategies became evident. One such strategy has been the combination of vinca alkaloids with BLM, an approach based on the in vitro investigations of BARRANCO and HUMPHREY [2], who demonstrated that sequential use of vincristine (VCR) and BLM could effect enhanced cell kill. The clinical translations of this study were carried out by LIVINGSTON et al. [33] and SAMUELS et al. [50] exploring dosage, schedule, and delivery modifications in patients with squamous and testicular cancer. Further application of vinca plus BLM combinations occurred; all these are presented in tables in this chapter.

A second popular approach has been the addition of BLM to already proven therapeutic regimens. Because of its almost complete lack of myelotoxicity when used independently, BLM has been incorporated in the combination chemotherapy of patients with head and neck tumors, lymphomas, and Hodgkin's disease.

A third approach has been the addition of BLM to standard, intensive radiation therapy (XRT). BLM is used to provide enhanced control of local as well as systemic disease. In patients with advanced local squamous cell disease of the head and neck [57], lung [13], and cervix, the addition of BLM has proven tolerable. The combination of other drugs with BLM and XRT is also currently of interest, especially in Hodgkin's disease and lung cancer.

With these strategies in mind, the protocols oriented to specific diseases can be conveniently grouped and discussed. Wherever appropriate, I have suggested the developmental evolution of these studies to help clarify current chemotherapeutic drug usage in the United States and intimate future directions.

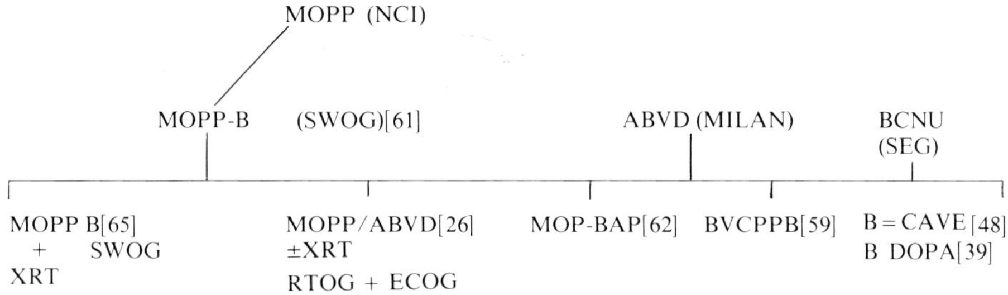

Fig. 1. Evolutionary development of chemotherapy in Hodgkin's disease

Hodgkin's Disease

The developmental flow of Hodgkin's disease (HD) protocols is shown in Fig. 1. The major source of this clinical research is, of course, the mechlorethamine, vincristine, procarbazine, prednisone (MOPP) program of De Vita et al. of the National Cancer Institute [21]. This program had strikingly effective clinical results; over half of the patients had a complete response and in a significant proportion of patients there was evidence of long-term control of disease. However, in an attempt to remedy MOPP treatment failure, Bonadonna et al. [6] demonstrated that a combination of doxorubicin (ADR), BLM, vinblastine (VLB), and imidazole carboxamide (DTIC) was an excellent noncross resistant combination. Also, the efficacy of both 1,3-bis(2-chloroethyl)-1-nitrosourea (BCNU) and 1-(2-chloroethyl)-3-cyclohexyl-1-nitrosourea (CCNU) in recurrent Hodgkin's disease was established. Therefore, from these sources, combinations of BLM with MOPP, MOPP with ADR, BLM, velban, and DTIC (ABVD), and new permutations of these elements for both primary and recurrent disease were described.

The specific protocols are listed in Table 1. One of the most interesting is the Southwest Oncology Group (SWOG) 774 (MOPP #4) study which compared MOPP with two combinations of MOPP + BLM [60]. The preliminary evaluation of this data indicates an apparent benefit with low dose BLM plus MOPP in terms of response rate. Whether this difference will effect long-term control of disease is yet to be known. Additionally, the current SWOG study is comparing MOPP plus BLM with a more complicated drug program, MOP-BAP (see Table 1). This protocol (SWOG 7406) [61] and the Southeast Group (SEG) study [13] represent attempts to induce more frequent and durable responses by including more drugs in the therapeutic schema.

Table 2 describes four programs for patients refractory to MOPP. Of interest is that these programs yield a high rate of complete response (CR) and partial response (PR) in these poor risk patients.

Finally, Table 3 describes three studies of combined chemotherapy and XRT. Case [12] reported that 19 out of 19 previously untreated cases and 34 out of 37 of his entire study group had a CR resulting from an aggressive combined modality approach. Two similar approaches are being studied by the Eastern Cooperative Oncology Group (ECOG) and SWOG.

The chief difficulty in evaluating the place of BLM in these protocols is that conventional MOPP or XRT are so effective that it will take many patients and many years of follow up to appreciate any beneficial activity.

Table 1. Protocols for Hodgkin's disease

Study	Chemotherapy (mg/m²)	N	CR	PR	Comments
SWOG 774 [60]	*MOPP* HN_2 6, VCR 1.4 } D1+D8 q 28 d × 6 PROC 100, PRED 50 } D1–D10	46	63%	15%	Stage III_B and IV Study closed Evaluation Ongoing
	MOPP + BLM 2 D1+D8	123	85%	11%	
	MOPP + BLM 10 D1+D8	41	73%	17%	Toxicity worse for BLM 10 mg/m²
SWOG 7406 [61]	MOPP + q 28 d ×10 BLM 2 D1+D8				Study in progress
	MOP-BAP #1 HN_2 6 D1 VCR 1.4, BLM 2 } D1 +D8 PROC 100, PRED 40 } D2–7, D9–12 ADR 30 D8				
	MOP-BAP #2 HN_2 3, VCR 1.4, BLM 2, ADR 15 } D1+D8 PROC 100, PRED 40 D2–7, D9–12				ARM closed 2/76
SEG [59]	BCNU 100, BLM 2, VLB 5, CYT 600 } D1 q 28 d PROC 50, PRED 60 } D1–10 Above alternating with ADR 60, DTIC 625, BLM 2 } D1 q 28 d				In progress

Lymphoma

The efficacy of BLM in the treatment of non-Hodgkin's lymphoma has led to its use in a variety of combinations. Fig. 2 outlines the developmental flow of these studies. Cytoxan (CYT), VCR, and prednisone (PRED) in combination (CVP) remain the backbone of all primary protocols. To this core of CVP both ADR and BLM were added with CHOP-B (SWOG) and BACOP (National Cancer Institute and Sidney Farber Center). Several of these primary treatment programs are described in Table 4 and clearly all are effective with

Table 2. Protocols for Hodgkin's disease after failure of Mopp treatment

Study	Chemotherapy (mg/m²)	N	CR	PR	Comments
Lokich [39]	*B-DOPA* BLM 4 D2+D5 DTIC 150 D1–5 q 21–28 d VCR 1.5 D1+D5 PRED 40 D1-6 ADR 50 D1	20	60%	20%	MOPP failures Median duration of response = 14+ months
Vinciguerra [70]	BLM 6, VLB 6 } D1+D8 q 28 d ADR 30, STRZ 1500 } D1	10	40%	10%	MOPP failures
PORZIG [48]	*B-CAVE* BLM 5 D1+D28+D35 CCNU 100, ADR 60, VLB 5 } D1	17	35%	29%	MOPP failures
LOH [37]	ADR 45, BLM 5, CCNU 50 } D1 DTIC 200, PRED 40 } D1-5	20	23%	45%	MOPP failures MST for CR = 12+ months MST for PR = 7+ months

Table 3. Combined chemotherapy and radiation therapy for Hodgkin's disease

Study	Chemotherapy (mg/m²)	N	CR	PR	Comments
CASE [12]	MOPP Alternate q 28 d + ADR 25 D29+D33 BLM 2 D33-41, D48-56 VLB 250 D19+D43 DTIC 250 D21+D43 + XRT to bulky decrease sites (month 5) 20004 in 2 wk.	37	89%	11%	100 % CR in previously untreated cases (19/19) Levamisole maintenance randomization
SWOG 7518 [64]	MOPP q 28 d × 10 + BLM 2 D1+D8 MOPP + BLM ×3→ XRT to bulky disease: CR; PR → MOPP + BLM × 4	—	—	—	In progress
EST 1476 [26]	MOPP + BLM ×6 → XRT, BCG ADR 25, BLM 2, VLB 6 } D1+D15 q 25 d DTIC 250 ×3	—	—	—	In progress

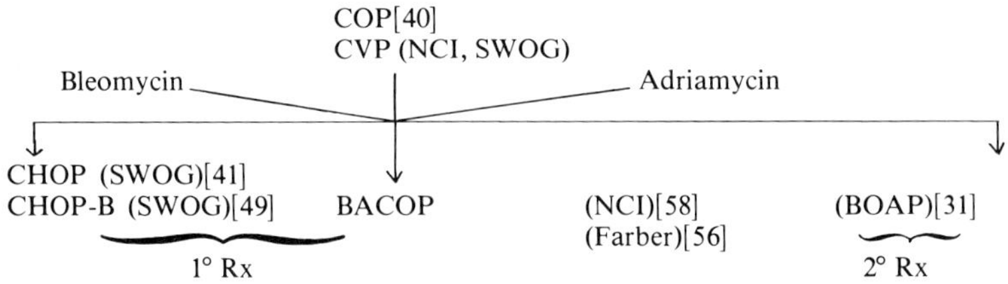

Fig. 2. Evolutionary development of chemotherapy in non-Hodgkin's lymphomas

Table 4. Protocols for non-Hodgkin's lymphoma

Study	Chemotherapy (mg/m²)	N	CR	PR	Comments
Rodriguez [49]	*CHOP-B* q 21 Until ADR = 450 then COP CYT 750 } D1 q 21 d ADR 50 } VCR 1.5 } D1+D5 BLM 15 } PRED 100 D1-5	35	66%	25%	Median duration of response > 1 year
Skarin [58]	*BACOP* BLM 4 D1, D4, D8, D12 . . . ADR 45 D1 CYT 600 q 21 d VCR 1.2 D1+D8+D15 PRED 40 D1-28	19	63%		
Schein [56]	*BACOP* BLM 5 D15+D22 ADR 25 D1+D18 CYT 650 } D1+D8 VCR 1.4 } PRED D15-28	21	43%	44%	
Cabanillas [9]	CHOP-BLM + Levamisole 150 D8, 9, 15, 16 ↓ COP + Levamisole	35	54%	43%	DHL = 11/21 CR
Steinhertz [69]	VAB III	6		5	Pediatric patients
Sarna [55]	*COMBAP* CYT VCR MTX 50 mg/kg Leukovorin BLM ADR PRED	5			Not encouraging initial report
Wilson [73]	CHOP × 2 ↓ ARAC + 6 TG ↓ BLOP +	11	9		MDR = 14 mo Childhood lymphoma

Table 4. (Continued)

Study	Chemotherapy (mg/m²)	N	CR	PR	Comments
SWOG 7426/27 [62]	VCR 1.4, CYT 125 D1+D8 PRED 60, BLM 10 D1-5				In progress
	CHOP-B CYT 750, ADR 50 D1 VCR 1.4, BLM 15 D1+D5 q 21-28 × 8 PRED 100 D1-5				
	CHOP + BCG				
EST 3734 [26]	BCNU 60, CYT 1000, VCR 1.2 D1 q 21 d PRED 100 D1-5				In progress
	COPA CYT 600, ADR 50, VCR 1.2 D1 PRED 100 D1-5				
	COPB CYT 1000, VCR 1.2, BLM 10 D1 PRED 100 D1-5				
	CPOB CYT 1000 D1 VCR 1.2, BLM 10 D1 + D5 PRED 100 D1-5				
Davis [30]	*BACO* CCNU 50, ADR 40, VCR 2 D1 BLM D2	8	62%	12%	Previous COP or XRT failures
Kerr [31]	*BOAP* ADR 60, VCR 0.5 D1 PRED 100 D1-5 BLM 10 D8+D11+D15+D18	9	44%	44%	Patients previously treated with MOPP, COP, BCNU
Steinberg [68]	*B-VAP* BLM 10, VLB 4, ADR 40 D1 PRED 60 D1-5 q 21 d	9		66%	COP or MOPP failures MDR = 4.5 months

response rates of 40%-60% lasting many months. The theoretical advantage of the BACOP programs is the use of the nonmyelosuppressive drugs (VCR, PRED, BLM) at the later portion of each cycle when the myelotoxicity of CYT and ADR would be in evidence. Thus, drugs can be administered throughout a longer cycle of therapy.

Unfortunately, more complicated programs (using 6 drugs or more) have not demonstrated greater benefit with the addition of each drug, but an ongoing evaluation of these programs is in process.

Finally, for patients in whom initial CVP or COP therapy fails, the use of second line protocols including BLM has evidenced some gratifying responses. Such programs as BACO[20] or BOAP[31] yield objective responses in the majority of cases.

Cervix

Until recently few systematic evaluations had been made of chemotherapy in squamous tumors of the cervix. However, one of the most extensively studied drugs in this type of tumor is BLM. Table 5 outlines the large organized experience of Baker et al. at Wayne State University with three serial studies of patients with disseminated disease using mitomycin C (MMC), VCR, and BLM in three schedules. Patients in the first study evidenced the most toxicity and the greatest number of responses, and in the third patients showed both toxicity that was acceptable and an overall response rate of 33%. Additionally, Conroy's preliminary data [16] and the Phase I-II study of BLM plus XRT as an adjuvant by Byfield [8] appear promising.

Table 5. Protocols for carcinoma of the cervix

Study	Chemotherapy (mg/m²)		N	CR	PR	Comments
Conroy [16]	BLM 10 MTX 10	wk. q 4 d	20		60%	Median duration of response = 7.5 months
Baker [1]	*A* MMC 20 VCR 0.5 BLM 6	 q 6 wk. 2 × wk. × 6 wk. 2 × wk. × 6 wk. (6 h later)	24	31%	25%	Severe toxicity MST = 24 wk.
	B MMC 20 VCR 0.5 BLM 6	 q 6 wk. q wk. × 6 q wk. × 6	27	4%	19%	Less toxicity than A MST = 12 wk.
	C NMC 20 VCR 0.5 BLM 20	 q 8 wk. D1+D4 infusion D1-5 × 2	49	10%	23%	Less toxicity than A MST = 28 + wk.
Byfield [8]	BLM + Local XRT	10 q wk. (Total/wk., 50 U)	10			Toxicity tolerable 5/10 patients with locally advanced tumor NED

Head and Neck

The utility of BLM in squamous cell head and neck malignancies derives from its activity both as a single agent and in combination with other drugs, XRT, and surgery. As shown in Fig. 3 the consistent core of almost all chemotherapy programs for head and neck cancer remains methotrexate (MTX), in either regular dosage or in high dosage (H.D., MTX) along with leukovorin rescue. To this significant activity of MTX as a single agent has been added

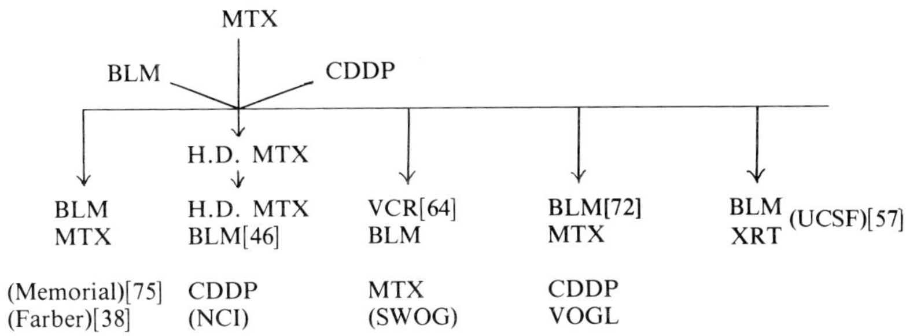

Fig. 3. Evolutionary development of chemotherapy in cancer of the head and neck

its activity with BLM, cis dichlorodiammine platinum (CDDP), and many other agents. Some of the larger studies are presented in Table 6. Although many programs have been evaluated, the majority of studies to date have not proven multiple agents to be more efficacious than MTX used maximally as a single agent. This is especially disappointing considering the aggressive approach employed. However, some of the newer programs using H.D. MTX, BLM, and CDDP, which appear to be markedly active in the preliminary reports, have been hopeful.

Table 6. Protocols for cancer of the head and neck

Study	Chemotherapy (mg/m²)		N	CR	PR	Comments
Yagoda [74]	BLM 15 MTX 15	q 4-14 d	15		52%	Failed previous XRT or surgery
Livingston [33]	COMB #3		21		28%	
Costanzi [17]	BLM 7.5 MTX 30 OHU 2	D1+D2 D3	17		59%	Median duration of response = 2+ months
Livingston [34]	CYT 1000 VCR 0.75-1 BLM 30 ↓ MTX 30 ↓ ADR 60 MECCNU 150	D1+D22 D2 D2 (6 h later) q wk. ×12 D1+D22 D1	17	17%	35%	
Donegan [22]	MTX 5-20 Daily i.a. 5 FU 31-125 Infusion ×5-72D BLM 0.08-32 mg/kg q d + leukovorin		15	20%	40%	
Bitter [3]	MTX 240 BLM 15 U	i.a. or i.v. with leukovorin i.a. or i.v. (300 u total)	17		100%	
Murphy [45]	CYT 600 ADR 40 VCR 0.75 BLM 30 ↓ MTX 30 ↓	D1+D12 D1+D22 } D1+D8 . . . D43 q wk. ×6	22	9%	9%	Poorer response than MTX alone

Table 6. (Continued)

Study	Chemotherapy (mg/m^2)	N	CR	PR	Comments
	CYT 600 } D1+D22 ADR 40 } ↓ Maintenance				
VOGL [71]	MTX 40 D1+D15 BLM 10 g wk. g 21d CDDP 50 D3 or D4	4		50%	Tolerable toxicity
SWOG 7517 [63]	VCR 2 mg } BLM 20 } D1 (6 h later) MTX 40 }				In progress
SWOG 7519 [65]	MTX 15 } D1-3 MTX 15 } MECCNU 200 D1 q 6 wk. BLM 12.5 D15+D22+D29+ D36				In progress
NCI [46]	BLM Infusion MTX—High dose + leukovorin CDDP				In progress
Silverberg [57]	BLM 15 mg 2 × wk.-2 mg 3 × wk. XRT	29	55%	45%	Tolerable toxicity with apparent enhanced local control

Head and neck tumors have such a high rate of local failure that attempts have been made to use BLM as an adjuvant to intensive XRT. These combined modalities appear to be tolerable and effective. In the future, considerable investigation will be directed toward interdigitating cytoreductive chemotherapy with definitive surgery or radiation or both. This approach seems most reasonable.

Testis

In no other cancer has BLM had such wide usage as in testicular cancer. The current era of highly effective protocols dates from the introduction of high dosage VLB plus BLM by Samuels et al. [52]. Fig. 4 outlines the evolution of the major protocols. Exploration of intermittent and continuous administration of BLM led to three consecutive trials by Samuels (VB_1, VB_2, and VB_3). Cvitkovic and coworkers began sequentially exploring more complicated programs including alkylators, antibiotics, VLB, and BLM. The identification of the efficacy of CDDP led to its incorporation into VAB II and VAB III as well as to Einhorn's VLB plus BLM plus CDDP program [27]. Because CR rates of 75% or more have been reported, these programs are being evaluated as adjuvant therapies to surgical procedures.
The specific dosages and response rates of these protocols are presented in Table 7. Of interest is not only the satisfying response rate, but also the long term disease control rate. It must be stressed that significant morbidity attends these therapies, but these toxicities become acceptable when the intent is "curative."

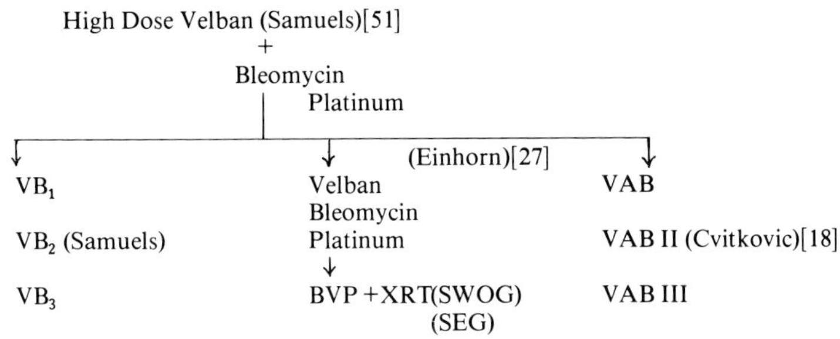

Fig. 4. Evolutionary development of chemotherapy in cancer of the testis

Table 7. Protocols for carcinoma of the testis

Study	Chemotherapy (mg/m²)	N	CR	PR	Comments
Samuels [52]	*COMF-BLM* CYT 200 D VCR 2 D1+D8 MTX 15 2× wk. 5FU 400 D1-5 BLM 30 mg/D1-8	35	43%	20%	Extragonadal
Samuels [53]	*VB-1* VLB 0.2-0.3 mg/kg D1+D2 BLM 15-20 2× wk.	26	27%		Survival better for VB-3 48 wk. > 72 wk. for embryonal tumors
	VB-3 VLB 0.2-0.3 mg/kg D1+D2 BLM 30 mg/d infusion D2-6	34	58%		
Samuels [54]	*VB-3*		65% 44%		Embryonal Teratoca (survival not different) Minimal pulmonary metastases = 18/20 CR Advanced pulmonary metastases = 15/31 CR Abdominal metastases = 9/20 CR
Cvitkovic [18]	*VAB* VAB II VAB III	71 51 80	14% 58% 63%	22% 17% 25%	NED=12% NED=23% NED=63% Only 2/192 fatal toxicities
Einhorn [27]	CDDP 20 D1-5 VLB 0.2 D2+D3 BLM 30 mg/wk. ×12 + (6 h post VLB) Maintenance VLB 0.3 mg/kg q 3 wk. + BCG	20	75%	25%	Median disease-free time > 9 months
Merrin [43]	BLM VLB CDDP Induction PRED ↓	28	68%	32%	16/28 NED at 3/18 months

Table 7. (Continued)

Study	Chemotherapy (mg/m²)		N	CR	PR	Comments
	ACTD ADM CYT ↓ ADM CYT	Consolidation Maintenance				
Daniels [19]	CYT 7 MITH 0.05 VLB 0.075 BLM 0.4	mg/kg D1–3 mg/kg D1+D3+D5 mg/kg D1–4 q 21–28 D mg/kg D1–5	11	36%		
	ACT D 0.01 MTX 0.5 CYT 10 VCR 0.025	mg/kg mg/kg D1–5 mg/kg D1 mg/kg D1 + D5	12	41%		
Blom [4]	ACT D 0.4	D1–5	42	12%	10%	Overall survival not significantly different
	ACT D 0.4 VCR 1 BLM 15	D1–5 D1 + D8 q 21 d D1+D8+D15	42	19%	50%	
Burgess [7]	ADM 75 VCR 1 BLM 30	D1 D1+D8+D15 q 21 d	25	28%	51%	
MEMO [42]	VLB 4 BLM 15 ↓ CDDP 20 VCR 1.4 ACT D 0.35 ↓ Surgical Resection	D1+D2 q 21 d 2× wk. × 7 D1–5 D1 D1–4	6	3	3	Chemotherapy preoperatively
SWOG [66]	VLB 7.5 BLM 15 XRT	D1 D2–5				Stage IB and II in progress Tolerable toxicity to date
	VLB 7.5 BLM 15	D1+22 D2–15 + D23–26				

Lung

Despite the relatively poor single agent activity of BLM against all cell types of lung cancer, its relative lack of myelosuppressive toxicity and the paucity of other active agents has led to an ordered succession of studies initiated by LIVINGSTON et al. and carried out by SWOG. Fig. 5 traces the evolution of these protocols. The use of timed sequential VCR plus BLM appeared initially promising and a series of four-drug protocols (the COMB series) [35] and a five-drug program (BACON) [36] were evaluated.

Table 8 outlines seven programs for non-oat-cell lung cancer. Disappointingly, none of these has proven significantly effective in increasing response rates or prolonging survival in the majority of patients. More critically, in a direct comparison, COMB proved more toxic and no more effective than CYT alone. Additionally, in a direct comparison between BACON and NAC, there was no superiority for the more aggressive program.

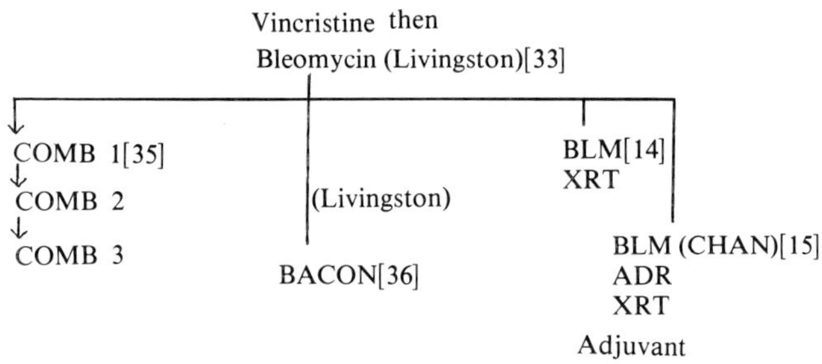

Fig. 5. Evolutionary development of chemotherapy in carcinoma of the lung

Table 8. Non-oat-cell tumors of the lung

Study	Chemotherapy (mg/m^2)	N	CR	PR	Comments
Hoogstraten [28]	CCNU 130 q 6 wk. BLM 10 × 2 wk. or 20 wk.	55		3%	
Livingston [35]	COMB CYT 800, MECCNU 100 } D1 q 4 wk. VCR 0.5–75 mg D2 2 × wk. × 48 BLM 7.5 mg D2 (6 h post VCR) 2 × wk. × 48	61		24%	11/33 squamous 3/28 adeno-carcinoma MST = 12.5 wk. PR 8.5 wk. NR
Wilson [72]	CYT	27		4%	
	COMB	20		5%	worse toxicity with COMB median survival = 11–14 wk.
Livingston [36]	*NAC*	54		23%	36+wk. median duration
	BACON CCNU 65 q 8 wk. ADR D1+D29 HN_2 8 D1+D29 VCR 0.75–1 D1+D8+D15 +D22+D29+D36 BLM 30 D1–D36	56		27%	24 wk. significant toxicity noted 4% fatality 9% severe
Lanzotti [32]	CYT 200, 5 FU 450 } D6–10 MTX 20, VCR 2 } D6+D9 BLM 15–30 infusion D1–4	38		39%	Med. survival = 36 wk. for responders (vs. 12.5 non-responders) 5/14 squamous 6/17 adenocarcinoma 4/7 large cell
CARR [10]	VCR 1.2, BLM 12 } D1+D5 (6 h post VCR) ADR 50 D2 q 4 wk.				0/12 squamous 3/18 large cell ca. 2/16 adeno ca. responses
IHDE AACR [29]	BLM 2×wk. ×6 MTX 25 2×wk. STRP 1000/wk.	14		36%	MDR = 1.5 month MST = 3.5 month Nonmyelosuppres-sive

Table 9 outlines three adjuvant trials of chemotherapy + XRT. These studiès are too preliminary to demonstrate long term effectiveness, but therapies do appear to be tolerable. Finally, Table 10 outlines two trials of combination therapy including BLM for oat cell cancer. Although both these programs are encouraging, this tumor is known to be a highly responsive one and this fact must temper any enthusiasm for a new protocol.

Table 9. Non-oat-cell tumors of the lung

Study	Chemotherapy (mg/m^2)	N	CR	PR	Comments
Samuels [50]	BLM 15 mg/wk. ×3 VCR 2 mg/wk. ×3 MTX 25–30 mg/wk. ×3 Split + course XRT 3000 r	27	19%	37%	Median survival = 70 wk. for responders
CHAN [14]	BLM 10 2× wk. + XRT 2000 r in 5 d rest 3 wk. then repeat	15		46%	Med. survival = 13 months
CHAN [15]	ADR 40 D1+D18 BLM 10 2× wk. XRT 4000 r in 5 wk. ↓ ADR BLM	40	23%	35%	22% significant esophagitis MST = 10 months responders 5 months nonresponders

Table 10. Oat-cell tumors of the lung

Study	Chemotherapy (mg/m^2)	N	CR	PR	Comments
Skarin [58]	BLM 4 mg 2× wk. ×6 ADM 45 } D1+D22+D43 CVT 600 } VCR 1.2 mg/wk. ×6 PRED 40 d ×28 wk. 8–14 XRT 6000r to BULK 3000r to CNS	9	45%	45%	Significant BLM lung toxicity led to discontinuing BLM
Eagan [23]	VCR 1.2 } D1+D5 BLM 12.5 (6 h later) } ADR 50 D2	13		38%	Median survivals 249 d

Miscellaneous

Combinations employing BLM have been used in a variety of other tumors. Table 11 outlines some of these attempts. In general the numbers of patients studied are small and these are either ongoing or proposed studies.

Table 11. Miscellaneous studies

Study	Chemotherapy (mg/m^2)	N	CR	PR	Comments
Kaufman [30]	BLM 50 infusion D1-5 ↓ VCR infusion D5 (2 h later) ↓ MTX 225 infusion D6 (18 h later) leukovorin	8	25%	36%	Anorectal cancer ½ had prior XRT
Mosende [44]	BLM 12 D1+D2 CYT 600 q 14 d ACT d 450 mcg/m^2	14		64%	Osteogenic sarcoma 6/6 response in previously untreated patients
Paladine [47]	VLB 10 } q wk. BLM 15 }	5		2	Breast cancer
SWOG 7608 [67]	BLM 25 mg/d infusion D1-4 BCNU 200 D8-12 DTIC 200 D12-16				Melanoma proposed
EST 1273 [24]	6000 r 6000r + BLM 15 q d				Esophageal cancer proposed

Summary

As bleomycin has up to now proved effective when used alone, the main thrust of current clinical investigations predominantly concerns its use in combination with other drugs. This has occurred along three broad patterns: 1) combination with vinca alkaloids which has been mainly in testicular carcinoma; 2) as part of multidrug regimens where bleomycin added for its lack of myelosuppression. This has occurred in the malignant lymphomas, lung cancer, and head and neck cancer; 3) in combination with radiotherapy which has taken place mostly in head and neck and cervix cancer. To date, the combination of velban and bleomycin has had a major impact in improving the ability to induce complete remissions in advanced testicular carcinoma. Other drugs such as cis-platinum diaminedichloride and actinomycin D have been added and no definitive combination has been established. In the lymphomas the addition of bleomycin to the MOPP or CVP regimen has given higher complete response rates, but long-term survival data are still awaited.

References

1. BAKER, L. H., OPIPARI, M.: Mitomycin C, vincristine and bleomycin in disseminated squamous cell cancer of the uterine cervix. Proc. Am. Ass. Cancer Res. **18**, No. C-21 (1977).
2. BARRANCO, S. C., HUMPHREY, R. M.: The effects of bleomycin on survival and cell progression in Chinese hamster cells *in vitro*. Cancer Res. **31**, 1218-1223 (1971).
3. BITTER, K.: Immunity suppression by bleomycin-methotrexate combined treatment in patients with epidermoid carcinoma of the oral cavity. J. Maxillofac. Surg. **2**, 35-39 (1974).

4. BLOM, J., BRODOVSKY, H. S.: Comparison of the treatment of metastatic testicular tumors with actinomycin-D or actinomycin-D, bleomycin, and vincristine. Proc. Am. Ass. Cancer Res. **17**, No. C-213 (1976).
5. BLUM, R. H., CARTER, S. K., AGRE, K.: A clinical review of bleomycin—a new antineoplastic agent. Cancer **31**, 903–914 (1973).
6. BONADONNA, G., ZUCALI, R., MONFARDINI, S., DELENA, M., USLENGHI, C.: Combination chemotherapy of Hodgkin's disease with adriamycin, bleomycin, vinblastine, and imidazole carboxamide versus MOPP. Cancer **36**, 252–259 (1975).
7. BURGESS, M. A., EINHORN, L. H., GOTTLIEB, J. A.: Treatment of metastatic germ cell tumors with adriamycin, vincristine, and bleomycin. Proc. Am. Ass. Cancer Res. **16**, No. 1094 (1975).
8. BYFIELD, J. E., SEAGREN, S. L., WEINTRAUB, I.: Combined bleomycin (Bl) and X-radiation therapy (XRT) for advanced cervix carcinoma (ACC). Proc. Am. Ass. Cancer Res. **17**, No. C-31 (1976).
9. CABANILLAS, F., RODRIGUEZ, V. M., HERSH, G., MAVLIGIT, G., BODEY, G. P., MIDDLEMAN, E. L.: Chemoimmunotherapy of advanced non-Hodgkin's lymphoma (NHL) with CHOP-BLEO + Levamisole. Proc. Am. Ass. Cancer Res. **18**, No. 248 (1977).
10. CARR, D. T., LEE, R. E., COLES, D. T.: ICRF-159 vs. poly-chemotherapy in non-oat cell lung cancer. Proc. Am. Ass. Cancer Res. **17**, No. 73 (1976).
11. CARTER, S. K.: A survey of bleomycin in multiple drug therapy in the United States. In: GANN Monograph on Cancer Research 19. Carter, S. K., Ichikawa, T., Mathé, G., Umezawa, H. (eds.). Tokyo: University of Tokyo Press 1976, pp. 285–299.
12. CASE, D. C. Jr., YOUNG, C. W., NISCE, L., LACHER, M. J., LEE, B. J. III.: Eight drug combination chemotherapy (MOPP and ABDV) and local radiotherapy for advanced Hodgkin's disease. Proc. Am. Ass. Cancer Res. **17**, No. C-71 (1976).
13. CHAN, P. Y. M., KAGAN, A. R., BYFIELD, J. E., ARONSTAM, E. M.: Combined therapy of bleomycin and external irradiation in inoperable lung cancer—a pilot study of the Western Cancer Study Group. Proc. Am. Ass. Cancer Res. **16**, No. 1085 (1975).
14. CHAN, P. Y. M., BYFIELD, J. E., KAGAN, A. R., ARONSTAM, E. M.: Unresectable squamous cell carcinoma of the lung and its management by combined bleomycin and radiotherapy. A clinical study of the enhanced results. Cancer **37**, 2671–2676 (1976).
15. CHAN, P. Y. M., BYFIELD, J. E., ARONSTAM, E. M., KAGAN, A. R.: Adriamycin (AD), bleomycin (BL) and external radiation therapy (XRT) in the treatment of advanced unresectable lung cancer. Proc. Am. Ass. Cancer Res. **18**, No. C-324 (1977).
16. CONROY, J. F., LEWIS, G. C., BRADY, L. W., BRODSKY, I., KHAN, S. B., ROSS, D., NUSS, R.: Low dose bleomycin and methotrexate in cervical cancer. Cancer **37**, 660–664 (1976).
17. COSTANZI, J.: Bleomycin (Bleo) infusion as a potential synchronizing agent in carcinoma of the head and neck. Proc. Am. Ass. Cancer Res. **17**, No. 42 (1976).
18. CVITKOVIC, E., CHENG, E., WHITMORE, W. F., GOLBEY, R. B.: Germ cell chemotherapy update. Proc. Am. Ass. Cancer Res. **18**, No. C-232 (1977).
19. DANIELS, J. R.: Testis carcinoma. Combination chemotherapy. Proc. Am. Ass. Cancer Res. **17**, No. C-181 (1976).
20. DAVIS, L. K., SHAW, M. T., SKEEL, R. T.: Bleomycin, adriamycin, CCNU and oncovin combination (BACO) in advanced and recurrent lymphomas. Proc. Am. Ass. Cancer Res. **18**, No. C-26 (1977).
21. DEVITA, V. T., SERPICK, A. A., CARBONE, P. P.: Combination chemotherapy in the treatment of advanced Hodgkin's disease. Ann. Intern. Med. **73**, 881–895 (1970).
22. DONEGAN, W. L., HARRIS, P.: Regional chemotherapy with combined drugs in cancer of the head and neck. Cancer **38**, 1479–1483 (1976).
23. EAGAN, R. T., CARR, D. T., COLES, D. T., RUBIN, J., FRYTAK, S.: ICRF-159 versus poly-chemotherapy in non-small cell lung cancer. Cancer Treat. Rep. **60**, 947–948 (1976).
24. Eastern Cooperative Oncology Group: Protocol No. EST 1273.
25. Eastern Cooperative Oncology Group: Protocol No. EST 1476.
26. Eastern Cooperative Oncology Group: Protocol No. EST 3734.
27. EINHORN, L. H., FURNAS, B. E., POWELL, N.: Combination chemotherapy of disseminated testicular carcinoma with cis-platinum, diammine dichloride (CPDD), vinblastine (VLB), and bleomycin (Bleo). Proc. Am. Ass. Cancer Res. **17**, No. C-13 (1976).
28. HOOGSTRATEN, B., HAAS, C. D., HAUT, A., TALLEY, R. W., RIVKIN, S., ISAACS, B. L.: CCNU and bleomycin in the treatment of cancer: a Southwest Oncology Group study. Med. Pediat. Oncol. **1**, 95–106 (1975).
29. IHDE, D. C., COHEN, M. H., BRODER, L. E., MINNA, J. D.: Non-myelosuppressive chemotherapy of non-small cell carcinoma of the lung with bleomycin, methotrexate and streptozotocin. Proc. Am. Ass. Cancer Res. **18**, No. 389 (1977).
30. KAUFMAN, J. H., WEBER, A., ADAMS, A., KHAN, T., MITTELMAN, A., EVANS, J. T.: Chemotherapy of advanced squamous cell carcinoma of the anus (S.A.) with high dose methotrexate (H.D. Mtx) or

continuous infusion bleomycin, vincristine and methotrexate (BOM). Proc. Am. Ass. Cancer Res. **18**, No. C-204 (1977).

31. KERR, R. O., ROSSOF, A. H., COLTMAN, C. A.: Combination chemotherapy of advanced lymphoma with BOAP. Proc. Am. Ass. Cancer Res. **17**, No. C-210 (1976).
32. LANZOTTI, V. J., THOMAS, D. R., HOLOYE, P. Y., BOYLE, L. E., SMITH, T. L., SAMUELS, M. L.: Bleomycin (NSC-125066) followed by cyclophosphamide (NSC-26271), vincristine (NSC-67574), methotrexate (NSC-740), and 5-fluorouracil (NSC-19893) for non-oat cell bronchogenic carcinoma. Cancer Treat. Rep. **60**, 61-68 (1976).
33. LIVINGSTON, R. B., BODEY, G. P., GOTTLIEB, J. A. FREI, E. III: Kinetic scheduling of vincristine (NSC-67574) and bleomycin (NSC-125066) in patients with lung cancer and other malignant tumors. Cancer Chemother. Rep. **57**, 219-224 (1973).
34. LIVINGSTON, R. B., BURGESS, M. A., HART, J. S., GOTTLIEB, J. A.: Sequential combination chemotherapy for head and neck squamous cancer. Proc. Am. Ass. Cancer Res. **16**, No. 1026 (1975).
35. LIVINGSTON, R. B., EINHORN, L. H., BODEY, G. P., BURGESS, M. A., FREIREICH, E. J., GOTTLIEB, J. A.: COMB (cyclophosphamide oncovin, methyl-CCNU, and bleomycin): a four-drug combination in solid tumors. Cancer **36**, 327-332 (1975).
36. LIVINGSTON, R. B., FEE, W. H., EINHORN, L. H., BURGESS, M. A., FREIREICH, E. J., GOTTLIEB, J. A., FARBER, M. O.: BACON (bleomycin, adriamycin, CCNU, oncovin and nitrogen mustard) in squamous lung cancer. Experience in fifty patients. Cancer **37**, 1237-1242 (1976).
37. LOH, K. K., GAMBLE, J. F., SHULLENBERGER, C. C., FULLER, L. M.: Combination chemotherapy in MOPP resistant Hodgkin's disease. Proc. Am. Ass. Cancer Res. **18**, No. C-3 (1977).
38. LOKICH: J., FREI, E. III.: Phase II study of concurrent methotrexate and bleomycin chemotherapy. Cancer Res. **34**, 2240-2242 (1974).
39. LOKICH, J. J., FREI, E. III, JAFFE, N., TULLIS, J.: New multiple-agent chemotherapy (B-Dopa) for advanced Hodgkin's disease. Cancer **38**, 667-671 (1976).
40. LUCE, J. K., GAMBLE, J. F., WILSON, H. E., MONTO, R. W., ISAACS, B. L., PALMER, R. L., COLTMAN, C. A. Jr., HEWLETT, J. S., GEHAN, E. A., FREI, E. III.: Combined cyclophosphamide, vincristine, and prednisone therapy of malignant lymphoma. Cancer **28**, 306-317 (1971).
41. MCKELVEY, E. M., GOTTLIEB, J. A., WILSON, H. E.: Hydroxyldaunomycin (Adriamycin) combination chemotherapy in malignant lymphoma. Cancer. **38**, 1484-1493 (1976).
42. MEMO, R., WISE, H., METZ, E., NEIDHART, J.: Intensive sequential chemotherapy and surgery for stage III non-seminomatous testicular cancer. Proc. Am. Ass. Cancer Res. **18**, No. 368 (1977).
43. MERRIN, C.: Multimodal treatment of advanced testicular tumor with cis di amine di chloro platinum (CPDD), bleomycin (Bleo), vinblastine (VLB), vincristine (VCR) and actinomycin D (ACT D). Proc. Am. Ass. Cancer Res. **18**, No. C-128 (1977).
44. MOSENDE, C., GUTIERREZ, M., ROSEN, G.: Bleomycin, cyclophosphamide, and dactinomycin combination chemotherapy in osteogenic sarcoma. Proc. Am. Ass. Cancer Res. **18**, C-351 (1977).
45. MURPHY, W. K., LIVINGSTON, R. B., BEHAN, E., BODEY, G. P.: Sequential chemotherapy in the treatment of cancer of the head and neck. Proc. Am. Ass. Cancer Res. **18**, No. 758 (1977).
46. NCI Protocol.
47. PALADINE, W., USBORNE, C., CUNNINGHAM, T. J., OLSON, K., SPONZO, R.: Treatment of advanced breast cancer with vinblastine and bleomycin. Proc. Am. Ass. Cancer Res. **17**, No. C-147 (1976).
48. PORZIG, K., ROBERTSON, A.: Treatment of advanced Hodgkin's disease (HD) with B-CAVe following MOPP failure. Proc. Am. Ass. Cancer Res. **18**, No. C-303 (1977).
49. RODRIGUEZ, V., CABANILLAS, E., BURGESS, M. A.: Combination chemotherapy ("CHOP-Bleo") in advanced (non-Hodgkin's) malignant lymphoma. Blood **49**, 325-333 (1977).
50. SAMUELS, M. L., JOHNSON, D. E., HOLOYE, P. Y.: The treatment of stage 3 metastatic germinal cell neoplasia of the testis with bleomycin combination chemotherapy. Proc. Am. Ass. Cancer Res. **14**, No. 89 (1973).
51. SAMUELS, M. L., BARKLEY, H. T., HOLOYE, P. Y., ROSENBERG, P. J., SMITH, T. L.: Combination chemotherapy with bleomycin (NSC-125066), vincristine (NSC-67574) and methotrexate (NSC-740) plus split-course radiotherapy in the treatment of non-oat-cell bronchogenic carcinoma. Cancer Chemother. Rep. Part 1. **59**, 377-383 (1975).
52. SAMUELS, M. L., HOLOYE, P. Y., JOHNSON, D. E.: Bleomycin combination chemotherapy in the management of testicular neoplasia. Cancer **36**, 318-326 (1975).
53. SAMUELS, M. L., BOYLE, L. E., HOLOYE, P. Y., JOHNSON, D. E.: Intermittent versus continuous infusion bleomycin in testicular cancer: A comparison of response and survival in embryonal carcinoma (class 2) and teratocarcinoma (class 3 & 4). Proc. Am. Ass. Cancer Res. **17**, No. 392 (1976).
54. SAMUELS, M. L., LANZOTTI, V. J., HOLOYE, P. Y., HOWE, C. D.: Stage III testicular cancer: Complete response by substage to velban plus continuous bleomycin infusion (VB-3). Proc. Am. Ass. Cancer Res. **18**, No. 584 (1977).
55. SARNA, G. P., HASKELL, C. M.: Combination chemotherapy including methotrexate and rescue for

non-Hodgkin's lymphomas. Proc. Am. Ass. Cancer Res. **18**, No. C-213 (1977).
56. SCHEIN, P., DEVITA, V., CANELLOS, G., CHABNER, B., YOUNG, R.: A new combination chemotherapy program for diffuse histiocytic (DHL) and mixed (DML) non-Hodgkin's lymphoma: BACOP. Proc. Am. Ass. Cancer Res. **16**, No. 1108 (1975).
57. SILVERBERG, I. J., PHILLIPS, T. L., FU, K. K., CHAN, P. Y. M.: Bleomycin with radiation therapy in the treatment of head and neck malignancies. Proc. Am. Ass. Cancer Res. **17**, No. C-170 (1976).
58. SKARIN, A., ROSENTHAL, D., MOLONEY, W., FREI, E. III.: Treatment of advanced non-Hodgkin's lymphoma (NHL) with bleomycin (B), adriamycin (A), cyclophosphamide (C), vincristine (O) and prednisone (P) (BACOP). Proc. Am. Ass. Cancer Res. **15**, No. 531 (1974).
59. Southeast Oncology Group Protocol 75HD0103.
60. Southwest Oncology Group Protocol 774 (MOPP #4).
61. Southwest Oncology Group Protocol 7406.
62. Southwest Oncology Group Protocol 7426/27.
63. Southwest Oncology Group Protocol 7517.
64. Southwest Oncology Group Protocol 7518.
65. Southwest Oncology Group Protocol 7519.
66. Southwest Oncology Group Protocol 7527.
67. Southwest Oncology Group Protocol 7608.
68. STEINBERG, D., SPARKS, J. T.: Bleomycin, velban, adriamycin and prednisone (B-VAP) in advanced resistant non-Hodgkin's lymphoma and Hodgkin's disease (HD). Proc. Am. Ass. Cancer Res. **18**, No. 223 (1977).
69. STEINHERZ, P., TAN, C., GHAVINI, F., HELSON, L., ROSEN, G., WOLLNER, N.: VAB III combination chemotherapy in childhood malignancies. Proc. Am. Ass. Cancer Res. **18**, No. C-231 (1977).
70. VINCIGUERRA, V., COLEMAN, M., DEGNAN, T. J., JAROWSKI, C. I., SILVER, R. T.: BVDS—A polychemotherapy regimen for MOPP refractory Hodgkin's disease. Proc. Am. Ass. Cancer Res. **17**, No. C-266 (1976).
71. VOGL, S. E., KAPLAN, B. H.: Methotrexate, bleomycin, and cis-diaminedichloroplatinum in combination for squamous cancer. Proc. Am. Ass. Cancer Res. **18**, No. C-200 (1977).
72. WILSON, H., LAGAKOS, S., BODEY, G., GUTIERREZ, A., SELAWRY, O., SEALY, R., RYALL, R. D.: Therapy of advanced epidermoid carcinoma: Lung. Proc. Am. Ass. Cancer Res. **17**, No. C-232 (1976).
73. WILSON, J. A., MOTT, M. G., WILBUR, J. R.: Intensive combination chemotherapy of childhood non-Hodgkin's lymphoma (NHL). Proc. Am. Ass. Cancer Res. **18**, No. C-202 (1977).
74. YAGODA, A., LIPPMAN, A. J., WINN, R. J., SCHULMAN, P., COHEN, F. B.: Combination chemotherapy with bleomycin (BLM) and methotrexate (MTX) in patients with advanced epidermoid carcinomas. Proc. Am. Ass. Cancer Res. **16**, No. 1105 (1975).

Combined Use of Bleomycin with Radiation in the Treatment of Cancer

M. ABE, Y. SHIGEMATSU, and S. KIMURA

In August 1974, a cooperative study was started by 18 institutions in the Kansai district to evaluate the effect of bleomycin combined with radiotherapy in the treatment of esophagal, bronchogenic and intra-oral carcinomas. The objective of this study was to determine whether the combined use of bleomycin with radiotherapy would yield results superior to those of radiotherapy alone. This report presents the preliminary data accumulated in this study up to the present time.

During the period 1974-1976, a total of 189 cancer patients who had not received any previous treatment were enrolled in this study: 72 with esophagal carcinoma, 50 with bronchogenic carcinoma and 67 with intra-oral carcinoma. These patients were studied by controlled trial and thus were randomized into two option groups by enveloped numbers distributed to the institutions. The option groups were: 1. Combined treatment by bleomycin plus radiotherapy, and 2. control treatment by radiotherapy alone.

Radiotherapy consisted of a total dose of 3000 rad of supervoltage radiation using either ^{60}Co or Linac administered in 200 rad doses five times weekly over a 3 week period. Bleomycin, given along with radiotherapy, consisted of a total dose of 67.5 mg administered intramuscularly in 7.5 mg doses three times a week over a three week period. In the case of intra-oral carcinoma, however, the program consisted of a total dose of 90.0 mg administered intravenously in 15 mg doses twice a week over a 3 week period. On the basis of previous clinical experience, it was suggested by several participating doctors that this modified program be adopted because of its advantages in terms of enhancing local control of intra-oral carcinoma.

The bleomycin program was determined from experimental and clinical data published previously. In an experimental study by TERASHIMA [5], mouse fibroblastic cells and lymphatic leukemia cells were treated with varying concentrations of bleomycin. Survival response, indicated by an upward concave curvature, consists of a steep portion as well as a more gradual portion. The gradual portion has been shown to be the result of resistance induced by bleomycin. This resistance disappeared 4 h after removal of the drug. It should be noted then, that in view of this finding, it can be considered a more reasonable clinical procedure to administer smaller doses of bleomycin in greater frequency rather than less frequent and larger doses of the same cumulative amount. Clinically, with regard to the timing of bleomycin administration in conjunction with irradiation, little difference has been reported in the overall effectiveness of combined treatment. The scheduling of bleomycin, therefore, whether it was to be given before or after irradiation, was not especially defined.

The entire treatment program was divided into two phases. In the first phase, patients followed the 3 week fixed treatment schedule mentioned above. In the second phase, beginning one week after the end of the first phase, patients were assigned to subsequent treatment programs—i.e., operation or further radiotherapy—whichever was considered best by the participating doctors. This study could thus proceed without any ethical problems. Summary of the treatment schedule in the controlled trial is shown in Fig. 1.

Local effects of treatment were evaluated at the end of the first phase of treatment and upon the completion of the entire treatment. Crude survival rates up to 18 months after treatment were also calculated. Stage grouping of esophagal, bronchogenic and intra-oral carcinomas was made according to the UICC classification proposed in 1973.

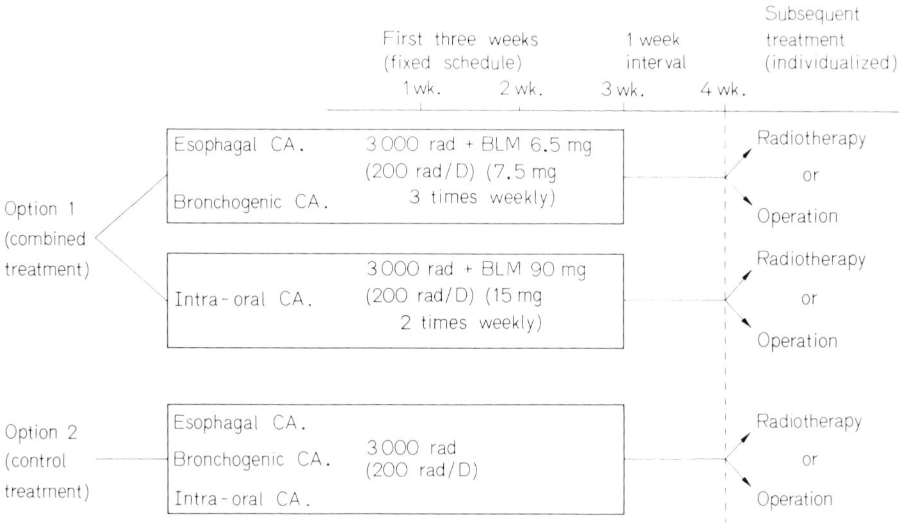

Fig. 1. Treatment schedule of controlled trial

Esophagal Carcinoma

Criteria of Ineligibility for the Trial

Patients excluded from the study were those a) over 70 years of age, b) having marked fibrosis or active tuberculosis in the lung, c) having fistula of the esophagus, d) having marked stenosis requiring gastrostomy, e) having distant metastasis.

Materials

Of the 72 patients originally assigned to the two treatment groups, 13 had to be excluded because of incomplete data. Of the remaining 59 patients, 27 received combined treatment and 32 received radiotherapy alone. As shown in Table 1, stage distribution is practically identical in both groups.

Results

a) Tumor Response

In order to compare the direct effect of combined treatment on the primary lesion with that of radiotherapy alone, the tumor regression rate was calculated from the tumor size measured weekly after treatment. The tumor size was estimated by the length of its longitudinal axis on X-ray film. The tumor regression rate was expressed as the percentage of residual tumor size over initial tumor size. In the second phase of treatment, six patients in the combined treatment group and 12 in the control group received operations, and hence, evaluation for tumor response in these patients could only be made up to the end of the first phase of treatment.

As shown in Table 2, residual tumor size at the completion of the entire treatment was found to be about 7% smaller in the combined treatment group than in the control group. For the polypoid type, the effect of combined treatment was found to be significant. The tumor disappearance rate in the combined treatment group was 33.3% (7/27), while in the control group it was 15.6% (5/32).

b) Survival Rate

Table 3 shows the crude survival rate up to 18 months after treatment. The survival rate of patients in the control group was about 10% higher than that of the combined treatment group.

Bronchogenic Carcinoma

Criteria of Ineligibility of the Trial

Patients excluded from this study were those a) over 70 years of age, b) having heart disease, inflammatory lesions or marked fibrosis in the lung, c) with carcinoma diagnosed as oat cell, d) having pleural effusion, e) having undergone an operation other than an exploratory one, f) having a lesion classified as T_4, g) having distant metastasis.

Materials

Of the 50 patients enrolled in this study, 23 belonged to the combined treatment group and 27 to the control group. Stage distribution in both groups is shown in Table 4. The number of cases in which the tumor size could be measured from X-ray film was 12 in the combined treatment group and 17 in the control group. Histologic distribution, which may play the most important role in determining tumor response to radiation, can be considered to be practically identical in both groups (Table 5). Stage distribution between groups was also almost equivalent.

Results

a) Tumor Response

Tumor regression rate was calculated from changes in tumor size which was computed as the product of maximum length times maximum width, as measured from X-ray film. The percentage of residual tumor after treatment is shown in Table 6. After 3 weeks, combined treatment resulted in an 18% reduction in tumor size compared to 42% in the control group. At the completion of the entire treatment, combined treatment resulted in a 48% reduction compared to 58% in the control group.

b) Survival rate
The crude survival rate of patients with bronchogenic carcinoma is shown in Table 7. At 6 months, the survival rate for the combined treatment group exceeded that of the control group by about 10%; at 12 months, by about 15%; and at 18 months, by about 6%.

Intra-oral Carcinoma

Criteria of Ineligibility for the Trial

Patients excluded from this study were those a) over 70 years of age, b) having marked fibrosis or active tuberculosis in the lung, c) having a histologic diagnosis other than squamous cell carcinoma, d) having a lesion classified as T_1, e) having a fixed lymphadenopathy in the neck, f) having distant metastasis.

Materials

Of the 67 patients entered in this study, 34 received combination treatment and 33 control treatment. Stage and site distributions are shown in Tables 8 and 9, respectively. Frequency of gingival carcinoma was considerably higher than that of other types. Stage distribution can be considered to be equivalent in both groups.

Results

a) Tumor Response
The effect of treatment was evaluated weekly in terms of tumor regression as well as at the completion of the entire course of treatment. Tumor response was classified as R_3 (complete or almost complete regression), R_2 (regression of more than 50%), R_1 (regression of less than 50%) and R_0 (no regression). As shown in Fig. 2, the combined treatment group had a significantly higher tumor regression rate than that of the control group. Complete tumor regression was achieved in a total of 15 out of 34 patients (44.1%) in the combined treatment group in contrast to five out of 33 patients (15.2%) in the control group.
b) Mucosal Reaction
In intra-oral carcinoma, the most undesirable side effect in radiotherapy is mucositis. This adverse effect was evaluated in terms of the degree of mucosal reaction and classified as S_3 (ulceration with bleeding or severe coating tongue), S_2 (intensive inflammation or moderate coating tongue), S_1 (edematous inflammation or slight coating tongue) and S_0 (no reaction). The mucosal reaction scored weekly after irradiation is shown in Fig. 3. Mucosal reaction was significantly high in the combined treatment group. In all cases, however, this reaction subsided within a 2-4 week period after treatment.
c) Survival Rate
Table 10 shows crude survival rates up to 18 months in both groups. The 18 month survival rate in the combined treatment group exceeded the rate for the control group by about 20%.

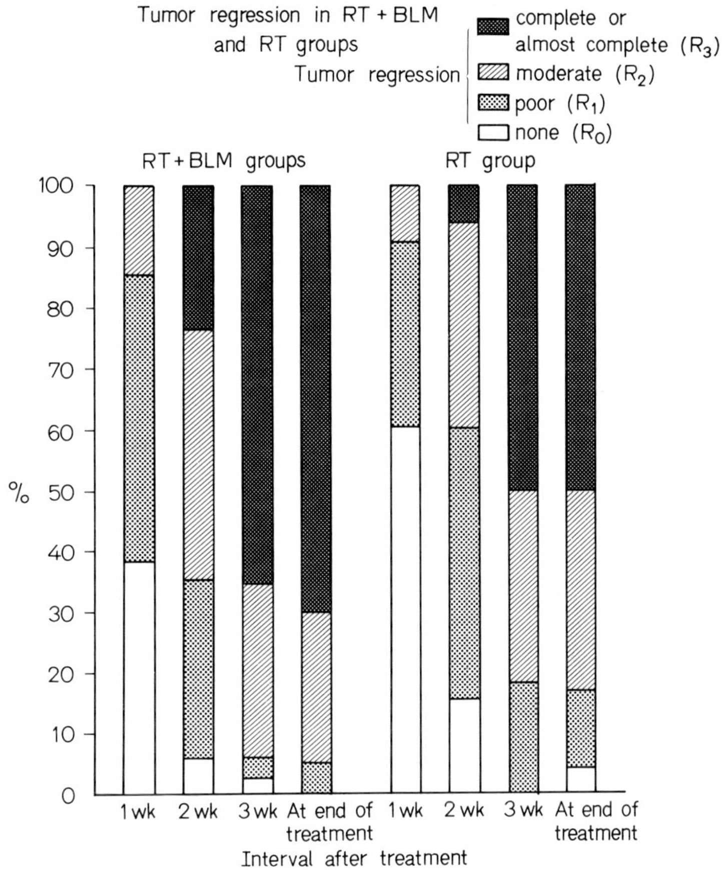

Fig. 2. Intra-oral carcinoma

Discussion

Recently the advantage of simultaneous combined treatment of bleomycin with radiation has been suggested by experimental studies. Bleomycin interferes with cell repair following radiation and this indicates the possibility of a synergistic action potential between the two agents [2, 6]. Encouraging results were reported in head and neck tumors [1, 4] as well as esophagal carcinoma [7]. However, it has also been pointed out that clinical response to bleomycin appears to vary among individuals and even among the same histologic lesions [3]. Our data, accumulated in this study up to the present time, has shown that in the case of intra-oral carcinoma, a significantly superior tumor response was obtained in the combined treatment group. However, in the case of bronchogenic and esophagal carcinomas, no significant difference was found except for esophagal carcinoma of polypoid type. This discrepancy may be considered to derive from differences among the diseases themselves as well as differences in the bleomycin treatment schedule. For most patients with intra-oral carcinoma, the simultaneous combination of a total radiation dose of 3000 rad plus a total

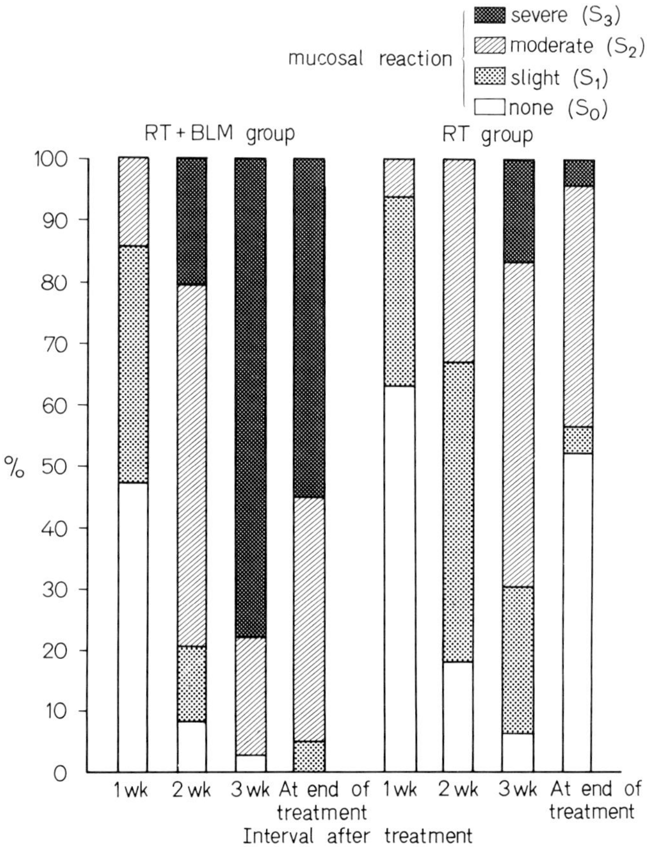

Fig. 3. Mucosal reaction in RT + BLM and RT groups

bleomycin dose of 90 mg over 3 weeks was found to be the tolerance limit of the mucosal membrane. On the other hand, combined treatment was adoptable for most bronchogenic and esophagal carcinoma patients.

Concerning survival response of esophagal and bronchogenic carcinoma patients, there seems to be no definite evidence derived from our study that combined use of bleomycin with radiotherapy significantly improves the survival rate in comparison with radiotherapy alone. In intra-oral carcinoma, the 18 month follow-up after combined treatment gave a survival rate higher by about 20% than after radiotherapy alone. To date, the follow-up of our patients is too premature to arrive at any conclusive evaluation. Our clinical trial is now working toward making a fuller assessment of the effectiveness of the combined use of bleomycin with radiotherapy in a more prolonged follow-up study.

Summary

1. The data accumulated in this study up to the present time shows that combined treatment of radiation and bleomycin in intra-oral carcinoma resulted in marked tumor regression and

a significantly higher tumor disappearance rate as compared with radiotherapy alone. The 18 month survival rate for the combined treatment group exceeded the rate for the control group by about 20%.

2. In esophagal carcinoma, bleomycin in combination with radiation markedly improved the regression rate of polypoid type tumor, while no significant improvement was observed in other types. The 18 month survival rate of the control group was about 10% higher than that of the combined treatment group.

3. In bronchogenic carcinoma, no significant difference was observed in tumor regression or survival rate of either group.

Tables

Table 1. Stage distribution of esophagal carcinoma

Stage	RT + BLM group		RT group	
	No. of pts.	Percentage	No. of pts.	Percentage
I	3	11.1%	6	18.8%
II	21	77.8%	24	75.0%
III	3	11.1%	2	6.2%
Total	27	100%	32	100%

Table 2. Comparison of tumor regression by radiotherapy plus bleomycin (RT+BLM) and by radiotherapy alone (RT) in the treatment of esophagal carcinoma

Morphological type	Mode of treatment	No. of patients	Average length of lesion	Percentage of residual tumor	
				At 3000 rad	At the end of treatment
Polypoid	RT + BLM	5	7.2 cm	55.4%	14.8%
	RT	7	5.0 cm	64.3%	33.3%
Saw	RT + BLM	6	6.3 cm	74.5%	58.8%
	RT	3	6.7 cm	76.3%	72.3%
Funnel	RT + BLM	7	7.9 cm	41.0%	37.9%
	RT	7	7.7 cm	60.7%	40.1%
Spiral	RT +BLM	16	7.9 cm	67.7%	42.4%
	RT	21	7.1 cm	70.7%	51.0%
Total	RT + BLM	34	7.5 cm	61.6%	40.3%
	RT	38	6.8 cm	68.0%	47.4%

Table 3. Crude survival rates of patients with esophagal carcinoma

Mode of treatment	6 months	12 months	18 months
RT + BLM	$19_{(5)}/27_{(6)}$ =70.4%	$19_{(4)}/25_{(6)}$ =36.0%	$2_{(2)}/22_{(6)}$ = 13.6%
RT	$22_{(9)}/32_{(12)}$ =68.8%	$15_{(7)}/30_{(10)}$ =50.0%	$6_{(2)}/25_{(8)}$ =24.0%

( ): Number of patients having received operation as subsequent treatment.

Table 4. Stage distribution of bronchogenic carcinoma

Stage	RT + BLM group		RT Group	
	No. of pts.	Percentage	No. of pts.	Percentage
I	5	21.7%	9	33.3%
II	10	43.5%	12	44.5%
III	8	34.8%	6	22.2%
Total	23	100%	27	100%

Table 5. Histological distribution of patients with bronchogenic carcinoma in whom tumor size could be measured from X-ray film

Histology	RT + BLM group		RT group	
	No. of pts.	Percent.	No. of pts.	Percent.
Squamous cell carcinoma	5	41.6%	8	47.1%
Adenocarcinoma	3	25.0%	6	35.3%
Undifferentiated cell carcinoma	2	16.7%	2	11.8%
Unestablished	2	16.7%	1	5.8%
Total	12	100%	17	100%

Table 6. Percentage of residual tumor in bronchogenic carcinoma after treatment.

Mode of treatment	At 3000 rad	At the end of treatment
RT + BLM	81.8% (12 cases)	51.9% (7 cases)
RT	57.5% (17 cases)	42.1% (10 cases)

Table 7. Crude survival rates of patients with bronchogenic carcinoma

Mode of treatment	6 months	12 months	18 months
RT+BLM	$19_{(5)}/23_{(5)}$ = 82.6%	$8_{(2)}/18_{(3)}$ = 44.4%	$2_{(1)}/15_{(2)}$ = 13.5%
RT	$19_{(4)}/27_{(4)}$ = 70.4%	$5_{(1)}/17_{(4)}$ = 29.4%	$1_{(0)}/14_{(3)}$ = 7.1%

( ): Number of patients having received operation as subsequent treatment.

Table 8. Stage distribution of intra-oral carcinoma

RT + BLM group (total 34 cases)			RT group (total 33 cases)		
	T_2	T_3		T_2	T_3
N_0	15	5	N_0	13	6
N_1	4	3	N_1	6	4
N_2	2	2	N_2	1	1
N_3	3	0	N_3	2	0

Table 9. Site distribution of intra-oral carcinoma

Site	RT + BLM group		RT group	
	No. of pts.	Percent.	No. of pts.	Percent.
Gingiva	14	41.2%	17	51.5%
Tongue	5	14.7%	6	18.2%
Mouth floor	7	20.6%	4	12.1%
Palate	7	20.6%	4	12.1%
Buccal mucosa	1	2.9%	2	6.1%
Total	34	100%	33	100%

Table 10. Crude survival rates of patients with intra-oral carcinoma

Mode of treatment	6 months	12 months	18 months
RT+BLM	$31_{(15)}/31_{(15)}$ = 100%	$18_{(9)}/32_{(14)}$ = 78.3%	$16_{(7)}/21_{(11)}$ = 76.2%
RT	$29_{(15)}/30_{(16)}$ = 96.7%	$19_{(12)}/24_{(12)}$ = 79.2%	$11_{(5)}/20_{(9)}$ = 55.0%

( ): Number of patients having received operation as subsequent treatment.

References

1. Berdal, P., Ekroll, T., Iversen, O. H., Weyde, R.: Treatment of squamous cell carcinomas in head and neck with bleomycin and with combined bleomycin and X-rays. Acta Otolaryngol. **75**, 318–320 (1973).
2. Jørgensen, S. J.: Time-dose relationship in combined bleomycin treatment and radiotherapy. Eur. J. Cancer **8**, 93–97 (1972).
3. Nabeya, K.: The use of bleomycin in the treatment of carcinoma of the esophagus. In: Fundamental and Clinical Studies of Bleomycin. Carter, S. K., Ichikawa, T., Mathé, G., Umezawa, H. (eds.) Tokyo: University of Tokyo Press 1976, Gann Monograph on Cancer Research No. 19, pp. 177–186.
4. Shanta, V., Rangakumar, G., Sattar, D. A.: Combined therapy of buccal mucosal cancers using ^{60}Co beam therapy and bleomycin: Preliminary report on a clinical trial. Jap. J. Clin. Oncol. **6**, 83–86 (1972).
5. Terashima, T., Takabe, Y., Katsumata, T., Watanabe, M., Umezawa, H.: Effect of bleomycin on mammalian cell survival. J. Natl. Cancer Inst. **49**, 1093–1100 (1972).
6. Terashima, T., Watanabe, M., Takabe, Y., Miyamoto, T.: Action of bleomycin on proliferative capacity of mammalian cells. In: Fundamental and Clinical Studies of Bleomycin. Carter, S. K., Ichikawa, T., Mathé: G., Umezawa, H. (eds.) Tokyo: University of Tokyo Press 1976, Gann Monograph on Cancer Research No. 19, pp. 63–82.
7. Yamashita, H., Nagase, T., Kamada, R., Chujo, H., Gomi, M., Honda, Y., Amino, S. Horiguchi, N., Kaneda, K., Yokoyama, T., Mikuriya, S., Matsumoto, K.: Combined treatment of malignant tumor with irradiation and bleomycin. J. Jap. Cancer Ther. **7**, 1–15 (1972). (in Japanese with English summary).

A Sequential Combination of Bleomycin and Mitomycin C in the Treatment of Advanced Squamous Cancers

T. MIYAMOTO

Summary

The 49 patients with squamous cell type of cervical, lung, esophagus and head and neck cancers were treated with a sequential combination of bleomycin (BLM) and mitomycin C (MMC) as follows; 5 mg of BLM daily for 5 or 7 days followed by a single injection of 10 mg of MMC on day 6 or day 8. After one week of rest period, this course was repeated two to five times depending on the response or adverse effects. For cervical cancer, 17 patients out of 18 (94%) responded with complete remission (CR) in 13 (72%) and partial remission (PR) in 4 (22%). For lung cancer, four patients out of five responded. In two of the responders, metastatic tumors disappeared completely, but primary tumors decrease to about 10% in volume. For esophagal cancer, one patient out of 3 had CR after combining the BLM and MMC treatment with radiotherapy. For head and neck cancer, these were some differences in the response rates between two hospitals. In one hospital, 12 patients out of 22 (53%) responded, with CR in 4 (18%), whereas in the other hospital, 10 patients out of 11 (94%) responded, including eight with CR (72%). Regarding the toxicity, the overall incidence was very low, although lung complications were frequent. These results are promising with hopeful prospects for the control of advanced squamous cancers with metastasis.

Introduction

Mitomycin C (MMC) and bleomycin (BLM) were discovered in Japan by Hata et al. in 1950 [6] and Umezawa et al. in 1966 [17], respectively. After a long term of clinical trials, both drugs have come to assume an important position in cancer chemotherapy.

MMC is one of the most reliable anti-cancer agents which is effective in various tumors such as cancers of the gastrointestinal tract, ovary, breast and lung. The dose-limiting toxicity of the drug is damage to hematopoiesis.

BLM is effective in various kinds of malignancy such as squamous cancer, lymphomas and testicular cancer. The dose-limiting toxicity is lung complications such as fibrosis.

The response rate of these sensitive tumors to both drugs was approximately 20%-30% with rare cases of complete remission. As described below, a combined use of BLM with MMC produced an excellent response in almost all advanced squamous cancers with metastasis. The unique combination of BLM and MMC, introduced in this paper, has been developed on the basis of information of the specific in vitro effect of MMC on the cells at G2, synchronized by successive administration of BLM. The clinical results obtained with our combined modality will be presented.

Materials and Methods

Drug Regimen

The protocol of the combined use of BLM with MMC is illustrated in Fig. 1. BLM at a dose of 5 mg is given every day for 5 or 7 days by drip infusion or intramuscularly followed by an injection of MMC at a dose of 10 mg on day 6 or 8. This is one course of bleomycin-mitomycin (B-M) therapy for induction. The course is usually repeated four or five times at an interval of one week rest period.

Evaluation of Response

Complete remission (CR) was defined as a disappearance of all clinical evidence of tumor. Partial remission (PR) was defined as a response in which all tumors were reduced in volume by more than 50%, but complete disappearance was not achieved. Other responses were classified as no remission (NR).

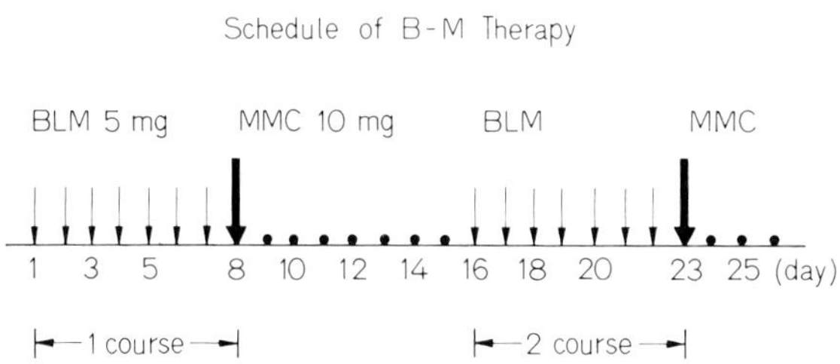

Fig. 1. Illustrated protocol of bleomycin and mitomycin-C (B-M) therapy

Results

Table 1 shows the response of cervical, lung, esophagus and head and neck cancers to B-M therapy. All cancers were the squamous cell type except for few in which no histology was available. The data for the first three types of cancer were obtained from the Division of Hospital, National Institute of Radiological Sciences (N.I.R.S.). The data for the head and neck cancer were from the Keio University and Miyazaki Prefectual Hospital, respectively.

In N.I.R.S., 21 patients with metastatic cervical cancer have been treated with this combination. 18 of them were objectively evaluated. All of the evaluated patients, except for one, 94% did respond; there were 13 complete responders (72%) and four partial responders (22%).

Table 2 shows the signs and symptoms of the complete responders before therapy and the number of B-M courses given. All of the signs and symptoms disappeared within two courses on average and in three courses at the longest.

Responses in some cases with CR are presented in Figs. 2 to 8. As shown in Figs. 2 to 6, lung tumors disappeared completely or changed into scar on roentgenogram after two to five courses of B-M therapy. Fig. 6 and 7 are from the same patient. Upper roentgenogram in

Fig. 7 shows the destruction of the 3rd proximal phalanx by a metastatic tumor. After four courses of B-M therapy, the finger became shorter because of tumor regression and subsequent shortening of the involved bone. As shown in left scan in Fig. 8, a space occupying lesion in a swollen liver disappeared completely with concomitant reduction in liver size after five courses (right scan in Fig. 8).

Table 1. Results of B-M therapy

	Number of patients	CR	PR: Complete disappearance of some tumors	PR: No disappearance	NR	% Remission (CR)
Cervical cancer	18	13	2	2	1	94 (72)
Lung cancer	5		3	1	1	
Esophagus cancer	3	1 (radiotherapy)			2	
Head and neck cancer	[a]22	4		8	10	54 (18)
	[b]11	8		2	1	90 (72)

[a] Keio university
[b] Miyazaki Prefectual Hospital

CR Complete remission
PR Partial remission

Table 2. Signs and symptoms and their response

Case No. (with complete remission)	Symptoms and signs before treatment	No. of B-M courses before disappearance of symptoms and signs
1	cough	1
2	cough	1
3	bloody sputum, cough	2
4	mild dyspnea	2
5	cough, dysphagia, lumbago	2
6	cough, dyspnea	1-2
7	bloody sputum, cough, bone pain	2-3
8	cough	1
9	cough	1
10	lumbago	2
12	paralysis of legs, incontinence leg pain, lumbago	1-3
14	lumbago, chest pain	2
15	leg and thigh pain	2-3
average		2

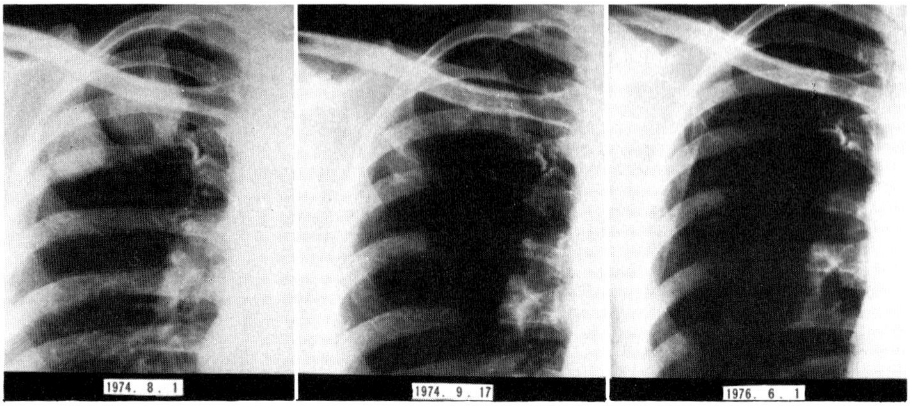

Fig. 2. A 61 year old woman with cervical cancer. Lung metastases appeared 1.5 years after the radiotherapy to the primary, at stage of III. Photographs show the chest roentgenograms before treatment (left), after the fifth course of B-M therapy (middle), and 1.5 years after the final (seventh) administration of MMC (right). Tomograms at the time of the right film show that the tumor changed into scar

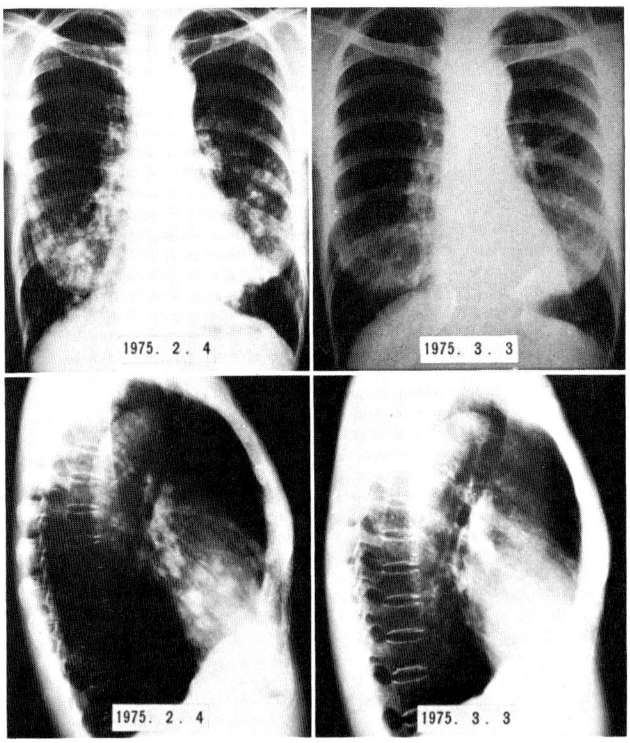

Fig. 3. A 69 year old woman who had cervical cancer with multiple lung metastases. Following the radiotherapy to the primary, the patient was treated with this combination. Left upper and lower chest films are before treatment and right upper and lower chest films are after the second course of B-M therapy. The tomograms after the treatment had tumor shadow

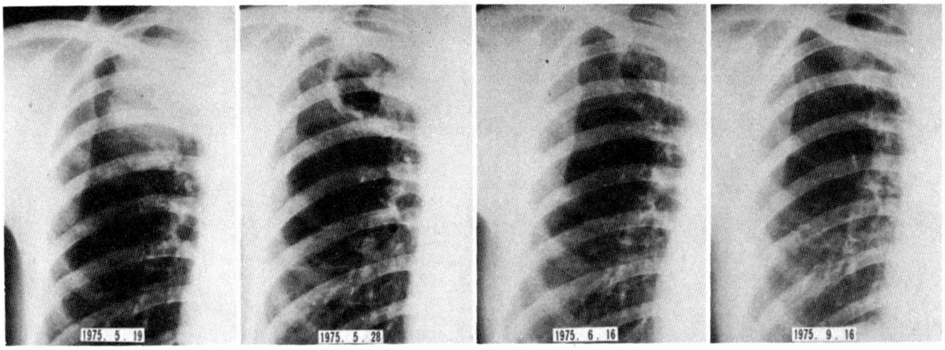

Fig. 4. A 44 year old woman with cervical cancer. Radical irradiation had been given to the primary 6 years before lung tumor appeared. From left to right, the chest films before treatment, after the first course, after the third and after the fifth. She had a fever of over 38°C for 2 days after the first shot of MMC. The second chest film shows a big cavity in collapsed tumor suggesting a casual relation to the fever

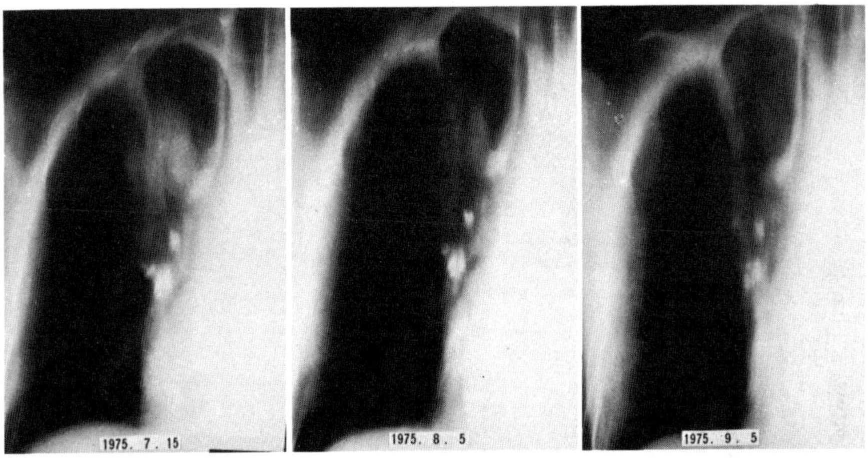

Fig. 5. A 51 year old woman with cervical cancer. She had successive recurrence in the Virchow's lymph-node, mediastinum and esophagus over 3 years after radiotherapy to the primary. These metastases were successfully controlled by irradiation. But finally metastases appeared in the lungs. The chest tomograms before treatment (left), after the first course (middle) and after the second (right) demonstrate a remarkable response

Five patients with lung cancer have been treated with B-M regimen. Four of them responded, but there was no CR. In one of them, in whom the primary tumor in the right upper lung had disappeared by neutron therapy, metastases in the skin, lymph nodes and bones were treated with the combination. After two courses, tumors in the skin and lymph node decreased to 10% in volume and the ossification occurred in the involved bones with relief of pain. In the patients shown in Figs. 9 and 10, the tumors regressed clearly after three courses. The metastatic tumors responded to a much greater extent than the primary, and disappeared completely.

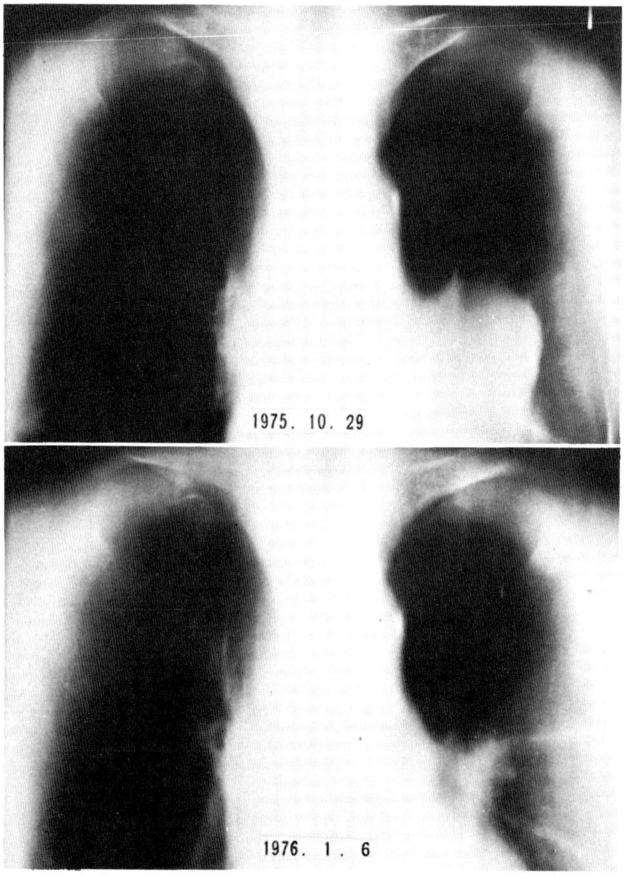

Figs. 6 and 7. A 54 year old woman with cervical cancer. Lung and bone metastases appeared 6 months after the radiotherapy to the primary at stage of II. She complained of severe bone pain caused by metastasis in the left scapula and the third proximal phalanx with swelling of the finger. Upper tomogram and bone film are before therapy, and the film below after four courses

Three patients with esophagus cancer metastasized to lung or supraclacular region were also treated. In one of them, primary and metastatic tumors in the supraclavicular region disappeared completely after four courses of B-M therapy combined with simultaneous radiotherapy.

Patients with head and neck cancer have been treated by this regimen at the Keio University and Miyazaki Prefectual Hospitals. As shown in Table 1, there was some difference in response rate between the two hospitals. 12 out of 22 patients (52%) responded, including four patients with CR (18%) in Keio University, whereas 10 out of 11 patients (94%) with relapsed and advanced cancer also responded, including eight with CR (72%) in Miyazaki Prefectual Hospital.

The dose-limiting toxicity was evaluated for the cases at N.I.R.S. and Keio University. At N.I.R.S. the evaluation was restricted to the patients with cervical cancer. As indicated in Table 3, the frequency of lung complications was clearly greater in comparison with that in single use of BLM (3), (19). Two patients died of lung fibrosis. The frequency of leucopenia

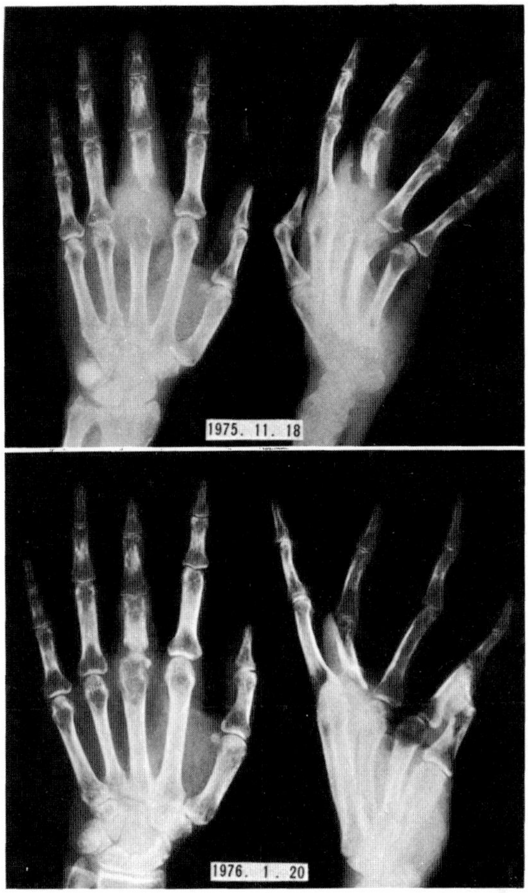

Fig. 7

($<2{,}000/mm^3$) was different between the two institutes. The higher frequency in N.I.R.S. may be due to the fact of that all the patients in the past had irradiation of over 3000 rads to the entire pelvis.

Discussion

The effect of BLM and MMC in a single and systemic use on metastatic cervical cancer was about 20%-30% in terms of response rate [4]. In contrast, the combined use of BLM with MMC produced a much higher response rate of 92%, with CR in 72%, which was superior to that of any other combination for this cancer [7].

For lung cancer of a squamous type, the response rate for each drug was less than 10% in single use [5]. No other combinations ever produced a response rate greater than 20% [5]. Although the number of patients with lung cancer treated with B-M therapy is not yet sufficient for evaluation, it seems that this combination will produce a much better response than others reported previously.

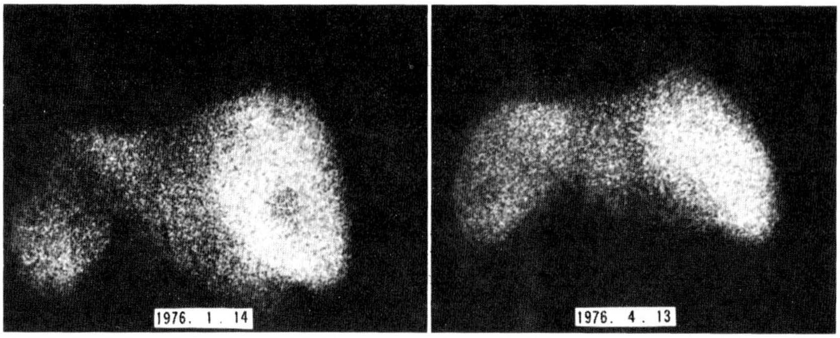

Fig. 8. A 49 year old woman with cervical cancer. She had metastases to the lung, bone and liver 1.5 years after radiotherapy to the primary at stage of II. After the fifth course of B-M therapy, the space occupying lesion, hepatomegaly and lung metastases disappeared. Photograph shows the liver scans with ^{99m}Tc phytate before treatment (left) and after the fifth course (right)

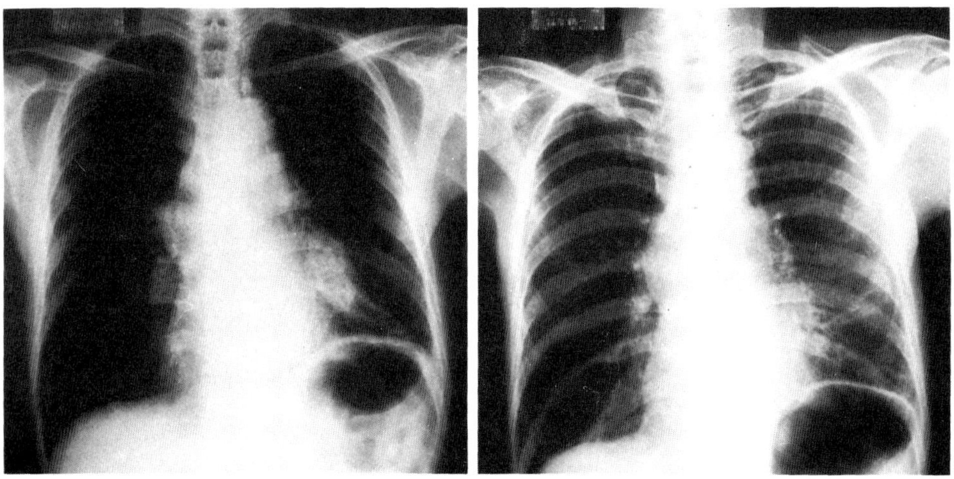

Fig. 9. A 65 year old man with lung cancer. He complained of dyspnea and hoarseness, which disappeared after the third course. Left chest film is before treatment and right after three courses

BLM in single use was fairly effective to head and neck cancer, but there were few patients with CR [3]. MMC was much less effective than BLM [11]. Despite the different response rates reported by the Keio University and Miyazaki Prefectual Hospitals, it is clear that the B-M therapy afforded a much better response in the treatment of the cancer.

Regarding the toxicity, the overall incidence was generally low although lung complications were fairly frequent. It was due mainly to the smaller total doses used in the B-M therapy. The average total dose of BLM and MMC administered in the B-M regimen was less than 150 mg and 50 mg, respectively.

The tumor response seen on chest roentogenograms for metastatic cervical cancer and lung cancer was evaluated quantitatively as a function of the number of B-M course. For a round tumor the cross sectional diameters were measured to obtain the volume as a spherical mass. The irregularly shaped ones were transcribed from a chest roentogenogram to a thick piece of

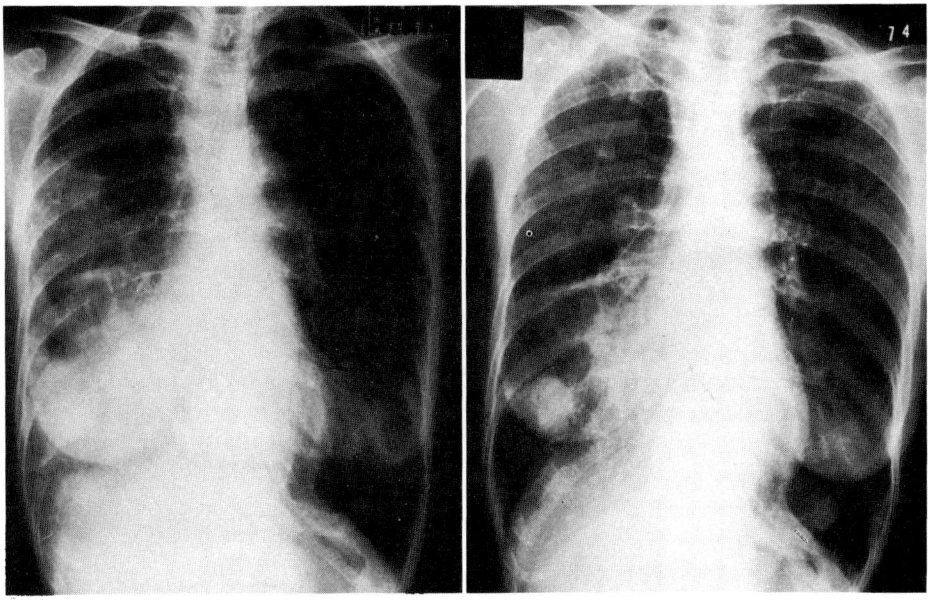

Fig. 10. A 69 year old woman with lung cancer. Left chest film is before treatment and right one after three courses

Table 3. Toxicity of B-M therapy

Adverse effects	Incidence (%)
Lung complications	11 (2/18) N.I.R.S.
	17 (4/23) Keio University
Leucopenia (<2000/mm^3)	27 (5/18) N.I.R.S.
	3 (3/18) Keio University

paper and weighed. The weight (W) multiplied by its square root ($\sqrt{W}$) was taken as a relative tumor volume. These volumes, measured during and after treatment, were normalized to the value obtained at the beginning of treatment and plotted on a semilogarithmic scale to obtain the tumor regression curve.

The tumor regression curves shown in Fig. 11 have been drawn for each patient with metastatic cervical cancer. All tumors regressed almost exponentially. The tumors of complete responders (bold solid lines) decreased to below 10% in volume within three to five courses. It was demonstrated, in a more detailed analysis, that the effect of MMC was enhanced about 10 times by pretreatment with BLM compared with single use [7]. In partial responders, some tumors regressed as remarkably as those in complete responders (fine solid lines), but others regressed less effectively (fine dotted lines).

There were two type of tumor regression in CR as seen in this figure after the first course of B-M therapy. One is the drastic decrease in tumor volume immediately after the first

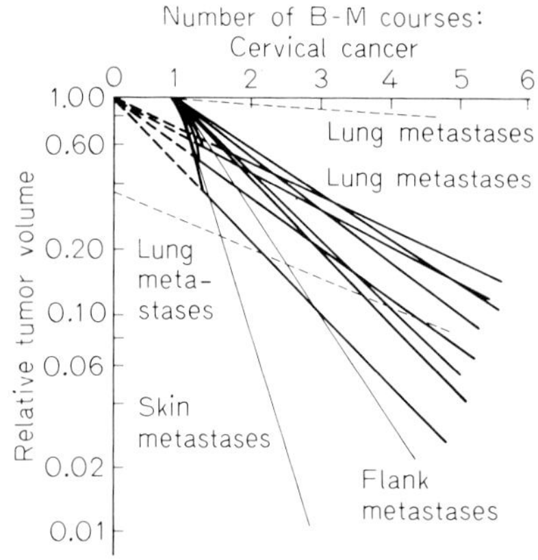

Fig. 11. Curves showing tumor regression against the number of B-M course. All curves are from the patients with cervical cancer. Bold lines show the curves for the lung tumors of the patients with CR. The exponentially declining curves following drastic decrease in volume soon after the first shot of MMC are extrapolated to the ordinate at the beginning of treatment (dotted lines). Fine lines show the curves from the metastases of the lung (dotted) and skin and in the abdomen palpable from the flank (solid) of the patients with PR

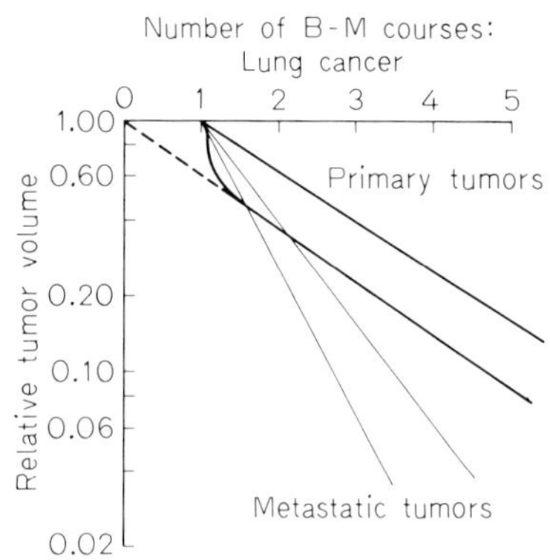

Fig. 12. Curves showing tumor regression against the number of B-M course. The curves are from the patients presented in Figs. 9 and 10. and one other patient with lymth node metastasis in addition to skin and bone. Primary tumors in the lung (solid lines) regressed more slowly than metastases (fine lines)

administration of MMC followed by a more gradual decrease in exponential function (bold solid line). The other is a decrease which is exponential throughout. These observations suggested that there may be two different actions of B-M therapy on tumor. As shown in Fig. 12, similar features were observed in the tumor regression curve for lung cancer. In addition, it was noted that the primary tumors responded to a lesser extent than metastatic tumors. It may be necessary, therefore, to combine another means such as surgery or radiotherapy with B-M therapy in the treatment of primary tumor.

Judging from the response to each of BLM and MMC of cervical, lung, and head and neck cancers, it is clear that the effect of B-M therapy on these cancers would be superior to the additive effect of each agent. Furthermore, a quantitative observation of regressing tumors on chest films revealed that none of the patients showed regression of tumor during BLM treatment, or before administration of MMC after the treatment with BLM in the tumor. The possible explanations for the enhanced response are: 1) MMC may exert preferential killing effect on the proliferating cells which were blocked at G2 [12] by successive administration of BLM [1, 15, 18]; 2) tumor cells may be potentiated by unknown combined action of the two agents on cellular DNA, which BLM breaks [14] and MMC cross-links [13]; 3) a preferential lethal effect of BLM [2, 66] and MMC on nonproliferating cells [8, 9, 10] may not be dismissed. Studies on cell biology as the basis of the present modality are now under way.

Acknowledgments

The author thanks Drs. Takabe, Watanabe, Nakagima, Tanabe and Terasima for their useful advice from a clinical and basic viewpoint, Dr. Inuyama at the Keio University and Dr. Ohno at Miyazaki Prefectual Hospital for their kind information on the patients with head and neck cancer, Prof. Okuda at the Chiba University for his useful English advice and Mrs. Furuya and Miss Matzuda for their help in the preparation of the manuscript.

References

1. Barranco, S. C., Luce, J. K., Romadahl, M. M., Humphrey, R. M.: Bleomycin as a possible synchronizing agent for human tumor cells *in vitro*. Cancer Res. **33**, 882–887 (1973).
2. Barranco, S. C., Novak, J. K., Humphrey, R. M.: Response of mammalian cells following treatment with bleomycin and 1.3 bis (2-chloroethyl)-1-nitrosourea during plateau phase. Cancer Res. **33**, 691–694, (1973).
3. Blum, R. H., Carter, S. K., Agre, K.: A clinical review of bleomycin: A new antineoplastic agent. Cancer **31**, 903–914, (1973).
4. Clarysse, A., Kenis, Y., Mathé, G.: Cancer Chemotherapy. Its Role in the Treatment Strategy of Hematologic Malignancies and Solid Tumors; p481 Berlin-Heidelberg-New York: Springer 1976.
5. Clarysse, A., Kenis, Y., Mathé, G.: Cancer Chemotherapy. Its Role in the Treatment Strategy of Hematologic Malignancies and Solid Tumors; pp408–412. Berlin-Heidelberg-New York: Springer-1976.
6. Hata, T.: Mitomycin, a new antibiotic from Streptomyces. J. Antibiot. **9**, 141 146 (1956).
7. Miyamoto, T., Takabe, Y., Watanabe, M., Terasima, T.: Drastic remission effect of a sequential combination with Bleomycin and Mitomycin C on an advanced cervical cancer. (in preparation).
8. Miyamoto, T., Takabe, Y., Watanabe, M., Terasima, T.: Effect of bleomycin on Burkitt lymphoma and mouse L cells: Comparison of the sensitivity of cells in exponential and stationary phase to bleomycin. Proc. Jap. Cancer Assoc., 33th Annu. Meet. **94** (1974) (abstr.).
9. Miyamoto, T., Takabe, Y., Watanabe, M., Terasima, T.: Kinetic analysis of metastatic lung cancer treated with mitomycin-C. Proc.Jap. Cancer Assoc., 34th Annu. Meet. **81** (1975) (abstr.).
10. Miyamto, T., Takabe, Y., Watanabe, M., Terasima, T.: Effect of Futraful on metastatic adenocarcinomas and proposal for some principle of single and combined chemotherapy. Gan to Kagaku Ryoho (Cancer Chemother.) **3**, 1225–1235 (1976).
11. Moor, G. E., Bross, I. D. J., Ausman, R.: Effects of mitomycin-C (NSC-26980) in 346 patients with cancer. Cancer Chemother. Rep. **52**, 675 (1968).
12. Ohara, H., Terasima, T.: Lethal effect of mitomycin-C on cultured mammalian cells. Gann **63**, 137–327 (1972).
13. Szybalski, W., Iyer, V. N.: The mitomycines and porfiromycins. In: Antibiotics. Gottib, I. D., Shaw, P. D. (eds.). New York-Berlin-Heidelberg: Springer—Verlag 1967 Vol. I, pp211–245.
14. Terasima, T., Takabe, Y., Katsumata, T., Watanabe, M., Umezawa, H.: Effect of bleomycin on mammalian cell survival. J. Natl. Cancer Inst. **49**, 1093–1100 (1972).
15. Tobey, R. A.: Arrest of Chinese hamster cells in G2 following treatment with the anti-tumor drug bleomycin. J. Cell Physiol. **79**, 259–266 (1975).

16. Twentymann, P. R., Bleehem, N. M.: Changes in sensitivity to radiation and to bleomycin occurring during the life history of monolayer cultures of a mouse tumor cell line. Br. J. Cancer **31**, 68–74 (1975).
17. Umezawa, H., Maeda, K., Takeuchi, T., Okami, Y.: New antibiotics, bleomycin A and B. J. Antibiot. (Tokyo) **19**, 200–209 (1966).
18. Watanabe, M., Takabe, Y., Katsumata, T., Terasima, T.: Effect of bleomycin on progression through the cell cycle of mouse L cells. Cancer Res. **34**, 878–881 (1974)
19. Yagota, A., Mukheryi, B., Young, C., Eticubanas, E., Lamonte, C., Smith, J. J. R., Tan, C. T. C., Krakoff, I. H.: Bleomycin, an antitumor antibiotic. Clinical experience in 274 patients. Ann. Intern. Med. **77**, 861–870 (1972).

Fundamental and Clinical Studies on New Bleomycin Analogs

A. MATSUDA, O. YOSHIOKA, T. YAMASHITA, and K. EBIHARA
H. UMEZAWA, T. MIURA, K. KATAYAMA, M. YOKOYAMA and
S. NAGAI

In the last 15 years, there has been great progress in the study of antitumor antibiotics. Professor UMEZAWA in his early study on bleomycin (BLM) proposed the following principle: Even a cytotoxic agent may exhibit therapeutic action against certain types of tumors if it is distributed in the tumor in a higher concentration than in other tissues, or if it is not inactivated or activated in those tumors. This principle has been exemplified by the study of BLM.

As already reported [4, 5], about 300 BLM analogs, differing from one another in their terminal amine moiety, have been produced by fermentation, chemical modification or semisyntheses.

In this paper we will report on the fundamental and clinical characteristics of new BLMs.

Screening of New Bleomycins for Antitumor Activity

For the selection of new BLMs most useful in cancer treatment, the first step was to test for anti-HeLa cell activity. In this test, ID_{50} (μg/ml) was determined by counting the cells detached from the sheet of growth. About 150 of the new BLMs were thus selected.

In the second step, selected BLMs were tested for their inhibiting effect on Ehrlich ascites carcinoma and the therapeutic indices (LD_{50} by daily injection for 10 days/ED_{50} by daily injection for 10 days) were estimated. In the third step, 100 BLMs which had shown therapeutic indices of not less than 16 were further tested for the ability to inhibit Ehrlich solid carcinoma. Those which had ID_{50} values smaller than 1 mg/kg/day for 10 days, were selected.

In the fourth step, the organ distribution was tested in brain, lung, stomach, liver, spleen, kidney, skin, and tumor (Ehrlich solid) 1 h after i.p. injection of 100 mg/kg of the 75 new BLMs selected above.

The concentrations of each BLM in the organs were determined by usual microbiologic method.

Summarized results of the most interesting BLMs are shown in Table 1. Some of the BLMs were distributed in higher concentrations in stomach, skin, and lungs, than the natural BLM clinically used at present. (Hereafter, this BLM is described as present BLM).

Among new BLMs there were four which, excepting BLM-BAPP and BLM-A5033, showed 1.6–5.0 times higher concentrations in the stomach. Concentrations in the stomach of five new BLMs and present BLM were as follows: present BLM: 2.6 μg/g, BLM-PYP: 6.3 μg/g, BLM-PEP: 7.5 μg/g, BLM-BAPP: 0.3 μg/g, BLM-A5196: 13.2 μg/g, BLM-M5196: 4.1 μg/g, and BLM-A5033: O. These four BLMs were tested for their effect on chemically induced gastric cancer in rats and dogs, as described in Section IV.

Examination of Pulmonary Toxicity of New Bleomycins

Professor UMEZAWA has suggested that the compounds which have the same or stronger antitumor activity and lower pulmonary toxicity than present BLM might be more effective in cancer treatment. We, therefore, endeavored to establish a pulmonary toxicity test method using small experimental animals. Professor UMEZAWA et al. [6] had previously reported that the activity of lung and skin to inactivate BLMs, was much weaker in old mice (28 weeks) than in young mice (3 weeks). Based on this result, we succeeded in the development of a test method for pulmonary toxicity.

Male ICR-SLC mice of 15 weeks (S.P.F.) were used. The test was carried out in a conventional animal room. Each group consisted of 20 mice to which 5 mg/kg test BLM was injected i.p., daily for 10 days. The control group was injected with physiologic saline. To examine the development of pulmonary toxicity, 5 weeks after the last injection all mice were sacrificed, the lungs fixed with neutral formaline solution, and the histologic specimens prepared. Usually the whole left lung, and the superior and inferior lobe of the right lung were examined by light microscopy. Mice which had infectious bronchitis and bronchopneumonia were discarded from the test.

The examination was focused on the presence of fibrosis, although interstitial pneumonitis and pleural inflammation were examined. The degree of congestion and interstitial and intraalveolar edema, the number of alveolar macrophage, morphologic changes in bronchiolar and alveolar epithelial cells and in blood vessel walls were also examined.

The degree of pulmonary fibrosis was divided into five classes as follows:

Grade
+ (0) absence of figrosis
± (1) presence of areas with questionable fibrosis in alveolar septae
+ (2) a few foci of fibrosis, often in subpleural area
++ (4) scattered foci of fibrosis
+++ (6) diffuse fibrosis

The data were expressed as follows:

$$\text{Incidence (percent)} = \frac{\text{Number of mice in group with fibrosis}}{\text{Number of mice tested in group}} \times 100$$

$$\text{Grade (mean score)} = \frac{\text{Total score of specimens in group}}{\text{Number of specimens in group}}$$

For the evaluation of pulmonary toxicity of various BLMs, present BLM was taken as the control and the data were expressed with relative value to present BLM.

The dose response relationship was observed in dose range from 2.5–10 mg/kg present BLM. Incidences of fibrosis were 2.5 mg/kg: 40%, 5.0 mg/kg: 60%, 10 mg/kg: 90%. The experimental results are shown in Fig. 1.

Among the various BLMs, the incidence of pulmonary toxicity was lowest [1/12] with BLM-M5196 and highest with BLM-TMD (2x). The grade of BLM-M5196 was the lowest and that of BLM-HPE was the highest. As compared with present BLM, values of other BLMs were as follows (incidence and grade): BLM-PEP: 0.36 and 0.25, BLM-PYP: 0.80 and 1.24, BLM-BAPP: 0.35 and 0.22, BLM-A5196: 0.71 and 0.42, and BLM-A5033: 0.31 and 0.21.

As shown in Fig. 1, it is apparent that pulmonary fibrosis can be produced in old mice by BLMs and the magnitude of the toxicity varies among various BLMs which are different in the terminal amine moiety.

The magnitude of pulmonary fibrosis of various BLMs is not parallel to the antitumor activity as shown by BLM-A5196.

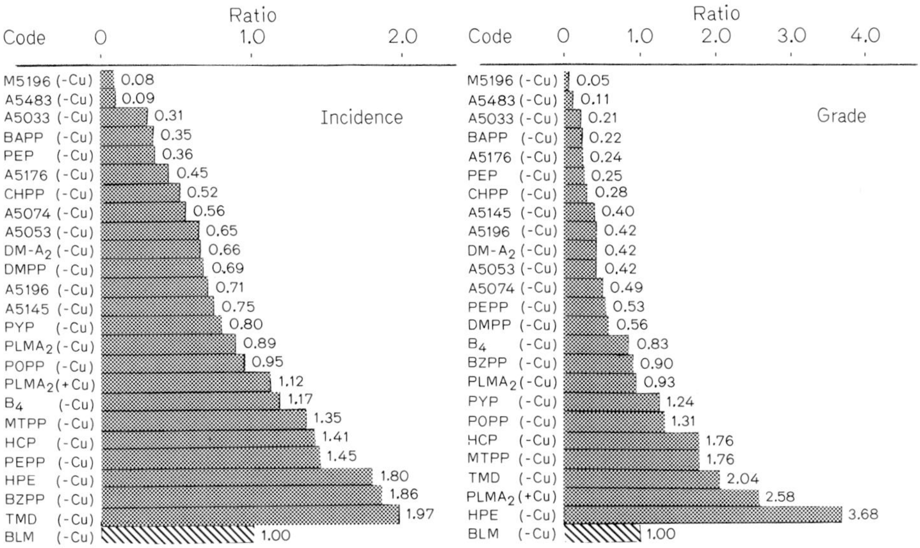

Fig. 1. Magnitude of pulmonary fibrosis of new bleomycins [compared with bleomycin (5 mg/kg)]

Effect of New Bleomycins on Methylcholanthrene (20-MC) Induced Squamous Cell Carcinoma of Mice

In order to confirm the effect of various BLMs on squamous cell carcinoma which was induced by 20-MC in mice [1], female dd/Y-S 10 week old mice were used. Each group consisted of 12 mice. The hair on the application area of 20-MC was cut and saturated 20-MC solution in acetone was applied twice a week for 18 weeks. The doses of each BLM were 62.5 and 250 μg/mouse, i.p., twice a week for 15 weeks after the first painting of 20-MC. Evaluation of the result was performed within a week of the last injection of the compound. Cancerous lesion of skin was fixed with formaline solution and histologic specimens were prepared and examined for the presence of squamous cell carcinoma.

The result was expressed as follows:

$$\frac{\text{Number of mice in group with cancer}}{\text{Number of mice in group}} = \text{Cancerization \%}$$

Summarized data are presented in Table 2.

Some BLMs have shown almost the same activity as present BLM in suppression of squamous cell carcinoma. In a dose of 62.5 μg/mouse, BLM-A5196, BLM-PYP and BLM-PEP showed stronger effect than present BLM and the effect of BLM-BAPP was the same as present BLM. The effect of 250 μg/mouse BLM-A5196, BLM-PEP and BLM-BAPP could not be evaluated because of toxic death during the treatment.

Therapeutic Effect on Chemically Induced Gastric Cancer in Rats and Dogs

Effect on Chemically Induced Gastric Cancer in Rats

Several new BLMs which had been selected by testing antitumor activity, organ distribution and pulmonary toxicity were tested for the ability to inhibit gastric cancer chemically induced in rats by Dr. Sugimura's method [3].

190 male Wistar rats 6 weeks old were used. N-methyl-N'-nitro-N-nitrosoguanidine (MNNG) was dissolved (83 μg/ml in 0.4% Tween 60 solution) and the solution given to rats instead of drinking water for 32 weeks and thereafter replaced with water. In 18–19 weeks after the cessation of administration of MNNG, all rats were operated on to examine the incidence of gastric cancer. The stomach was opened along the greater curvature of the forestomach and washed with physiologic saline. The tumor was usually localized on the pylorus region of the glandular stomach.

Localization, size and number of tumor were recorded and the forestomach and abdominal wall were closed successively. The operation mortality was less than 10%. Thereafter, all rats were divided into five groups. Each group consisted of 20 rats with tumor and 10 rats without tumor, macroscopically.

If treatment with BLMs or 5-FU was started immediately after cessation of administration of MNNG, it caused a high frequency of deaths by hemorrhagic obliteration of the intestine. This death was avoided by starting treatment 21 weeks after the cessation of MNNG administration. In this case, the death rate was only 3%. The test compounds were given three times a week, totalling 37 times. The doses of each compound were 1–2 mg BLM-BAPP/kg, 1.5 mg BLM-PEP/kg, 0.5 mg BLM-A5196/kg and 5 mg 5-FU/kg. Total doses of these drugs were roughly 50% of LD_{50}. Physiological saline was administered to the control group instead of drug solution. After the end of treatment, all rats in each group were sacrificed and the stomach was examined for the localization, number and size of tumor, and other histopathologic findings. The number of rats with persistent tumor and the number of rats with a tumor at the end of treatment are shown in Table 3.

In the control group (17 survivors) which had tumors before treatment, the size of all tumors increased (see Table 4). The ratio of the number of rats with persistant tumor to the number of surviving rats were as follows: BLM-BAPP: 2/9 (22%), BLM-PEP: 5/16 (31%), BLM-A5196: 11/19 (58%), and 5-FU: 14/16 (88%).

Tumor persistence ratio in BLM-BAPP and BLM-PEP groups was significantly lower than control and 5-FU groups.

In the control group of rats which had no tumor before treatment, tumors appeared in five out of 10 surviving rats. Tumor appearance in each drug treatment group was as follows: BLM-BAPP: 1/6 (17%), BLM-PEP: 0/9 (0%), BLM-A5196: 4/7 (57%), and 5-FU: 5/10 (50%). Thus, the BLM-PEP group showed a statistically significant low rate of tumor progression, compared with the control and 5-FU groups. Almost same results were observed in rats which died during treatment.

The number and the size of tumors before and after treatment are shown in Table 4.

Summation of the number of rats with tumor and the number of tumor in the control and 5-FU group were increased after treatment but decreased in BLM-BAPP, BLM-PEP, and BLM-A5196 groups.
Conforming with these results, summation of tumor sizes indicated the same trend in each group. In the BLM-A5196 group, there were two extremely large tumors and as a result, the summation of size of all tumors increased and was larger than that of the control. The effectiveness of BLM-PEP treatment in the tumor size was statistically significant, compared with control and 5-FU groups, compared with that in other groups and the control.
All stomachs of rats which survived at the end of treatment or which died were examined histopathologically but stomachs which had undergone strong autolysis could not be examined.
This examination was done by Professor Makoto Enomoto, Department of Pathology, School of Medicine, St. Marianna University.
The criteria of diagnosis was based on "The general rules for the gastric cancer study in surgery and pathology. Part III. 1974. Japanese Research Society for Gastric Cancer."
For the evaluation of chemotherapeutic effect of drugs, special attention was given to the rate of incidence of adenocarcinoma and suspicious adenocarcinoma. Rats which had adenocarcinoma together with suspicious adenocarcinoma were counted as those having adenocarcinoma. The results on histologic findings are shown in Table 5.
Incidence of adenocarcinoma, including suspicious ones in the control group, was 79% of rats examined.
The incidences in drug-treated groups are as follows: BLM-BAPP: 25%, BLM-PEP: 30%, BLM-A5196: 36%, and 5-FU: 52%.
Conforming to the lower rate of incidence of adenocarcinoma and suspicious adenocarcinoma in drug-treated groups, incidence of gastritis, which was one of the evidences of tumor healing, was increased as follows: BLM-BAPP: 54%, BLM-PEP: 44%, BLM-A5196: 39%, 5-FU: 19%, and saline: 14%. The effectiveness of treatment shown macroscopically confirmed that shown by histopathologic examination.
Among BLMs, BLM-BAPP and BLM-PEP showed stronger therapeutic effects than BLM-A5196 in gastric cancer of rats. 5-FU showed less effect than all BLMs tested in the incidence rate of adenocarcinoma.

Chemoprophylactic Effect on Chemically Induced Gastric Cancer in Dogs

Chemoprophylactic effect of BLM-PYP and present BLM against chemically induced gastric cancer in dogs was examined by Dr. Kurihara's method [2] using 30 male beagle dogs 7–11 months old.
N-ethyl-N'-nitro-N-nitrosoguanidine (ENNG) was dissolved at 150 μg/ml in 2% Tween 60 solution. Just before administration, 250 ml of ENNG solution was mixed with defatted milk powder (20 g) and the pellet diet was given to the dogs twice a day for 8 months, except Sundays. By this method, gastric cancer was produced in 87% of dogs [26/30]. 1.5 months before the end of administration of ENNG, six out of the 30 dogs were selected, by endoscopically biopsied examination for atypism of stomach, and divided into three groups. Each group consisted of two dogs with almost the same grade of atypism. Test compounds were given twice a week for 6 months and the doses of each compound was 0.3 mg/kg.
During and after the treatment, endoscopic observation of tumor progression in all dogs was continued monthly until the present time. The results of the chemoprophylactic effect of BLM-PYP and present BLM are shown in Fig. 2.
Gastric cancer was detected in two dogs of the control group by biopsy during the saline administration. The date of tumor detection in drug-treated groups was various, as indicated in Figure 2.

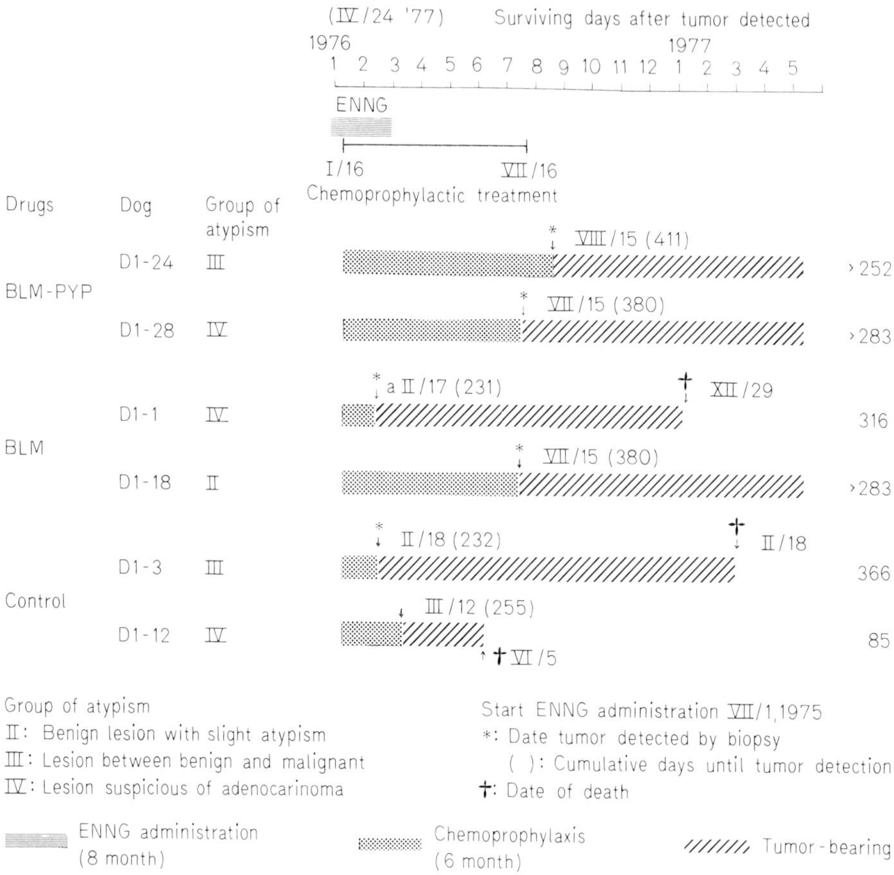

Fig. 2. Chemoprophylactic effect of BLM-PYP and present BLM on dog gastric cancer

Cumulative days until tumor detection in each group were as follows: control: 232,255, BLM-PYP: 411,380, and present BLM: 231,380 days. Detection of canceration of two dogs in BLM-PYP group and one of present BLM group were delayed by the treatment.
Observation on tumor progression in surviving dogs of each group is being continued.

Effect on Human Gastric Cancer Heterotransplanted to Nude Mice

The value of an animal tumor system for screening depends on its ability to select new compounds of greater efficacy against human tumor.
In addition to chemically induced carcinoma, we have tested compounds for the effect on human gastric cancer heterotransplanted in nude mice. Female nude mice nu/nu-BALB/c/A/BOM (S.P.F.) 6–8 weeks old (bred at the Laboratory Animals Breeding and Research Centre, Ry, Denmark) were used in groups of 3–5 mice. Tumors used were taken from various patients in National Hospital Medical Center (Emeritus Director, Prof. T. Ichikawa) and Department of Surgery, Tokyo Medical and Dental University (Prof. T.

Murakami). Since 1974, we have successfully transplanted six cases of gastric adenocarcinoma. Moreover, in four of these cases lymphatic metastasis were also successfully transplanted.

Five of these 10 tumors could be serially transplanted and have been established as tumor lines.

Solid tumor blocks of about 1 × 2 × 2 mm^3 were excised and implanted subcutaneously to bilateral axillary part of nude mouse.

Following inoculation, the animals were weighed and tumors measured in two dimensions with a slide caliper.

Treatment with drugs was started when tumor grafts had been accepted and measured about 30 mm^2. The drug was injected i.p. daily for 10 days. The doses of each drug were as follows: BLM-PEP, BLM-PYP, and present BLM: 3 mg/kg, and 5-FU: 15 mg/kg.

One day after the last treatment, animals were sacrificed and the tumors weighed. An example [7] of the results is shown in Fig. 3. Each curve represents the mean value from four mice.

The growth curves in groups of BLM-PEP, BLM-PYP and present BLM showed clear regression whereas in 5-FU it showed only slight retardation.

	Dose mg/kg/Day × 10 (i.p.)	Relative tumor size Exp. 1	Exp. 2
Control		2.40 (1.00)	2.36 (1.00)
Bleomycin	3.0	1.59 (0.66)	
PYP-BLM	3.0	1.70 (0.71)	
PEP-BLM	3.0		1.54 (0.65)
5-FU	15.0		2.06 (0.87)

( ): Ratio to control

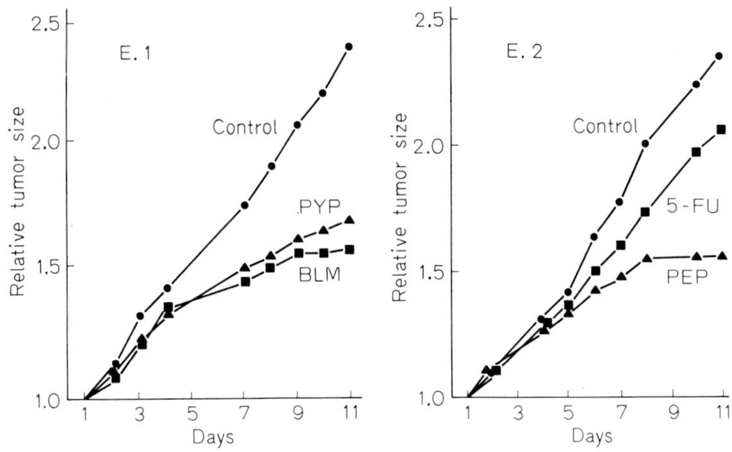

Fig. 3. Effect of bleomycins on heterotransplanted human gastric carcinoma in nude mice

Patient: M. W., Male, 59 Tumor strain: G/W
Diagnosis: Advanced carcinoma of stomach with metastasis to lymph nodes
Histology: Tubular adenocarcinoma, well differentiation, scirrhous
(Prof. T. Murakami: Dept. of Surgery, Tokyo Medical and Dental University
Experimental animal: nu/nu-BALB/c/A/BOM (S.P.F.) 6–7 weeks

In this experiment, present BLM, which was confirmed to be of no effect on chemically induced gastric cancer, showed an effectiveness against human gastric cancer in nude mice similar to BLM-PEP and BLM-PYP.

The cause of this discrepancy may be the preferential distribution of present BLM in skin. In the case of 5-FU, doses over 15 mg/kg caused toxic death in all mice, while at lower doses of 10 and 5 mg/kg, the tumor growth was not retarded. Thus we could not see the efficacy of 5-FU in this tumor system.

Phase I Study of Bleomycin-PEP

As described in the previous chapters on the screening of new bleomycins, BLM-PEP was selected because of the following results: a) higher antitumor activity, b) lower pulmonary toxicity, c) stronger effect on chemically induced squamous cell carcinoma and gastric cancer of experimental animals, and was launched into the phase I clinical study. Application of BLM-PEP [N-(3-aminopropyl)-α-phenethylamine bleomycin] to the phase I study on a variety of advanced and recurrent cancers was investigated during the period from August 1976 to February 1977 in the following institutions.

1) The Second Department of Surgery,
   Faculty of Medicine,
   University of Tokyo
2) Department of Clinical Cancer Chemotherapy,
   The Research Institute for Tuberculosis, Leprosy and Cancer,
   Tohoku University
3) The First Department of Surgery,
   School of Medicine,
   Tokyo Medical and Dental University

This paper reports the preliminary results on the toxicities and clinical effects of BLM-PEP in the selected 32 cases where the response of the disease to BLM-PEP was evaluable.

Materials and Methods

Phase I study of BLM-PEP was carried out with 32 cases which involved the various cancers shown in Tables 6, 7, 8.

Initially, BLM-PEP was given twice weekly at a dose of 2.5 mg, i.v. or i.a. The doses were gradually increased and schedules were varied paying attention to the occurrence of acute toxic symptoms such as the disorder of liver and kidney functions. Clinical features and effects of BLM-PEP were examined at least once a week.

Laboratory studies including white blood cell and platelet counts and determination of hematocrit, blood urea nitrogen, alkaline phosphatase and serum transaminase (S-GOT, S-GPT) levels were carried out before, during and after the BLM-PEP therapy.

The dose ranges of BLM-PEP in these 32 cases were as follows: single dose: 2.5–10 mg twice or three times weekly in most patients, except those cases in Table 6 for which the dose should be 5–7.5 $\sim$ 20–30 mg; weekly: 7.5–70 mg (average: 35 mg), total dose: 32.5–435 mg (average: 153 mg).

BLM-PEP was administered in the following routes: i.v. injection only: 17 cases, i.a. infusion only: five cases, i.v. plus i.a.: 10 cases.

Toxicity and Side Effects

The occurrence of toxic reaction in 32 cases are recorded in Table 9. Of all the 32 cases, no adverse symptom was observed in 17 cases (53%) and in all cases no abnormality was found in hematologic nor biochemical tests.

a) Fever: Body temperature was observed after every administration of BLM-PEP. When the temperature rise was 1°C or more, it was regarded as fevered. Fever as a side effect was found at the highest rate as nine out of 32 cases (28%), but there were no cases where the medication was discontinued because of fever. No correlation was found between fever, weekly dose and total dose of BLM-PEP.

It seems that incidence and severity of the fibrile response to BLM-PEP was lower than that to present BLM.

b) Pulmonary Change: Abnormal shadow was found radiographically in two cases, and so the medication was discontinued though the change was very slight. These pulmonary changes could not be confirmed as interstitial pneumonia because pulmonary function tests could not be performed on these advanced stages of cancer. The dosage, where the pulmonary changes were recorded, was in total 51–100 mg, while in the other 22 cases to whom 101–450 mg were accumulatively administered, no sign of pulmonary toxicity was observed. We are proceeding with the further study with some expectation of less pulmonary toxicity.

c) Other Symptoms: Stomatitis, alopecia, nausea and fatigue were observed to a slight degree but the medication was not discontinued in any of these cases.

Clinical Effect

Clinical effects of BLM-PEP are presented in Tables 10 and 11.

Objective improvement was found in nine out of 32 cases (28%). All nine patients also showed some subjective improvement. There were five other subjectively improved cases (four cases of lung cancer and one case of leiomyosarcoma), while no objective improvement was found among them. As shown in Table 12, i.a. infusion of BLM-PEP produced higher antitumor effect than i.v. injection.

a) Lung Cancer. Both subjective and objective improvements were found in one out of six cases. In four cases there was subjective improvement concerning cough, expectoration, and chest pain etc., while no objective improvement was found radiographically.

b) Gastro-intestinal Cancer. Neither subjective nor objective improvement was found in any of the 14 cases of gastrointestinal cancer.

c) Prostatic Cancer. It is noticeable that both subjective and objective improvements were found in both cases of prostatic cancer, but both of the two patients who had received hormone therapy died of heart disease after the cessation of treatment.

d) Reticulum cell Sarcoma. Both subjective and objective improvements were found in all three cases, and in two of these the patients are still living in a state of complete remission.

e) Hepatoma. Some temporary improvement was found not only subjectively but also objectively. The objective improvement was proved by liver scintigraphy, palpation and liver function tests. However, this patient died from a great hemorrhage due to a duodenal ulcer in the course of treatment.

f) Choriocarcinoma: The recurrent focus in the retroperitoneum disappeared, while the metastatic focus in the lung had progressed.

g) Metastasis of Tongue Cancer in the Neck: After the operation of tongue cancer, a metastatic lesion as large as 10×10 cm^2 was found in the cervical lymph node. When the total dose of BLM-PEP reached 100 mg, a remarkable shrinkage of the tumor was found. When the dose reached 360 mg, the size of the tumor had already been reduced to less than 10% of the initial size.

The cases with objective tumor response are listed in Table 12.

Discussion and Conclusion

Phase I clinical trial of BLM-PEP carried out in 32 advanced or recurrent cancer patients was reported preliminarily. The toxicity and antitumor effect of BLM-PEP are briefly summarized as follows from the results obtained.

a). Toxicity. The patients tolerated BLM-PEP treatment well. The incidence and degree of fever after injections were somewhat less, but not significantly than corresponding doses of present BLM.

b) Antitumor activity. Favourable responses were seen in cases of types sensitive to present BLM. Furthermore, in cases where present BLM has not clearly been evaluated, some patients with prostatic cancer and hepatoma responded. Therefore BLM-PEP may possess a wider antitumor spectrum than present BLM, although little response was observed in patients with gastric cancer.

Tables

able 1. Biologic properties of new bleomycins

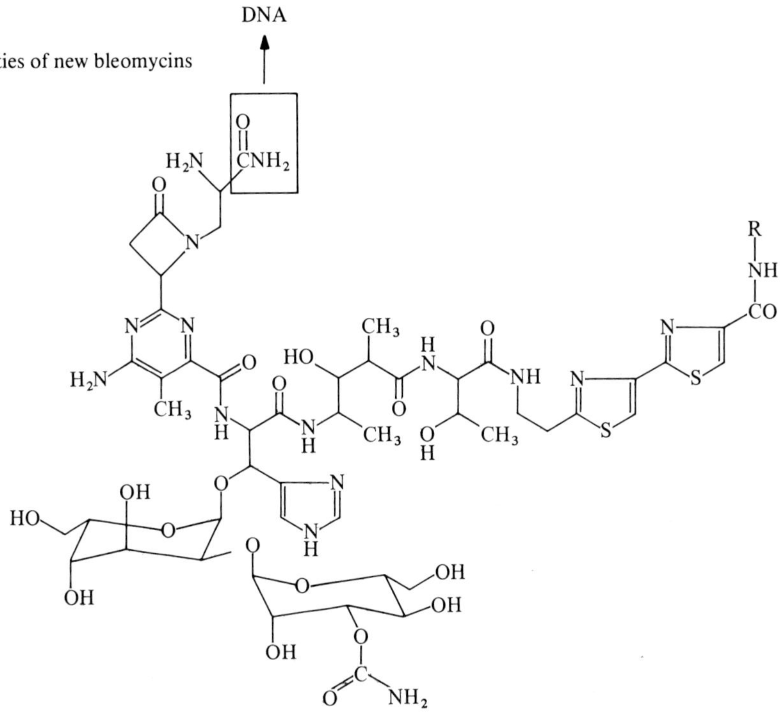

	Cu M.607 / B.Sub (u/mg)	E.Ascites $\frac{LD_{50}}{ED_{50}}$ = INDEX (mg/kg)	E.Solid ID_{50} (mg/kg)	Hela ID_{50} (mcg/ml)	Distribution Serum	Stomach	100 mg/kg, s.c., 1h Skin	Lung	Solid
	— $\frac{1234}{886}$	$\frac{13.1}{0.19}$ = 68.9	0.49	3.2	38.0	2.6	18.5	9.7	12.9
- + + NH–CH_2CH_2–(N-ring)	– $\frac{3120}{1180}$	$\frac{18.75}{0.39}$ = 48.1	0.61	2.4	65.0	6.3	37.7	7.4	10.1
- + + NHCH(CH_3)–(phenyl)	— $\frac{5570}{1550}$	$\frac{6.56}{0.39}$ = 16.8	0.41	3.2	83.0	7.5	26.6	14.1	22.1
P - + + NH + + + NH + + + CH_3	— $\frac{8470}{19180}$	$\frac{8.44}{0.39}$ = 21.6	0.72	1.2	33.0	0.32	13.7	0.5	3.1
6 - + + NH + + + NH–C(NH)–CH_2–(ring)–Cl	— $\frac{17588}{14367}$	$\frac{9.40}{0.19}$ = 49.5	0.74	1.6	93.3	13.2	25.5	15.3	18.9
6 - + + N(CH_3) + + + NH–C(NH)–CH_2 Cl	— $\frac{19639}{12735}$	$\frac{6.1}{0.19}$ = 32.1	0.41	0.95	85.0	4.1	21.0	23.5	21.8
3 - + + NH + + + $NHCOCH_2CH_2COOH$	— $\frac{122}{52}$	$\frac{>25.0}{3.12}$ = >8.0	0.38	8.0	25.0	0	18.5	0	0

Table 2. Effect of various bleomycins on squamous cell carcinoma induced by 20-MC in mice

Bleomycins	Dose (mcg/mouse)	Died/Treated	Cancerized/ Treated	Cancerization %	Inhibition %
PEP-BLM	250.0	12/12	—	—	—
	62.5	1/12	5/11	45.4	47.8
PYP-BLM	250.0	4/12	1/8	12.5	85.6
	62.5	0/12	5/12	41.6	52.1
BAPP-BLM	250.0	12/12	—	—	—
	62.5	0/12	6/12	50.0	42.5
A5033	250.0	1/12	4/11	36.4	68.1
	62.5	1/12	6/11	54.5	37.3
A5196	250.0	12/12	—	—	—
	62.5	4/12	2/8	25.0	71.3
	15.6	1/12	2/11	54.5	37.3
BLM	250.0	1/12	2/11	18.1	79.2
(clinical)	62.5	2/12	5/10	50.0	42.5
Control	0	1/24	20/23	86.9	0

Table 3. Effect of bleomycins and 5-FU on chemically induced gastric cancer in rats (I)

Drug	Number of rats	Survivors: Number of Survivors	Survivors: Number of rats [a] with persistant tumors	Survivors: Number of rats [b] with appearance of tumors	Dead: Number of rats [a] with persistant tumors	Dead: Number of rats [b] with appearance of tumors
BAPP	30	15/30 (50%)	2/9 (22%) △△ □□	1/6 (17%)	5/11 (45%)	0/4 (0%)
PEP	29	25/29 (86%)	5/16 (31%) △△ □□	0/9 (0) △ □	0/3 (0%)	0/1 (0%)
A5196	29	26/29 (90%)	11/19 (58%) △△	4/7 (57%)	1/1 (100%)	0/2 (0%)
5-FU	29	26/29 (90%)	14/16 (88%)	5/10 (50%)	0/2 (0%)	0/1 (0%)
Saline	30	27/30 (90%)	17/17 (100%)	5/10 (50%)	2/2 (100%)	1/1 (100%)

△,△△ Significantly different from control ($P < 0.05$) △ ($P < 0.01$) △△

□,□□ Significantly different from 5-FU ($P < 0.05$) □ ($P < 0.01$) □□

[a] Rats which had tumors before treatment.

[b] Rats which had no tumors before treatment.

Table 4. Effect of bleomycins and 5-FU on chemically induced gastric cancer in rats (II)

Drug	Total number of rats	Chemotherapy	Number of rats with tumors	Sum of number of tumors	Sum of tumor size (mm^2)	Mean tumor size (mm^2)
		Before	20	24	289	12 ± .43
BAPP	30				+ 132	
		After	7	8	421	53 ± 27.0
		Before	19	24	316 △, □	13 ± 5.2
PEP	29				− 201	
		After	5	5	115	23 ± 10.8
		Before	20	25	397	16 ± 4.6
A5196	29				+1876	
		After	16	18	2273	126 ± 83.8
		Before	18	24	365	15 ± 4.0
5-FU	29				+628	
		After	19	35	993	28 ± 6.0
		Before	19	30	323	11 ± 3.5
Saline	30				+1547	
		After	25	40	1870	46 ± 11.7

△ Significantly different from control ($P < 0.01$) Mean ± S.E.
□ Significantly different from 5-FU ($P < 0.05$)

Table 5. Results of histological observation of stomach after treatment with bleomycins and 5-FU

		BAPP	PEP	A5196	5-FU	Saline
Number of rats examined		24	27	28	27	28
Group	V. Adenocarcinoma	4 (17%)	7 (26%)	8 (29%)	14 (52%)	19 (65%)
	IV. Lesion suspicious of adenocarcinoma	2 (8%)	1 (4%)	2 (7%)	0 (0%)	3 (11%)
	III. Lesion between benign and malignant	2 (8%)	3 (11%)	2 (7%)	3 (11%)	0 (0%)
	II. Benign lesion with slight atypism	2 (8%)	4 (15%)	3 (11%)	4 (15%)	1 (4%)
	Sarcoma	0 (0%)	0 (0%)	2 (7%)	0 (0%)	1 (4%)
	Gastritis	13 (54%)	12 (44%)	11 (39%)	5 (19%)	4 (14%)
	Normal	1 (4%)	0 (0%)	0 (0%)	1 (4%)	0 (0%)

From: The General Rules for the Gastric Cancer Study in Surgery and Pathology Part. III. 1974. Sept. (The 9th edition) Japanese Research Society for Gastric Cancer.

Table 6. Patients treated with bleomycin-PEP (University of Tokyo)

Sex/Age	Diagnosis	Previous treatment	Dose (mg/week/patient)	Total dose (mg)	Fever
M/49	Gastric cancer (recurrent)	MMC, 5-FU	35–70	200	0
F/69	Gastric cancer (recurrent)	OPE.	70	120	0
M/27	Choriocarcinoma (recurrent) + lung meta.	OPE., MMC, 5-FU	35–70	150	0
F/63	Gastric cancer	None	20	60	0
M/57	Leiomyosarcoma	5-FU	20	100	++
M/53	Hepatoma	None	30	160	0
M/65	Prostatic cancer + lung meta.	Hormone	15–30	110	0
M/56	Prostatic cancer + bone meta.	Hormone	40	120	+
M/65	Cervical lymphnode meta. of tongue cancer	Radio-therapy, vaccine	70	360	+
M/52	Reticulum cell Sarcoma (recurrent)	Radio therapy, chemotherapy	70	235	0
M/31	Reticulum cell sarcoma (recurrent)	MMC, 5-FU	70	435	0
M/74	Lung cancer	None	30	270	0
M/69	Lung cancer	MMC, 5-FU	50–60	205	0
F/63	Lung cancer	None	35	190	0
F/41	Lung cancer	Radiation, 5-FU, MMC	10–20	165	0
M/60	Lung cancer	None	35–70	205	0
M/55	Kidney cancer (clear cell Ca.)	None	35–70	300	0

Toxicity						Response	
Skin Change	Stoma-titis	Alo-pecia	Nausea	Pulmonary change	Fatigue	Objective (%)	Subjective
0	0	0	0	0	0	0	0
0	0	0	0	0	0	0	0
0	0	++	0	0	0	>80	Improvement
0	0	0	0	0	0	0	0
0	0	0	0	0	0	0	Improvement
0	0	0	0	0	0	>80	Improvement
0	0	0	0	0	0	>50	Improvement
0	+	0	0	0	0	>50	Improvement
++	0	0	0	0	0	>80	Improvement
0	++	0	0	0	0	>80	Improvement
0	0	0	+	0	0	>80	Improvement
+++	0	0	0	0	0	0	Improvement
0	0	0	0	0	0	0	Improvement
0	0	0	0	0	0	>50	Improvement
0	0	0	0	0	0	0	Improvement
0	0	0	0	0	0	0	Improvement
0	0	0	0	0	0	0	0

Table 7. Patients treated with bleomycin-PEP (Tohoku University)

Sex/Age	Diagnosis	Previous treatment	Dose (mg/week/ patient)	Total dose (mg)	
					Fever
F/51	Esophagus cancer	None	7.5-20	137.5	0
F/74	Gastric cancer	Non	7.5-10	57.5	0
M/72	Gastric cancer	Adriamycin, ACNU, 5-FU	7.5-10	77.5	0
M/55	Gastric cancer (recurrent)	MMC, 5-FU, CQ, CTX, FT-207	7.5-10	32.5	0
M/70	Gastric cancer	None	15-20	95	+
M/51	Gastric cancer (recurrent)	5-FU, Chromomycin A_3, ACNU	7.5-20	192.5	+
M/50	Lung cancer	BLM, radiation, FT-207, MMC, 5-FU	7.5-20	107.5	0
F/67	Reticulum cell sarcoma	Adriamycin, ACNU, 5-FU, NK-5033, VLB	01.5-20	52.5	+
M/44	Cervical lymphnode meta. (primary unknown)	None	10.5-20	67.5	+

Table 8. Patients treated with bleomycin-PEP (Tokyo medical and Dental University)

Sex/Age	Diagnosis	Previous treatment	Dose (mg/week/ patient)	Total dose (mg)		
					Fever	Skin Change
F/55	Gastric cancer	None	15-20	105	0	+
M/69	Gastric cancer (recurrent)	OPE., 5-FU	15-20	95	++	0
M/62	Gastric cancer	OPE., 5-FU	30-40	140	++	0
M/67	Rectum cancer (recurrent)	OPE., 5-FU	70	200	0	0
M/71	Gastric cancer	OPE.	10-20	50	0	0
M/46	Colon cancer	OPE., 5-FU	70	130	0	0

Toxicity						Response	
Skin Change	Stoma-titis	Alo-pecia	Nausea	Pulmonary change	Fatigue	Objective (%)	Subjective
0	0	0	0	0	0	0	0
0	0	0	0	+	0	0	0
0	0	0	0	0	0	0	0
0	0	0	0	0	0	0	0
0	0	0	0	0	0	0	0
0	0	+	0	0	+	0	0
0	0	0	0	0	0	0	0
0	0	0	0	0	0	>50	Improvement
0	0	0	0	+	0	0	0

Toxicity					Response	
Stoma-titis	Alo-pecia	Nausea	Pulmonary change	Fatigue	Objective (%)	Subjective
0	0	0	0	0	0	0
0	0	0	0	0	0	0
0	0	0	0	0	0	0
0	0	0	0	0	0	0
0	0	0	0	0	0	0
0	0	0	0	0	0	0

Table 9. Toxic reaction versus total dose

Total dose (mg)	Number of cases	Toxic reaction						
		Fever	Skin change	Alopecia	Stomatitis	Nausea	Fatigue	Pulmonary change
0- 50	2							
51-100	8	4						2
101-150	9	3	1		1			
151-200	6	1		2			1	
201-250	3				1			
251-300	2		1					
301-350	0							
351-400	1	1	1					
401-450	1					1		
Total Cases (%)	32	9 (28)	3 (9.4)	2 (6.3)	2 (6.3)	1 (3.1)	1 (3.1)	2 (6.3)

Table 10. Therapeutic effect on various recurrent and advanced cancers

Diagnosis	Number of cases	Objective Responses (Tumor Regression)				Subjective Response	
		>80%	80-50%	<50%	None	Improvement	None
Gastric cancer	12				12		12
Lung cancer	6		1		5	5	1
Reticulum cell sarcoma	3	2	1			3	
Prostatic cancer	2		2			2	
Rectum cancer	1				1		1
Colon cancer	1				1		1
Leiomyosarcoma	1				1	1	
Esophagus cancer	1				1		1
Hepatoma	1	1				1	
Choriocarcinoma with meta. in lung	1	1				1	
Cervical lymphnode meta. of tongue cancer	1	1				1	
Cervical lymphnode meta. (primary unknown)	1				1		1
Kidney cancer	1				1		1
Total cases	32	5	4	0	23	14	18

Table 11. Antitumor effect versus total doses

Total doses (mg)	Objective response (tumor regression)				Subjective response	
	>80%	80-50%	<50%	None	Improvement	None
0-100		1		8	1	8
101-200	2	3		6	7	7
201-300	1			5	4	2
301-400	1			4	1	1
401-500	1				1	
Total cases	5	4	0	23	14	18

Table 12. Patients with objective tumor response

Diagnosis	Age	Administration method	Therapy duration (days)	Total dose (mg)	Response		Survival time from start of therapy (days)
					Objective (%)	Subjective	
Lung cancer	63	5 mg 7×/w i.v.	76	345	>50	Improvement	111 still alive
Reticulum cell sarcoma	67	2.5, 10 mg 2×/w i.v.	30	52.5	>50	Improvement	30
Reticulum cell sarcoma	52	5–10 mg 7×/w subselective one shot i.a. and i.v.	25	235 i.a. 65, i.v. 170	>80	Improvement	87 still alive
Reticulum cell sarcoma	31	5–10 mg 7×/w subselective one shot i.a. and i.v.	119	435 i.a. 140, i.v. 295	>80	Improvement	156 still alive
Prostatic cancer	65	10, 5 mg 3×/w selective one shot i.a.	26	110	>80	Improvement	27
Prostatic cancer	56	5–10 mg 7×/w selective one shot i.a. and i.v.	17	120	>50	Improvement	20
Hepatoma	53	10 mg 3×/w selective one shot i.a.	30	160	>80	Improvement	39
Choriocarcinoma	27	5–10 mg 3×/w Subselective one shot i.a. and i.v.	32	150 i.a. 25, i.v. 125	>80 p[a]	Improvement	40
Cervical lymph-node meta. of tongue cancer	65	10 mg 7×/w i.v.	62	360	>80	Improvement	110 still alive

p[a]: Progress in lung metastasis.

References

1. Ichikawa, T.: Bleomycin, a new antitumor antibiotic. J. Jap. Med. Assoc. **61**, 487–497 (1969).
2. Kurihara, M., Shirakabe, H., Murakami, T., Yasui, A., Izumi, T., Sumida, M., Igarashi, A.: A new method for producing adenocarcinoma in the stomach of dogs with N-ethyl-N'-nitro-N-nitrosoguanidine. GANN. **65**, 163–177 (1974).
3. Sugimura, T., Fujimura, S., Baba, T.: Tumor production in the glandular stomach and alimentary tract of rat by N-Methyl-N'-nitro-N-nitrosoguanidine. Cancer Res. **30**, 455–465 (1970).
4. Umezawa, H.: Bleomycin: Discovery, Chemistry, and Action In: Fundamental and clinical studies of bleomycin. GANN Monograph on Cancer Research No. 19, Carter, S. K., Ichikawa, T., Mathé, G., and Umezawa, H. (ed.) 3–36, University of Tokyo Press (1976).
5. Umezawa, H.: Chemistry and mechanism of action of bleomycin. Federation Proc. **33**, 2296–2302 (1974).
6. Umezawa, H., Takeuchi, T., Hori, S., Sawa, T., Ishizuka, M., Ichikawa, T., Komai, T.: Studies on the mechanism of antitumor effect of bleomycin on squamous cell carcinoma. J. Antibiotics **25**, 409–420 (1974).
7. Yoshioka, O., Yamaguchi, S., Matsuda, A., Umezawa, H.: The role of nude mice as new assay system in research on cancer chemotherapeutic agents. Jap. J. Cancer Clin. **22**, 707–713 (1976).

Experimental Results with the Combination of Bleomycin Plus Mitomycin C

N. YAMANAKA, M. FUKUSHIMA, T. KATO, K. KOIZUMI, and K. OTA

Introduction

Bleomycin, a water-soluble basic glycopeptide antibiotic, is well known for treatment against human squamous cell carcinoma and malignant lymphoma [4, 5, 14, 17]. Recently, MIYAMOTO et al. reported that a sequential combination of bleomycin and mitomycin C induced a drastic remission effect on advanced cervical cancer [7].

Bleomycin induces DNA chain breakage and the action is enhanced by free radical producing systems such as sulfhydryl compounds and other oxidizing or reducing agents [8, 9, 11]. Free radical involvement has been implicated for the action of mitomycin C and other quinone-containing anticancer agents [3, 10, 12].

The mechanism of action of bleomycin in relation to free radical reactions and biologic systems is not well understood [18, 19]. Therefore, in the present study, we have addressed the following questions:

1. Is bleomycin in combination with mitomycin C or other quinone-containing anticancer agents effective on cells in cultures or on tumor-bearing animals?
2. Does the physiologic free radical producing system such as microsomal NADPH-dependent electron transport system enhance the DNA chain breakage by bleomycin and/or mitomycin C?
3. Are the free radical mediated reactions directly involved or related to the side effects of bleomycin?

Combination of Bleomycin and Mitomycin C or Other Quinone-Containing Anticancer Agents

The concentration of bleomycin required to kill cancer cells was lowered in the presence of other agents as shown in Table 1.

Quinone-containing anticancer agents such as mitomycin C, carbazilquinone, daunomycin, adriamycin and aclacinomycin A were demonstrated to be effective in increasing the sensitivity for bleomycin. However, other anticancer agents with different structures from quinones were without effect, even though they are known to be powerful anticancer agents by themselves. Bleomycin was more effective in combination with quinone-containing anticancer agents or oxidizing and reducing vitamins such as vitamin C and vitamin K_2.

The cooperative effect of different concentrations of bleomycin plus mitomycin C was also examined on AH66 tumor-bearing rats (Fig. 1). Among the combinations, the simultaneous treatment of bleomycin plus mitomycin C was found to be most effective in increasing the lifespan of tumor-bearing rats. Five days' injection of bleomycin (20 mg/kg/day) and

Table 1. Effect of combination of bleomycin and other agents on KB culture cells.
KB cells were cultured using Eagle's with Hank's salts, supplemented with 10% fetal calf serum and examined microscopically. Plus (+) signs represent cells killed by the treatment. Minus (-) signs indicate no effect

Anticancer agents	Conc. (μg/ml)	Bleomycin	(conc. μg/ml)	
		250	125	62.5
Mitomycin C	0.5	+	+	-
Carbazilquinone	0.1	+	-	-
Daunomycin	0.25	+	+	-
Adriamycin	0.25	+	+	-
Aclacinomycin A	0.25	+	+	-
Macromomycin	0.1	-	-	-
Neocarzinostatin	10	-	-	-
5-Fluorouracil	25	-	-	-
Cytosine arabinoside	5	-	-	-
Vinblastine	0.00025	-	-	-
Vincristine	0.001	-	-	-
Vitamin C	250	+	+	+
Vitamin K_1	10	+	−	−
Vitamin K_2	5	+	+	+
Vitamin K_3	5	+	-	-
Coenzyme Q_{10}	250	-	-	
Cepharanthin	10	+	+	+

Table 2. The stimulation of bleomycin-induced DNA chain breakage by NADPH and microsomes.
DNA chain breakage was estimated by acid-soluble radioactive products from [^{3}H]-thymine-labelled *E. coli* DNA. The standard reaction system contained microsomes (0.2 mg protein/ml), 0.24 mM NADPH, 6μg/ml [^{3}H]-thymine-labeled DNA (2805 cmp/μg DNA), 0.12 M KCI and 40 mM potassium phosphate buffer (ph 7.4 at 37°C) (total 0.5 ml). The reaction was terminated by the addition of 0.1 ml 35% trichloroacetic acid after 30 min incubation. After centrifugation, an aliquot of the supernatant was taken for determination of radioactivity using a liquid scintillation counter

Addition	cpm	DNA chain breakage (%)
None[a]	1670	59.5
—BLM -NADPH-mic	7	0.2
—BLM	4	0.1
—mic	19	0.7
—NADPH	16	0.6
+40 μg/ml Vit K_2	1756	62.6
+40 μg/ml Vit K_2-BLM	6	0.2
+ 8 μg/ml MMC	1536	54.8
+ 8 μg/ml MMC-BLM	3	0.1
+ Hydralazine hydrochloride		
50.0 μM	1272	45.3
0.5 mM	910	32.4
1.0 mM	740	26.4
+ Ecarazine hydrochloride		
35.0 μM	1574	56.1
0.35 mM	1552	55.3
0.7 mM	1479	52.7

[a] Abbreviations: BLM, bleomycin; mic, microsomes; Vit K_2, Vitamin K_2; MMC, mitomycin C.

mitomycin C (0.5 mg/kg/day) showed an increase in lifespan of more than 230%. Under these conditions, bleomycin or mitomycin C alone was not effective. The sequential combination of bleomycin and mitomycin C did not extend the lifespan of tumor-bearing rats markedly.

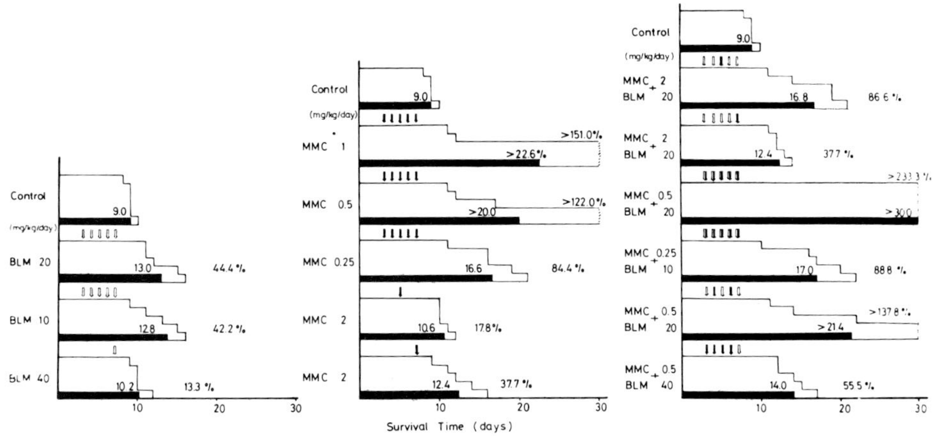

Fig. 1. Effect of combination of bleomycin and mitomycin C on AH66. AH66 (10^6 cells) were inoculated to Donryu rats (90-110 g). Injections i.p. with bleomycin and/or mitomycin C were carried out as indicated. ⇦ : bleomycin treatment; ⬅ : mitomycin C treatment; ⇦ : bleomycin plus mitomycin C treatment. % represents increase of lifespan

Enhancement of DNA Chain Breakage by Bleomycin in the Presence of Microsomes and NADPH

In the presence of bleomycin and/or NADPH-dependent microsomal electron transport systems (Table 2), broken pieces of [^{3}H]-thymine-labeled DNA were detected in acid-soluble fraction. NADH was ineffective and 0.2 mM PCMB inhibited the enhancement completely.

The enhancement of bleomycin-induced DNA chain breakage on isolated nuclei was observed by the additions of NADPH and microsomes (Table 3). In this system, additions of bleomycin and NADPH also stimulated the DNA chain breakage to some extent. NADH and the copper chelating form of bleomycin (bleomycin-Cu^{2+}) did not enhance the breakage effectively.

The DNA breakage was examined by using AH66 cells which were labeled by [^{3}H]-thymidine (Table 4). The addition of bleomycin and NADPH were effective in stimulating the DNA chain breakage. Under cellular conditions, bleomycin alone also stimulated the production of acid-soluble products. The effectiveness of exogenous NADPH on cellular levels was in agreement with the results obtained by McCay [16].

The DNA breakage was also shown by alkaline sucrose gradient analysis. The analysis was done by using isolated intact nuclear DNA. It is quite evident that the bleomycin-induced breakage was enhanced by NADPH and microsomes (Fig. 2).

Table 3. The stimulation of isolated nuclear DNA chain breakage by NADPH-dependent microsomal electron transport system with bleomycin.
AH66 cells were DNA-labeled with [^{3}H]-thymidine before purification. Labeled nuclei were isolated essentially according to Fukushima et al. (2). The standard reaction system contained 2.1×10^5 nuclei ml [^{3}H]-thymidine-labeled nuclei, 89514 cpm/1.05×10^5 nuclei), 5 mM $MgCl_2$, 0.15 M Tris-HCl (ph 7.5 at 37°C) (total 0.5 ml). After 30 min incubation, the reaction was terminated and acid-soluble radioactive products were measured as described in Table 2

Additions	cpm	DNA chain breakage (%)
None	63	0.2
+ 100 μg/ml BLM	88	0.3
+ 0.24 mM NADPH + 0.4 mg/ml mic	99	0.3
+ 100 μg/ml BLM + 0.24 mM NADPH	643	2.2
+ 100 μg/ml BLM + 0.24 mM NADPH + 0.4 mg/ml mic	3093	10.4
+ 100 μg/ml BLM + 0.24 mM NADH + 0.4 mg/ml mic	230	0.8
+ 100 μg/ml BLM-Cu + 0.24 mM NADPH + 0.4 mg/ml mic	122	0.4

Table 4. The stimulation of DNA chain breakage in AH66 cells by bleomycin and NADPH.
AH66 cells were labeled with [^{3}H]-thymidine. The standard reaction system contained 200 μg/ml BLM, 0.6 mM NADPH, 2 x 10^6 AH66 cells/ml ([^{3}H]-thymidine-labeled cells, 387160 cpm/1.0×10^6 cells) in 0.5 ml phosphate buffer saline solution, pH 7.4 at 37°C (total 0.5 ml). After 60 min incubation, the reaction was terminated and acid-soluble radioactive products were measured as described in Table 2

Addition	cpm	DNA chain breakage (%)
None	11,170	8.7
—BLM-NADPH	325	0.2
—BLM	308	0.2
—NADPH	1765	1.4
+ 20 μg/ml MMC	12,047	9.3
+ 40 μg/ml Vit K_2	13,070	10.1
+ Hydralazine hydrochloride 0.5 mM	6316	4.9
+ Ecarazine hydrochloride 0.7 mM	11,326	8.9

Effect of Mitomycin C or Vitamin K_2 on Bleomycin-Induced DNA Chain Breakage

The production of acid-soluble compounds was examined by the addition of mitomycin C or vitamin K_2 to bleomycin and to the NADPH systems. No stimulation of the DNA breakage was observed by the addition of mitomycin C to the isolated DNA (Table 2). However, at the cellular level, mitomycin C or vitamin K_2 increased the DNA breakage by bleomycin (Table 4). In the case of isolated nuclei, vitamin K_2 stimulated the breakage, but mitomycin C was without effect. There are some differences in the stimulative response induced by mitomycin C or vitamin K_2.

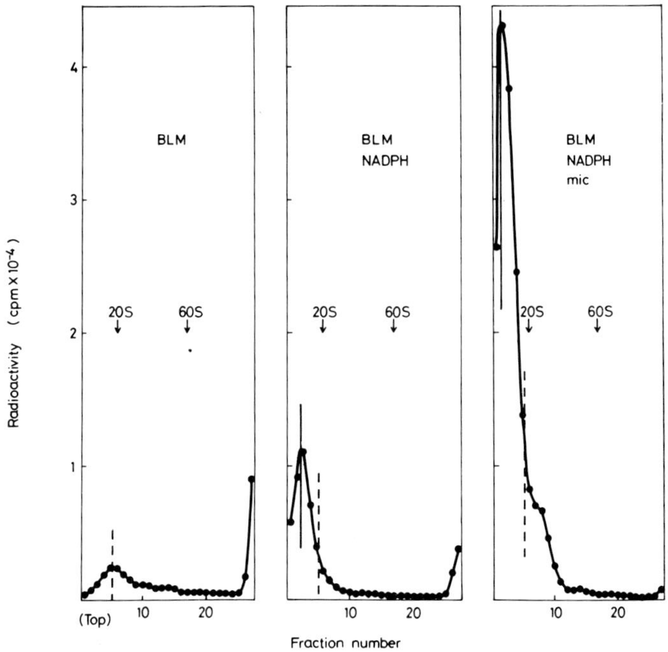

Fig. 2. Alkaline sucrose gradient analysis of isolated nuclear DNA treated by bleomycin and the microsomal NADPH-dependent electron transport system. The standard reaction system contained 1.4 × 10^5 [^{3}H]-thymidine-labeled nuclei/ml; microsomes (0.4 mg protein/ml); 100 μg/ml bleomycin; 0.24 mM NADPH; 0.15 M Tris-HCl buffer, pH 7.5; 5 mM $MgCl_2$. After 30 min incubation at 37°C, the reaction was terminated by diluting with cold Tris-HCl-Mg buffer and centrifuged nuclei were analyzed essentially according to WALTERS [15]. Centrifugation was done in an Hitachi ultracentrifuge at 15,000 γpm (Hitachi RP-40 rotor) for 15 h at 10°C

Production of TBA Reactive Compounds by Bleomycin or Bleomycin-Cu^{2+}

The formation of TBA (2-thiobarbituric acid) reactive compounds, which indicates the peroxidation reaction of lipids, was increased by bleomycin-Cu^{2+}, NADPH and microsomes (Fig. 3). The DNA addition was without effect on the bleomycin-Cu^{2+} system. However, the addition of bleomycin to an NADPH and microsome system inhibited the formation of TBA reactive compounds. In contrast, if DNA was added to the above system, TBA reactants were increased (Fig. 3). The involvement of TBA reactive compounds has been suggested in previous reports [5, 8] even though the spectral pattern of the products (not shown here) was slightly different from those of KUO et al. [6].

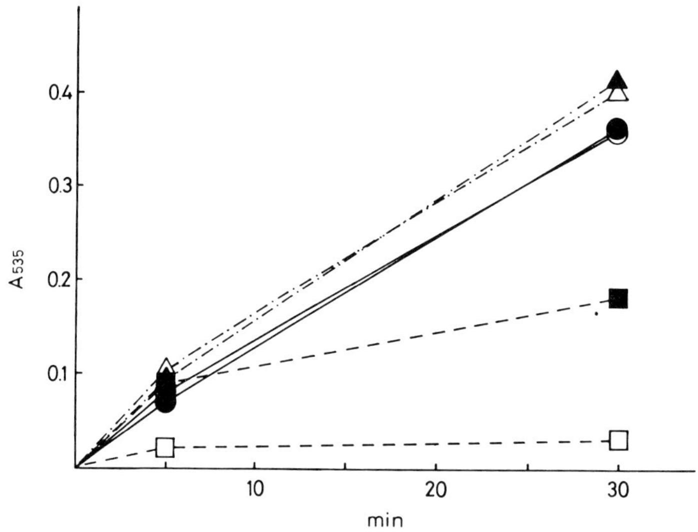

Fig. 3. Effect of bleomycin or bleomycin-Cu^{2+} on microsomal NADPH-dependent malondialdehyde formation. The standard reaction system contained microsomes (0.33 mg protein/ml); 0.2 mM NADPH; 0.12 M KCl; 40 mM potassium phosphate buffer, pH 7.4, 37°C (total 3.0 ml). Malondialdehyde formation was determined using TBA according to the method of TAPPEL except for n-butanol [1]. o—o: standard condition; •—•: plus 33 μg/ml DNA; □—□: plus 50 μg/ml bleomycin; ■—■: plus 50 μg/ml bleomycin and 33 μg/ml DNA; △—·—△: plus 50 μg/ml bleomycin-Cu^{2+}; △—·—△: plus 50 μg/ml bleomycin-Cu^{2+} and 33 μg/ml DNA

Inhibition of the Formation of TBA Reactive Compounds Induced by Bleomycin-CU^{2+} or Bleomycin

The formation of bleomycin-Cu^{2+}-stimulated TBA reactive products was accompanied by oxygen consumption and was effectively inhibited by antioxidants such as vitamin E or tinoridine (anti-inflammatory, membrane stabilizing drug) [18]. The results indicate that bleomycin-Cu^{2+} stimulates a lipid peroxidation reaction by the microsomal NADPH-dependent electron transport system. In contrast, the TBA reactants formation induced by bleomycin and DNA was not inhibited by the above antioxidants and the formation did not accompany oxygen consumption. The TBA reactants did not appear in the absence of DNA or in the presence of PCMB. This supports the suggestion that the breakage of DNA by bleomycin induces the aldehyde formation [5, 8]. Aldehydes such as malondialdehyde are highly toxic and it is very likely that the release of aldehyde compounds damages membranes and other tissue components. These facts have prompted us to attempt to scavenge these aldehydes by compounds such as hydralazine derivatives, homocysteine and penicillamine [13]. Hydralazine hydrochloride and isoniazid were effective in inhibiting the formation of TBA reactive compounds but homocysteine and ecarazine hydrochloride were not. As for acid-soluble product formation, hydralazine hydrochloride was inhibitory, but isoniazid and ecarazine hydrochloride were without effect. The effects of isoniazid and hydralazine on the bleomycin-induced DNA breakage by alkaline sucrose gradient analysis were studied by using isolated AH66 nuclei. Breakage was not inhibited by these reagents. Thus, the results suggest that isoniazid and hydralazine hydrochloride can scavenge aldehyde compounds released by DNA breakage induced by bleomycin without decreasing the antitumor effects of bleomycin. Aldehyde compounds are known to be related to collagen crosslinking [13] and bleomycin is also known to affect collagen tissue. From these facts, there is a possibility that the formation of aldehyde compounds by bleomycin and DNA is related to the side effect of bleomycin. Further studies are being carried out in our laboratory to prevent lung fibrosis by using antioxidants such as vitamin E and/or tinoridine and by hydralazine derivatives.

Summary

This investigation has established the following:

1. Bleomycin, in combination with mitomycin C or other quinone-containing anticancer agents, stimulated the damage to KB cells in culture.
2. In AH66 tumor-bearing rats, the simultaneous treatments of bleomycin plus mitomycin C extend the lifespan.
3. The bleomycin-induced DNA chain breakage was enhanced by the NADPH-dependent microsomal electron transport system. The enhancement was also observed at the level of isolated nuclei and cells. Vitamin K_2 and mitomycin C increased breakage at the cellular level by bleomycin and NADPH.
4. Bleomycin-Cu^{2+} had the tendency to increase the lipid peroxidation reaction by the microsomes. However, the reaction was effectively inhibited by antioxidants.
5. Bleomycin induced aldehyde formation from DNA breakage. The formation was effectively inhibited by scavenging reactions with hydralazine hydrochloride or isoniazid. The possibility of suppressing the side effect of bleomycin was discussed in relation to TBA reactive compounds.

Acknowledgement

We wish to thank Dr. M. Ogawa, Miss K. Nishida and Miss F. Matsumoto for many useful discussions and technical assistance. This work was supported in part by a Grant-in-Aid for Cancer Research from the Ministry of Health and Welfare.

References

1. Dillard, D. J., Tappel, A. L.: Fluorescent products of lipid peroxidation of mitochondria and microsomes. Lipids **6**, 715–721 (1971).
2. Fukushima, M., Okayama, H., Takahashi, Y., Hayaishi, O.: Characterization of NAD^+ glycohydrolase associated with the rat liver nuclear envelope. J. Biochem. (Tokyo) **80**, 167–176 (1976).
3. Handa, K., Sato, S.: Generation of free radicals of quinone group-containing anticancer chemicals in NADPH-microsome system as evidenced by initiation of sulfite oxidation. Gann **66**, 43–47 (1975).
4. Ichikawa, T., Matsumoto, K., Umezawa, H.: Clinical study of a new antitumor antibiotic,

bleomycin (preliminary report). Proc. 5th Int. Congr. Chemother., A IV-4/35, 507–516 (1967).
5. Kimura, K., Sakai, Y., Chikada, C., Kashimida, N., Inagaki, J., Mikuni, M., Sakano, T.: Chemotherapy of malignant lymphoma with special reference to effects of bleomycin. Cancer **29**, 58–60 (1972).
6. Kuo, M. D., Haidle, C. W.: Characterization of chain breakage in DNA induced by bleomycin. Biochim. Biophys. Acta **335**, 109–114 (1973).
7. Miyamoto, T., Takabe, Y., Watanabe, M., Terasima, T.: Drastic remission effect of a sequential combination of bleomycin and mitomycin C in advanced cervical cancer. Cancer & Chemotherapy (Tokyo) **4**, 273–291 (1977).
8. Müller, W. E. G., Yamazaki, Z., Berter, H. J., Zahn, R. K.: Action of bleomycin on DNA and RNA. Eur. J. Biochem. **31**, 518–525 (1972).
9. Nagai, K., Suzuki, H., Tanaka, H., Umezawa, H.: Decrease of melting temperature and single strand scission of DNA by bleomycin in the presence of 2-mercaptoethanol. J. Antibiot. (Tokyo) **22**, 569–673 (1969).
10. Nagata, C., Matsuyama, A.: On the mechanism of action of the carcinostatic antibiotic mitomycin C. Prog. Antimicrob. Anti-cancer Chemother. Proc. 6th Int. Congr. Chemother. **2**, 423–425 (1969).
11. Onishi, T., Iwata, H., Takagi, Y.: Effects of reducing and oxidizing agents on the action of bleomycin. J. Biochem. (Tokyo) **77**, 745–752 (1975).
12. Schwartz, H. S., Sodergren, J. E., Philips, F. S.: Mitomycin C: chemical and biological studies on alkylation. Science **142**, 1181–1183 (1963).
13. Siegel, R. C.: Collagen crosslinking. Effect of D-penicillamine on crosslinking *in vitro*. J. Biol. Chem. **252**, 254–259 (1977).
14. Umezawa, H. Maeda, K., Takeuchi, T., Okami, Y.: New antibiotics, bleomycin A and B. J. Antibiot. (Tokyo), Ser. A, **19**, 200–209 (1966).
15. Walters, R. A., Hildebrand, C. E.: A procedure for the rapid lysis of mammalian cells prior to alkaline sucrose density gradient centrifugation. Biochim. Biophys. Acta **407**, 120–124 (1975).
16. Weddle, C. C., Hornbrook, K. R., McCay, P. B.: Lipid peroxidation and alteration of membrane lipid in isolated hepatocytes exposed to carbon tetrachloride. J. Biol. Chem. **251**, 4973–4978 (1976).
17. Yagoda, A. Krakoff, I. H.: Observation of the use of bleomycin in the treatment of malignant lymphoma in the U.S.A. Japanese Cancer Assn., Gann Monogr. Cancer Res. **19**, 255–268 (1976).
18. Yamanaka, N., Kato, T., Ota, K.: Drug metabolism and side effect of anticancer agent—with special reference to mechanism of action and side effect of bleomycin. Cancer & Chemotherapy (Tokyo) **3**, 1139–1146 (1976).
19. Yamanaka, N., Ota, K.: Senescence, carcinogenesis, and cancer therapy in relation to free radical reactions. Cancer & Chemotherapy (Tokyo) **4**, 1–10 (1977).

Studies on the Clinical Pharmacology of Bleomycin*

S. T. CROOKE, R. I. COMIS, L. H. EINHORN, J. E. STRONG, A. BROUGHTON, and A. W. PRESTAYKO

Bleomycin is an antitumor antibiotic isolated from *Streptomyces verticillus* [9]. It is active in squamous cell carcinomas, lymphomas, and testicular carcinomas, and its most significant toxicity has been shown to be pulmonary fibrosis [1,3]. It has been suggested that it induces its antitumor effects by producing single and double stranded breaks in preformed DNA [8]. Until recently, little information concerning the clinical pharmacology of bleomycin has been available. Initial clinical pharmocokinetic studies employed a microbiologic assay using a *B. subtillis* AT6633 spore solution which was sensitive to approximately 0.2 mU/ml [5]. The elimination of bleomycin from blood was reported to vary, with some patients demonstrating first order kinetics and others not. The plasma half-life was reported in one study to vary from 16-45 min at doses in excess of 26 U/m^2 [7]. In another study, a dose of 15 U was reported to result in a maximum blood level of 3.3 μg/ml, and a serum half-life of 14 min [4]. Recently, a radioimmunossay for bleomycin was developed which proved to be more sensitive than previously reported microbiologic assays [2]. The antisera used in the radioimmunoassay were prepared with a bleomycin-bovine serum albumin conjugate. After the development of the radioimmunoassay, several studies were designed to determine a) the accuracy of the radioimmunoassay, b) the comparability of the radioimmunoassay to the microbiologic assay, c) the specificity of the radioimmunoassay, d) the pharmacokinetics of bleomycin administered to patients as an intravenous bolus, e) the effects of varying renal function on the pharmacokinetics of bleomycin, and f) the pharmacokinetics of bleomycin administered as a prolonged intravenous infusion. In this publication we present the results of the studies on the radioimmunoassay specificity and the pharmacokinetics of the intravenous bolus.

Material and Methods

Chemicals

Bleomycin (Blenoxane®), and BU-2231 were supplied by Bristol Laboratories, Syracuse, N.Y. Bleomycinic acid, bleomycin A_2, B_2, A_5, B_1, iso-bleomycin, desamidobleomycin A_2 were supplied by Nippon-Kayaku, Tokyo, Japan. Bleomycinic acid, bleomycin A_2, B_2, and A_5 were copper chelates, BU-2231A, BU-2231B, iso-bleomycin A_2 and bleomycin (Blenoxane®) were copper free.

---

* These studies supported in part by Bristol Laboratories and in part by N. I. H. Grant 5MOLRR.00750.

Assay Procedures

The microbiologic assay was performed employing a *B. subtillis* ATC6633 spore solution as previously described [5]. The radioimmunoassay was performed as previously described [2]. Competitive experiments were performed as previously described [2]. Replicates of each concentration were performed, and the results were found to be readily reproducible.

Sample Collection

Venous and arterial blood specimens were obtained in heparinized tubes at specified intervals up to 72 h after a dose of bleomycin. When serum was to be assayed, blood specimens were collected in nonheparinized tubes. Specimens were refrigerated, centrifuged, the plasma or serum obtained, and stored frozen (−20°C) until analyzed. Urine specimens were collected for varying periods of time, stored on ice, and frozen immediately at the termination of the collection period.

Blood and urine for pharmacologic studies from patients being treated with bleomycin, vinblastine and cis-platinum, were obtained after a dose of bleomycin approximately 72 h after completion of the cis-platinum infusion.

Patient Selection

To minimize variables, all patients enrolled in the intravenous bolus pharmacokinetics study had disseminated testicular carcinomas and were treated with bleomycin, vinblastine, and cis-platinum according to the regimen developed by Dr. Einhorn (table 1). The patients were selected because of the relative homogeneity of this group of patients. Moreover, since all patients were treated with the same regimen, potential pharmacokinetic differences due to drug interactions occuring in patients treated with varying regimens were obviated.

Additionally, since a major goal of the study was to determine the effect of varying renal function on bleomycin pharmacokinetics, the nephrotoxicity of this regimen allowed evaluation of patients in whom creatinine clearance varied during the study and resulted in a more rapid accrual of patients with varying creatinine clearances than possible with other regimens.

Table 1. Treatment regimen for metastatic testicular cancer

Bleomycin	30 u/wk. for 12 wk.
Cis-platinum II	20 mg/m^2 d 1-5 q 3 wk. for 9 wk.
Vinblastine	0.2 mg/kg/d ×2 q 3 wk.

Pharmacologic Calculations

A nonlin computer analysis was employed for treatment of the pharmacokinetic data. The method used is an adaptation of Hartley's modification of the Gauss-Newton method for linearizing equations and applying linear least squares [6].

Results

Radioimmunoassay Specificity

In Fig. 1, data obtained employing the radioimmunoassay are compared to the data obtained using the microbiologic assay. The coefficient of correlation between the methods within the range of sensitivity of the microbiologic assay was 0.987. Further, these studies demonstrated that both the radioimmunoassay and the microbiologic assays may be employed to assay either plasma or serum.

Fig. 2 shows the general structure of bleomycin, and the terminal amine groups for bleomycin A_2, A_5, and B_2. Bleomycinic acid does not contain a terminal amine structure, and bleomycin B_1 is the amide. Iso-bleomycin A_2 is the product of carbamoyl group migration in which the carbamoyl group is found on the 2-carbon rather than the 3-carbon position of the mannose sugar. Fig. 3 shows the structure of BU-2231B. The terminal amine, spermidine, is analogous to the terminal amine on bleomycin A_5.

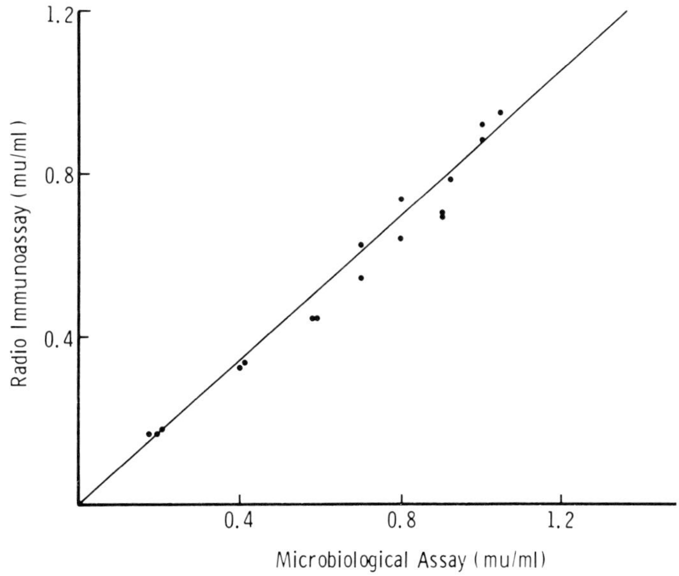

Fig. 1. Correlation of bleomycin determinations by radioimmunoassay and the microbiologic assay. Concentrations were determined as described in "Materials and Methods." The RIA results are plotted on the ordinate, and the microbiologic results on the abscissa. The points on the figure represent points of intersection of perpendiculars drawn to the data obtained with each assay

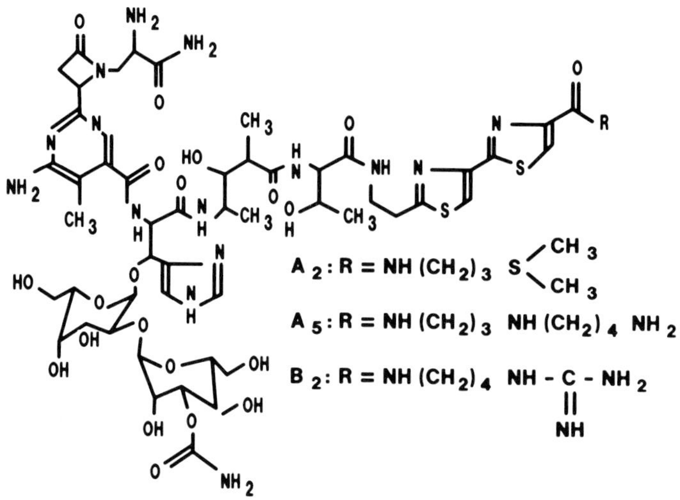

Fig. 2. Structure of bleomycin analogs. (R: Terminal amine)

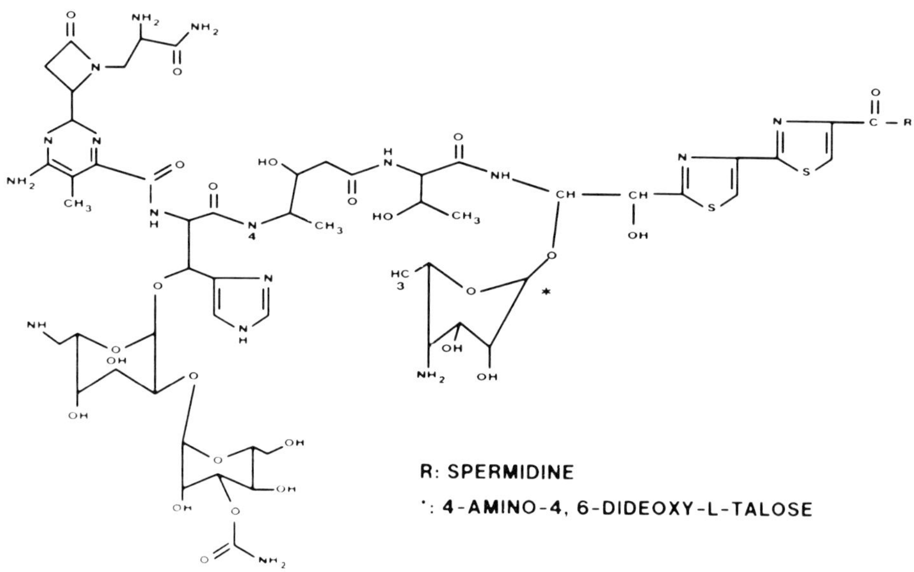

Fig. 3. Structure of BU-2231B. (R: Terminal amine)

Table 2. Bleomycin analog immunoreactivity

Bleomycin	Mean concentration (pM)	Standard deviation (pM)	Cross-reactivity (%)
Sulfate	3.45	±0.11	100
A_2	2.99	±0.22	115.4
B_2	4.63	±0.17	74.5
A_5	29.50	±5.14	11.7
Iso-A_2	13.70	±0.29	25.2
Acid	>100.00	—	<1.0
BU-2231B	>100.00	—	<1.0

The indicated quantity of bleomycin analog was required to produce a 50% inhibition of [I^{125}]-labeled bleomycin sulfate bound to antibody. Results are expressed as the mean pmolar concentration of the bleomycin analog determined in five separate analyses.

Table 2 shows that bleomycin (Blenoxane) competed successfully against labeled bleomycin indicating that the experimental procedure is valid. Bleomycin A_2, A_5 and B_2, members of the bleomycin mixture, competed to varying degrees. Iso-bleomycin A_2 competed at 20%-25% the efficiency of bleomycin A_2. Bleomycin B_1 competed at approximately the 1% level. Neither bleomycinic acid nor BU-2231 competed at any concentration.

Pharmacokinetics of Intravenous Bolus Injections

Table 3 shows the characteristics of patients enrolled in this study. The median age was 24 years. Ages varied from 18-47 years. With two exceptions, all initial performance statuses were 80 or greater. Initial creatinine clearances varied from 10.7-180 ml/min corrected to 1.73 m^2 body surface area. All patients had measurable disease. All evaluable patients achieved either partial (>50% decrease in the cross-sectional area of measurable lesions), or complete response. Two patients were not evaluable for response because of lack of measurable disease. One patient was not evaluable because of having received previous chemotherapy.

Table 4 presents the plasma terminal half-lives of bleomycin determined by the microbiologic and radioimmunoassays (RIA), relative to creatinine clearance. The data in this table demonstrate that, in general, the plasma or serum $t_{\frac{1}{2}}\beta$ of bleomycin determined with the radioimmunoassay agreed with the $t_{\frac{1}{2}}\beta$ determined with the microbiologic assay.

The data presented in Table 4 also demonstrate that the plasma clearance of bleomycin varied with the creatinine clearance. Fig. 4 shows the relationship of bleomycin plasma or serum $t_{\frac{1}{2}}\beta$ to creatinine clearance. These data conform to predictions for compounds cleared primarily by renal mechanisms. In Fig. 5, the log of the plasma or serum $t_{\frac{1}{2}}\beta$ is plotted against the creatinine clearance. This Figure demonstrates that the inflection point, i.e., the point at which the plasma $t_{\frac{1}{2}}\beta$ of bleomycin becomes prolonged, is at a creatinine clearance of approximately 25-35 ml/min. At creatinine clearances in excess of 25-35 ml/min, the mean $t_{\frac{1}{2}}\beta$ was 115 min. Below a creatinine clearance of approximately 25-35 ml/min, the plasma $t_{\frac{1}{2}}\beta$ of bleomycin increased exponentially as the creatinine clearance decreased. Fig. 6 shows similar data determined using the radioimmunoassay.

Fig. 7 shows data obtained on a patient in renal failure. These studies demonstrate a) at a creatine clearance as low as 10.7 ml/min, no bleomycin is detectable at 72 h post dose, b) bleomycin is probably not dialyzable, and c) that bleomycin clearance varied in a single patient as the creatinine clearance varied.

Bleomycin pharmacokinetics were evaluated sequentially in eight patients. These studies

Table 3. Patient characteristics

Patient's initials	Age	m²	Performance status	Initial creatinine clearance (ml/min)	Site of metastases	Tumor response
S.H.	24	2.0	90	10.7	Pulmonary	CR
R.S.	33	1.95	30	21.3	Pulmonary, CNS	PR
E.I.	29	2.3	80	62	Left inguinal node	CR
S.B.	25	1.8	80	64.6	Left cervical node, para aortic	PR
G.R.	27	1.65	90	78	Liver	
J.K.	46	1.6	80	88	Lung	CR
R.C.	21	2.3	80	89	Bone, lung, retroperitoneal nodes	PR (CR)
R.S.	24	1.9	60	98.6	Retroperitoneal mass	PR (CR)
B.C.	20	1.9	90	98.7	Pelvis, mediastinum, para aortic	N.E.
B.L.	47	2.1	90	107	Pulmonary, mediastinum	PR
K.R.	22	1.5	90	108.5	Skull, shoulder, elbow	N.E.
M.R.	22	2.1	90	109	Pulmonary, lymph node	CR
J.C.	25	1.76	90	110	Adjuvant therapy	N.E.
M.H.	26	2.08	90	115	Mediastinal mass	PR
G.R.	26	1.68	90	118	Pulmonary	CR
T.W.	26	1.88	90	123	Lung, retroperitoneal nodes	CR
R.S.	22	2.1	90	128	Large retroperitoneal mass, lung	PR (CR)
T.C.	18	1.84	90	140	Mediastinal mass, pulmonary	CR
S.R.	27	1.7	100	157	Lung	PR (CR)
R.S.	22	1.98	90	180	Pulmonary, liver nodes, para aortic	PR (CR)
Median	24	1.9				

Table 4. Plastma $t_{\frac{1}{2}}\beta$ Bleomycin versus creatinine clearance

Patient	Creatinine clearance (ml/min)	Microbiologie $t_{\frac{1}{2}}$ (min)	RIA $t_{\frac{1}{2}}$ (min)
S.H.	10.7	1260	1260
S.H.	15.2	660	660
R.S.	21	375	341
K.R.	35	276	178
R.C.	48	119	—
E.I.	62	157	114
S.B.	65	171	177
R.C.	89	158	117
G.R.	98	130	150
R.S.	99	92	68
B.C.	99	114	133
M.R.	105	123	103
B.L.	107	100	106
K.R.	108	41	25
M.R.	109	121	98
J.C.	110	85	74
M.H.	115	94	117
G.R.	118	173	129
R.C.	120	63	78.6
R.S.	122	134	209
T.W.	123	114	103
M.H.	127	115	98
T.C.	140	112	98
T.C.	146	121	98
R.S.	149	114	124
R.S.	180	95	140

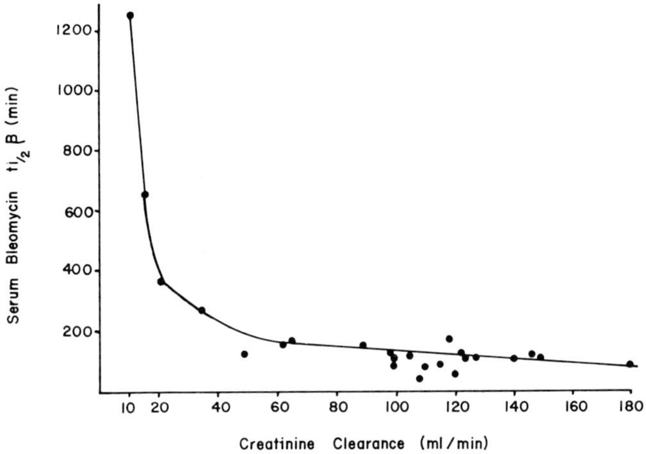

Fig. 4. The relationship of serum and plasma bleomycin $t_{\frac{1}{2}}\beta$ to creatinine clearance. Bleomycin concentrations were determined as described in "Materials and Methods." The elimination phase half-lives were calculated by a nonlin computer program

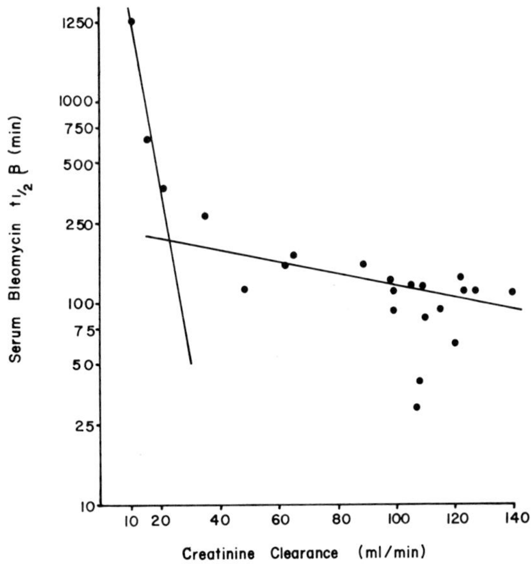

Fig. 5. Semilogarithmic plot of plasma and serum $t_{\frac{1}{2}}\beta$ of bleomycin versus creatinine clearance from values determined using the microbiologic assay

(Table 5) demonstrate that, in general, within a given patient the plasma half-life of bleomycin varied inversely with the creatinine clearance.

Table 6 shows that, with two exceptions, the volume of distribution varied from 14–35 liters. Two patients had volumes of distribution of 6.5 and 8.3 liters. Table 7 shows that the mean volume of distribution of bleomycin was equivalent in patients with creatinine clearances greater or less than 35 ml/min.

Table 8 shows data concerning the urinary excretion of bleomycin. A mean of approximately

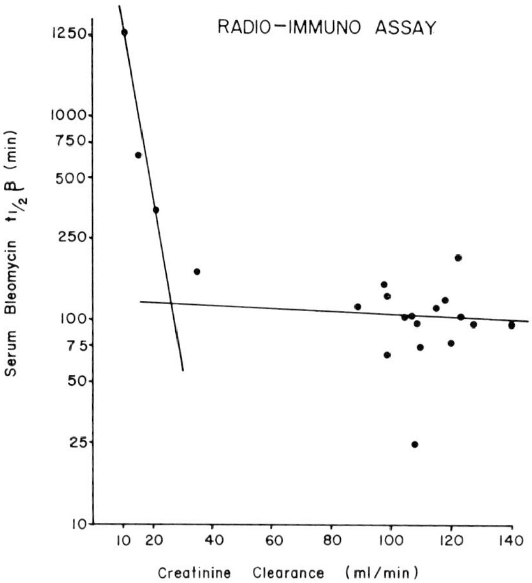

Fig. 6. Semilogarithmic plot of plasma and serum $t_{\frac{1}{2}}\beta$ of bleomycin versus creatinine clearance from values determined using the radioimmunoassay

50% of the total dose was excreted during the first 4 h post dose. Within 24 h post-dose, approximately 70% of the total dose was excreted in the urine.

Discussion

Radioimmunospecificity

The studies described demonstrate that changes in several areas of the bleomycin molecule alter the binding characteristics of bleomycin analogs. Clearly, the absence of a terminal amine results in a loss of cross-reactivity. Moreover, since bleomycin B_1, competed to only 1%, the length of the terminal amine is probably of significance. Migration of the carbamoyl group by one position resulted in a fourfold decrease in cross-reactivity suggesting that variations in this position of the molecule affect antibody recognition. That desamido-bleomycin A_2 cross-reacts at approximately 50% the level of bleomycin A_2 is a source of concern since this has been reported to be inactive. However, in our hands employing a PM-2 DNA assay, desamido-bleomycin A_2 is approximately 50% as active as bleomycin A_2. Since BU-2231B does not cross-react, it is clear that changes in the bleomycinic acid nucleus result in marked differences in antibody recognition.

Thus, these studies demonstrate that within the range of the microbiologic assay, the radioimmunoassay gives comparable results, and that in terms of closely related analogs, the assay is specific enough to be employed for clinical pharmacologic studies.

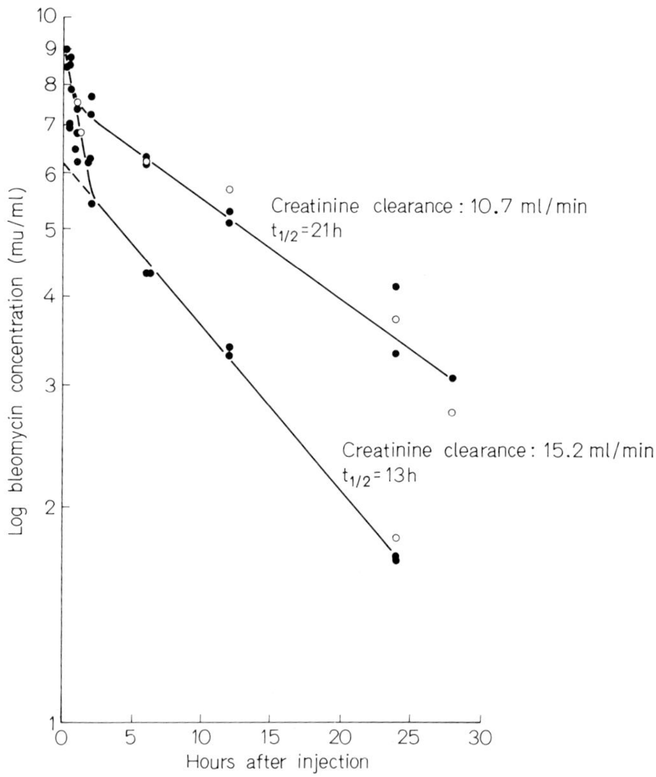

Fig. 7. Bleomycin concentrations in serum and plasma as determined by radioimmunoassay. Concentrations were determined by radioimmunoassay as previously described. The open circles indicate bleomycin concentrations in heparinized blood. The closed circles represent bleomycin concentrations in serum. (The open circle at 15 min corresponds to the curve for a creatinine clearance of 15.2 ml.)

Pharmocokinetics

The conclusions which may be derived from the pharmacokinetic study are: a) bleomycin is cleared principally by renal mechanisms; b) at creatinine clearances $\geq$25–35 ml/min, the $t_{\frac{1}{2}}\beta$ of bleomycin is approximately 115 min; c) at creatinine clearances <25–35 ml/min, the $t_{\frac{1}{2}}\beta$ increases exponentially as the creatinine clearance decreases; d) even in frank renal failure, no bleomycin was detectable in the blood 48–72 h after a bolus injection; e) in patients with creatinine clearances $\geqslant$ 50 ml/min, approximately 50% of a total dose of bleomycin is excreted in the urine in 4 h, and >70% in 24 h; f) the mean volume of distribution is approximately 20 liters, and does not vary with creatinine clearance; g) bleomycin is probably not dialyzable; h) the pharmacokinetic model describing bleomycin pharmacokinetics does not vary with varying renal function, i.e., a two-compartment model best explains the data in all patients; i) both the microbiologic and radioimmunoassays give comparable results in plasma or serum.

Thus, these studies demonstrate that there is no pharmacokinetic rationale for reducing the dose of bleomycin in patients with creatinine clearances in excess of 25–35 ml/min. Moreover, since in a patient in frank renal failure, no bleomycin was detectable in the blood 48–72 h after administration, a full dose semiweekly schedule is not unreasonable in these patients.

Table 5. Changes in renal status and plasma $t_{\frac{1}{2}}\beta$ Bleomycin during therapy

Patient	Week of therapy	Creatinine clearance (ml/min)	$t_{\frac{1}{2}}$ (min)
G.R.	0	118	129
G.R.	5	98	150
M.H.	0	115	117
M.H.	6	127	98
T.C.	0	140	98
T.C.	6	146	98
M.R.	0	109	86
M.R.	5	105	103
R.S.	0	180	95
R.S.	6	149	114
R.S.	9	122	134
K.R.	0	108	41
K.R.	9	35	276
R.C.	0	89	158
R.C.	3	120	63
R.C.	6	48	119
S.H.	0	10.7	1260
S.H.	1	15.2	660

Table 6. Creatinine clearance versus volume of distribution

Patient	Creatinine clearance (ml/min)	Volume distribution (liters)
S.H.	15	34.8
R.S.	21	16.3
K.R.	35	17.2
R.C.	48	33.1
E.I.	62	13.9
S.B.	65	6.5
R.C.	89	29.4
G.R.	98	18.8
B.C.	99	14.5
R.S.	99	19.1
M.R.	105	15.8
B.L.	107	23.6
K.R.	108	16.3
M.R.	109	22.9
J.C.	110	8.3
M.H.	115	30.1
G.R.	118	19.8
R.C.	120	18.1
R.S.	122	26.7
T.W.	123	29.4
M.H.	127	19.7
T.C.	140	18.8
T.C.	146	13.6
R.S.	149	23.4
R.S.	180	28.6

Table 7. Volume of distribution versus creatinine clearance

Creatinine clearance (ml/min)	Mean volume of distribution (liters)
$\leqslant 35$	22.7 ± 6.02
>35	19.8 ± 1.46

Table 8. Bleomycin excretion versus creatinine clearance

Patient	Creatinine clearance (ml/min)	$t_{\frac{1}{2}}\beta$ (min)	Cumulative bleomycin excreted in urine (%)			
			0-4h	0-8h	0-12h	0-24h
R.C.	48	200	50	58.3	59.9	60.6
E.I.	62	157	29	40.6	46.2	53.8
S.B.	65	171	35.3	46.9	52.9	58.2
R.C.	89	158	53	69.0	71.3	75.6
G.R.	98	150	54	70.0	75.0	77.6
M.R.	105	103	57.3	63.3	67.9	69.5
M.H.	115	117	62.6	76.6	80.6	82.1
R.S.	122	134	50	62.0	70.3	70.3
T.C.	140	98	47.6	63.6	66.4	67.9
Mean	93.7 ± 10.1	143 ± 11	48.7 ± 3.5	61.1 ± 3.7	65.6 ± 3.6	68.4 ± 3.1

References

1. Blum, R. H., Carter, S. K., Agre, K. A.: A clinical review of bleomycin—a new antineoplastic agent. Cancer **31**, 903-914 (1974).
2. Broughton, A., Strong, J. E.: Radioimmunoassay of bleomycin. Cancer Res. **35**, 1418-1421 (1976).
3. Crooke, S. T., Bradner, W. T.: Bleomycin—a review. J. of Med. **7**, 333-428, (1976).
4. Fujita, H.: Comparative studies on the blood level, tissue distribution, excretion and inactivation of anticancer drugs. Jap. J. Clin. Oncol. **12**, 151-162 (1971).
5. Fujita, H., Kimura, K.: Blood levels, tissue distribution, excretion and inactivation of bleomycin in progress in antimicrobial and anticancer chemotherapy. Proc. of the 6th Internat. Cong. of Chemother. Vol. **2**, 309-314 (1970), Baltimore: University Park Press.
6. Metzler, C. M., Nonlin, a computer program for parameter estimation in non-linear situations. Tech. Report 7292/69/7292/005, The Upjohn Co. 1969.
7. Ohnuma, T., Holland, J. F., Masuda, H., Waligunda, J. A., Goldberg, G. A.: Microbiologic assay of bleomycin: Inactivation, tissue distribution and clearance. Cancer **33**, 1230-1238 (1974).
8. Umezawa, H., Chemistry and mechanism of action of bleomycin. Fed. Proc. **33**, 2296-2302 (1974).
9. Umezawa, H., Maeda, K., Takeuchi, T., Akami, Y., New antibiotics bleomycin A and B., J. Antibiot. Ser. A **19**, 200-209 (1966).

Adriamycin and Other Anthracycline Antibiotics Under Study in the United States

R. S. BENJAMIN

Limitations of space prohibit a comprehensive review of the status of the anthracycline antibiotics in this paper. In fact, the extremely widespread use of adriamycin in current cancer chemotherapy makes a review of its use almost synonomous with a textbook of medical oncology. The present review, therefore, is highly selective, concentrating on recent developments in the use of adriamycin as a single agent, a summary of its use in combination chemotherapy of a number of malignant tumors emphasizing our own studies at M.D. Anderson Hospital and in the Southwest Oncology Group, and finally some of the newer anthracycline analogues which we have tested. Adriamycin has been the subject of a number of fine reviews [11, 12, 19, 33] and symposia [20, 21, 31, 73]. The reader is referred to these for further background data.

The widespread use of adriamycin is due to its extremely broad spectrum of antitumor activity. It is perhaps the most widely tested antitumor agent. Yet only in carcinomas of the esophagus and pancreas plus such rare tumors as carcinoid, islet cell tumors, and cloacagenic carcinoma have adequate trials not been reported. In fact, preliminary or anecdotal data suggest at least some activity in all of these tumors. In melanoma, renal carcinoma, colon carcinoma, and primary and secondary brain tumors responses have been infrequent enough to consider the drug inactive. In the brain tumors, lack of activity [82] is most likely due to the pharmacologic barrier to sufficient drug entering the tumor. On the other hand, adriamycin seems to be an essential part of primary chemotherapy of sarcomas, diffuse lymphomas, and carcinomas of the thyroid, lung, several GU, GYN, and pediatric tumors, and possibly carcinoma of the stomach. Data on the use of adriamycin in gastric carcinoma are presented elsewhere in this volume by Dr. Schein [71], and I shall therefore not consider it further.

Single agent adriamycin has recently been reported by Weiss and coinvestigators in the Central Oncology Group to be considerably less cardiotoxic when given on a weekly schedule (Table 1) [84]. These data are supported somewhat by a Western Cancer Study Group study analyzed by Paroly [59]. Although considerably fewer patients on the WCSG study reached doses likely to cause cardiac toxicity, observations in that study tend to confirm the Weiss report, although response rates for patients with sarcomas, breast carcinoma and lymphomas were somewhat higher in the COG study than in the WCSG study. It can certainly be concluded that adriamycin appears to have activity and probably decreased cardiac toxicity when given on a weekly schedule; however, the relative antitumor efficacy per unit of cardiotoxicity has not yet been fully established.

Many attempts have been made to define the cardiac toxicity of anthracyclines more fully using non-invasive techniques. Most recently described has been the quantitative measurement of the QRS voltage in the six limb leads on electrocardiogram as described by MINOW et al. [55, 56]. A 30% decrease in the value of this determination compared with a pretreatment electrocardiogram correlated significantly with the development of congestive heart failure. The most useful tool introduced for the study of anthracycline induced cardiomyopathy, however, is the cardiac biopsy which is discussed in detail by Dr. Daniels elsewhere in this symposium [28].

Table 1. Cardiotoxicity with weekly adriamycin

Author	Minow [55]	Weiss [84]	Paroly [59]
Affiliation	Pooled data	COG	WCSG
Schedule	3-weekly	weekly[a]	weekly[b]
Cumulative dose		No. with CMY/at risk (%)	
≤500	4/1254 (0.3)	1[c]/351 (0.3)	2[d]/313 (0.6)
501-600	7/66 (11)	0/23 (0)	0/13 (0)
< 600	19/61 (31)	4[c]/68 (6)	1[d]/10 (10)
< 1000	(not specified)	2[c]/31 (6)	

[a] 0.4 mg/kg (15 mg/m^2) d 1-3, 8-10, then q wk.
[b] 1 mg/kg (40 mg/m^2)/wk. × 1-2. Then ↓ to c. 0.5 mg/kg/wk.
[c] My interpretation from data provided.
[d] Preliminary data requiring confirmation.

The use of adriamycin had perhaps its most profound effects on the management of adults with soft tissue sarcomas. The drug was found to be active in many Phase I-II studies, and various combination regimens have been devised. The most effective regimens so far appear to be the combinations of adriamycin with DTIC with or without cyclophosphamide and vincristine in the studies designed by the late Dr. Jeffrey A. Gottlieb [34]. These studies demonstrated the major advantage of adding DTIC to adriamycin with or without vincristine or cyclophosphamide. In addition, they demonstrated the necessity for high-dose aggressive chemotherapy with adriamycin in this situation. The dose-response curve for adriamycin in sarcomas is quite steep, and modification of the adriamycin dosage because of the use of other myelosuppressive agents can compromise results. Thus, Creagan et al. had only a 10% response rate in 31 patients treated with vincristine, adriamycin and DTIC [26], whereas Gottlieb reported a 42% response rate with the same drugs in 107 patients (Table 2) [34]. In Creagan's study, however, adriamycin was used at a dose of 50 mg/m^2 on the third day of DTIC therapy and repeated every 5 weeks compared with Gottlieb's study where the adriamycin dose was 60 mg/m^2 every 3 weeks starting on the first day of DTIC therapy. Results of addition of other agents to adriamycin in the treatment of soft tissue sarcomas, particularly cyclophosphamide, have been disappointing. In our own studies, the addition of cyclophosphamide, vincristine and actinomycin-D to adriamycin (CYVADACT) was significantly inferior in a randomized study to CYVADIC [3, 4]. In addition, retrospective comparison of CYVADACT shows it to be inferior to the two-drug combination of adriamycin and DTIC, presumably because of the need to decrease the adriamycin dose in combination with the myelosuppressive cyclophosphamide [3]. Support for this contention is given by the ECOG study of Rosenbaum and Schoenfeld who compared single agent adriamycin with the combination of adriamycin with cyclophosphamide and vincristine [69]. They, too, found a lower response rate with the combination. The approach of increasing chemotherapy doses, utilizing intensive supportive care, with randomization into and out of a protective environment has been reported by Rodriguez to show a definitely increased response rate with the CYVADIC regimen in a small number of patients over that reported in a larger number in the SWOG study. In addition, remission duration and survival were prolonged in patients treated inside the protected environment where the highest doses of chemotherapy were obtained [3, 64].

The effects of cyclophosphamide, vincristine and adriamycin given as adjuvant therapy to patients with high-grade soft-tissue sarcomas showed no benefit [46]. In retrospect, the addition of cyclophosphamide to this regimen and the omission of DTIC were unfortunate. Our current study utilizes adriamycin-DTIC as adjuvant. In osteosarcoma, adjuvant adriamycin is an established form of treatment [24] comparing well with studies utilizing high-dose methotrexate [43]. Sutow has shown a 50% relapse-free survival without late

Table 2. Chemotherapy of metastatic sarcomas

Author	Affiliation	Regimen	Adria dose (mg/m²)	Cycle time (wk.)	No. pts.	% CR + PR
Creagan [26]	Mayo	VADIC	50	5	31	10
Gottlieb [34]	SWOG	VADIC	60	3	107	42
Benjamin [3]	SWOG	CYVADACT	50	3	225	39
Rosenbaum [69]	ECOG	CAV	50	3	38	13
Rosenbaum [69]	ECOG	Adria	70	3	37	28
Benjamin [3]	SWOG	CYVADIC	50	3	221	50
Rodriguez [64]	MDAH	CYVADIC (no PE)	70-90	3	12	59
Rodriguez [64]	MDAH	CYVADIC (PE)	70-90	3	15	74

recurrences after 2 years and follow-up extending 4-6 years utilizing an adriamycin-containing combination, CONPADRI-I [75, 76]. When the regimen was modified by adding high-dose methotrexate and decreasing the adriamycin, the initial proportion of patients surviving free of disease was higher; however, late relapses have occurred and the net result was no better [75]. Our own study of CYVADIC as adjuvant for osteosarcoma, although early, looks highly promising with a 57% relapse-free survival with follow-up ranging from 2-40 months [57]. The success of such adjuvant programs has led to the development of limb-saving procedures [68].

Adriamycin has undergone extensive trials in lung cancer. Results in small cell carcinoma with combinations of cyclophosphamide, vincristine and adriamycin appear to be as good as any therapy in these patients [49]. Our own studies in squamous lung cancer with the so-called BACON regimen (bleomycin, adriamycin, CCNU, vincristine and nitrogen mustard) have been reported showing a 45% objective response rate in terms of complete plus partial remissions with an additional 11% stable disease [48]. A subsequent study replacing the CCNU with methotrexate to form BAMON revealed only a 12% complete plus partial remission rate but a 39% stability rate. If responders and stable patients are considered together, the improvement rate was 55% on BACON and 52% on BAMON. The median survival for all patients on BACON was 15 w. whereas it was 18 w. on BAMON. Correcting for performance status, most patients fell into the performance status 5-7 category. Their survival on BACON was 20 w. compared with 18 w. on BAMON. While the toxicity of these regimens was too great to recommend their continued use, it appeared that stabilization of previously progressive disease or objective regression less than 50% was equivalent in its effect on survival to the more commonly accepted complete and partial remissions. A recent study by the V.A. lung group in squamous cell cancer randomized between four treatment regimens, cyclophosphamide, cyclophosphamide plus CCNU, cyclophosphamide plus adriamycin and adriamycin plus CCNU [41] (Table 3). Patients with well-differentiated tumors did best when treated with the adriamycin-cyclophosphamide regimen whereas either combination was superior to cyclophosphamide alone in patients with poorly-differentiated squamous carcinoma.

The study of Eagan at the Mayo clinic utilizing cyclophosphamide, adriamycin and CIS-platinum is of interest not only because of the remarkably good results but also because of the unique method of analysis [29]. Twenty patients with measurable disease were treated. Four of eight with squamous cell carcinoma, three of seven with adenocarcinoma and one of five with large-cell undifferentiated carcinoma had complete or partial remissions for an overall response rate of 8/20 or 40%. In addition, another 21 patients were treated whose disease could not be accurately measured. These patients were called evaluable. Four of 10 with squamous cell carcinoma, three of seven with adenocarcinoma and one of four with large cell carcinoma had objective regression confirmed by two observers although actual

Table 3. VALG squamous lung cancer study [41] median survival time in weeks

	CTX	CTX + CCNU	Adria + CTX	Adria + CCNU
138 pts., well dif.	10.7	10.0	24.0	13.9
82 pts., poorly dif.	12.5	24.4	23.3	25.8

tumor measurements could not be performed. The overall response rate was 8/21 or 38%. As an investigator frequently confronted with patients whose disease is unmeasurable, I heartily recommend widespread adoption of Dr. Eagan's approach to the evaluation of such patients. The alternatives of excluding the patients from the study or of including them only in the denominator both have major disadvantages.

In Hodgkin's disease, several investigators have followed the lead of Bonadonna [16] in devising non-cross resistant combination chemotherapy regimens including adriamycin primarily in the treatment of patients refractory to standard MOPP therapy. A complete remission rate of 67% has been observed in 149 patients collected from six series [22, 30, 50, 51, 61, 77]. In non-Hodgkin's lymphoma, on the other hand, adriamycin has become one of the major agents in primary combination chemotherapy. In a large SWOG study comparing CHOP (cyclophosphamide, adriamycin or hydroxyl daunomycin, vincristine or oncovin, and prednisone) with HOP (adriamycin, vincristine and prednisone) the complete remission rate of 71% of 204 evaluable patients on CHOP was superior to the 61% complete remission rate in 216 evaluable patients on HOP [54]. As in previous studies without adriamycin, complete remission rates were higher in patients with nodular lymphoma, 78% on CHOP and 67% on HOP. The most impressive results, however, were seen in the less responsive diffuse lymphomas, where a 67% complete remission rate was achieved with CHOP and a 60% complete remission rate with HOP. Of particular note were the complete remission rates in previously untreated patients with diffuse histiocytic lymphoma, 83% (29/35) on CHOP and 76% (22/29) on HOP. This tumor has an exceedingly aggressive course in the majority of patients treated with standard regimens, but is of major interest since many patients who achieve complete remission appear to be cured. Approximately 70% of patients achieving complete remission on this study remain in complete remission. In a subsequent study of CHOP plus low dose bleomycin, 69% 18/26 of patients with diffuse histiocytic lymphoma achieved complete remission and only three have relapsed, the remission-duration curve again leveling off at approximately 70% [67]. When systematic dose escalation was employed, sometimes in a protected environment, the disease-free survival curve appears flat with 83% of patients still in complete remission [66].

In breast cancer we have pursued a series of studies based on the combination of 5-FU, adriamycin and cyclophosphamide, the so-called FAC regimen [13]. Our initial study evaluated 44 patients of whom six achieved complete remission, 26 partial remission and the remainder stable disease. The complete+partial remission rate was 73%. Utilizing immunotherapy initially with BCG and later with Levamisole we have had similar results in terms of response rate. On FAC-BCG there were 105 patients with a 74% response rate [36] and on FAC-Levamisole, 111 patients with a 72% response rate [39]. The addition of immunotherapy was accompanied by a significant prolongation of remission duration and survival [36]. For this reason, FAC-BCG has become our standard regimen, and it has been incorporated in several studies at earlier stages of disease. Patients with inflammatory breast cancer have a high propensity for local recurrence and early dissemination. For this reason they are usually considered inoperable. In our own institution, these patients were previously treated with radiation therapy alone and had a median survival of 12 months. Dr. Blumenschein and his associates initiated a program utilizing FAC-BCG followed by radiation therapy in 18 patients. Their median duration of complete remission was 14 months compared with one of 5 months in our historical control series [15]. Extending the program still further, the FAC-BCG regimen was used in adjuvant treatment of patients with an isolated recurrence of breast cancer who had been rendered free of disease. These patients have an extremely poor prognosis usually relapsing within a year. Following adjuvant chemoimmunotherapy, disease-free survival is greater than 85% with a median follow-up of almost 2 years [14]. In patients with positive nodes following initial surgery, we have also utilized the FAC-BCG regimen [17]. Because of the higher probability of long-term cure in these patients, the cumulative adriamycin dose was limited to 300 mg/m² instead of our usual 450 mg/m² limit. As in all of our FAC studies, methotrexate replaced the adriamycin after the maximum cumulative dosage had been achieved. Disease-free survival in our patients on adjuvant FAC-BCG is 90% and is superior to that in our historical control patients regardless of menopausal status, stage, or the number of nodes involved. These differences are all significant with p values less than 0.03 except in premenopausal patients with 1-3 positive nodes where only one of 19 recurrences have been observed compared with six of 14 in the control group. Due to the small numbers, short follow-up and relatively good prognosis of our control group, the difference in disease-free survival in this group has a probability of 0.15. We have analyzed patients with regard to hazard ratio determined by forward logistic regression analysis of prognostic factors for length of disease-free survival. In all cases the superiority of adjuvant therapy is significant with p values inversely proportional to the hazard ratio of the control patients.

Daunorubicin has long been one of the most active agents in the treatment of acute leukemia. In childhood acute lymphocytic leukemia a 41% remission rate was observed in three series of 130 patients although some of these patients had prednisone as well [38, 44, 83]. Comparable data do not exist for adriamycin. In a single large series of 170 patients with far advanced disease, the complete remission rate was 14% [74]. In combination with vincristine, prednisone and other agents in four series of 210 patients, a complete remission rate of 95% was obtained when daunorubicin was used in the initial induction regimen [1, 37, 60, 72]. In adult leukemia (primarily AML) daunorubicin has been shown to have a 47% complete remission rate in 307 previously untreated patients recently reviewed by Wiernik et al. [87]. Considering all U.S. studies, the complete remission rate falls to 37% in 621 patients [8, 9, 10, 35, 47, 62, 83, 86, 87, 88]. Adriamycin has been studied in two series totalling 53 patients with an overall complete remission rate of 11% [25, 85]. Again, however, the adriamycin-treated patients had more extensive prior therapy and were less likely to respond. In combination chemotherapy, however, adriamycin appears to have equal activity to that of daunorubicin when combined with Ara-C given by continuous infusion. In fact, it is the difference between the use of Ara-C as a continuous infusion and its administration by i.v. push which accounts for the major difference in response rates in these studies. Either adriamycin [52, 53, 63] or daunorubicin [23, 27, 58, 65, 80, 81, 89] in combination with continuous infusion of Ara-C is significantly more effective than daunorubicin in combination with ara-C given by i.v. push with or without other drugs [18, 32, 58, 70, 86, 87] Table 4). In the original Ad-OAP series reported by McCredie et al. 41 of 59 patients achieved complete remission for an overall CR rate of 69% [52]. 80% [31/35] of patients under the age of 50 achieved complete remission, and with a 4 year follow-up, eight of the 31 complete responders remain alive and free of disease off chemotherapy.

Based on the promising data of Jacquillat et al. [42], we instituted studies with rubidazone, a semi-synthetic derivative of daunorubicin. Pharmacologically, rubidazone differs from daunorubicin in quantitative aspects of its metabolism [6]. When daunorubicin is injected, the principal plasma species within 1 h is its major metabolite daunorubicinol [40]. In contrast, rubidazone and daunorubicin levels following rubidazone administration exceed those of daunorubicinol for 24 h [6]. This is due in part to the fact that the rubidazone remaining inhibits the reduction of daunorubicin to daunorubicinol. Thus rubidazone is more than simply a depot form of daunorubicin. In our phase I study of rubidazone we

Table 4. Anthracycline-ARA-C combinations for adult acute leukemia

	No. of series	No. of pts.	No. CR	% CR	
DNA-Ara-C push	6	469	223	48	
				p=.0001	
DNA-Ara-C infusion	7	174	113	65	p=.0002
				p=0.27	
Adr-Ara-C infusion	4	418	251	60	

determined the optimal dose for antileukemic activity was 450 mg/m² [5, 6]. 13 of 39 patients with acute leukemia, all of whom had had prior therapy, achieved complete remission. We have now studied 48 patients at Phase II doses of 300 and 450 mg/m². Complete remission rate at 450 mg/m² dose is 54% in 24 patients with 2/7 (29%) achieving complete remission at the 300 mg/m² dose. Of interest, five of nine patients over the age of 50 (56%) achieved complete remission. The doses which could be tolerated by patients in remission where myelosuppression was dose-limiting were considerably lower than those utilized in induction therapy. Consolidation therapy with 300 mg/m² was severely myelosuppressive with a median lowest granulocyte count of 12/μl and median lowest platelet count of 27,000/μl. During maintenance, a median dose of 200 mg/m² produced a median lowest granulocyte count of 420 and a platelet count of 67,000 [5]. Based on these findings we suggested appropriate doses for solid tumor patients would be between 150 and 200 mg/m², a finding borne out in our Phase I study [7].

Since leukemic patients older than 50 are less likely to achieve a complete remission, we instituted a trial with rubidazone, vincristine, ara-C and prednisone (ROAP) in patients over the age of 50 and those who had relapsed without showing resistance to either anthracyclines or Ara-C [45]. Five of seven previously treated patients have achieved complete remission, and in previously untreated patients over the age of 50 treated with 200 mg/m² of rubidazone and 70 mg/m² of Ara-C per day as a continuous infusion for 7 days, 11/15 (73%) of the patients achieved complete remission, a significantly superior response rate to that seen in patients treated with a lower dose regimen (160 mg/m² rubidazone, 55 mg/m² Ara-C) where 4/12 or 33% of patients achieved complete remission. The results are also superior to our results in patients over the age of 50 treated with Ad-OAP, our standard regimen, analyzed in previous studies (p=0.04). With Ad-OAP the complete remission rate in patients over the age of 50 was 49% in 71 patients. The only difference between the Ad-OAP and high dose ROAP regimen is the use of 40 mg/m² adriamycin in place of the 200 mg/m² rubidazone dose.

We have recently performed studies utilizing adriamycin-DNA complex in an attempt to avoid the cardiac toxicity associated with adriamycin. In those studies we attempted to follow the precise preparation techniques of Trouet et al. who demonstrated an improved therapeutic index for the DNA complex in preclinical studies [78, 79]. European studies with adriamycin-DNA complex have suggested decreased cardiac toxicity [78]. In our own study we did observe cardiac toxicity, proven by endomyocardial biopsy [2]. In fact, both activity and toxicity were similar to those of free adriamycin although our pharmacologic studies demonstrated increased peak plasma levels of the DNA complex together with delayed early clearance from plasma. More recently, we have noted differences in intrinsic viscosity of our DNA solutions from those of Trouet. It is possible, therefore, that other preparations of adriamycin-DNA complex may indeed be less cardiotoxic.

In comparing the various anthracycline antibiotics, it is apparent that these are among the most active antineoplastic drugs. Daunorubicin is usually given at a single agent dose of 180 mg/m²/course, usually divided in 3 days. This dose was developed in patients with acute leukemia, and solid tumor studies with daunorubicin have found the drug highly myelosuppressive. Adriamycin, in contrast, was developed in solid tumor patients. The usual dose is 75 mg/m²/course, usually as a single dose. When this dose was translated into acute leukemia in heavily pretreated patients, less satisfactory results were obtained than those with daunorubicin. In our studies with adriamycin-DNA complex, we attempted to increase the dose of drug in patients with acute leukemia up to 120 mg/m² [2]. Unfortunately, at those doses, mucositis became the dose-limiting toxicity. Rubidazone was tried initially in patients with acute leukemia. The single dose recommended is 450 mg/m²; however, in patients with solid tumors doses are limited to 150–200 mg/m² because of myelosuppression. Daunorubicin never had extensive adequate testing in patients with solid tumors, although it is highly active in acute leukemia. Similarly, rubidazone, which is also extremely myelosuppressive, is also very active in acute leukemia. Its activity in solid tumors is currently being evaluated, but it is possible that it may be less effective than adriamycin in the treatment of patients with solid tumors. Adriamycin, the most widely used of these agents, is somewhat less myelosuppressive. It appears to be the most active in solid tumors but may be somewhat less active in acute leukemia. Thus it seems that the more myelosuppressive anthracyclines may have advantages in the treatment of acute leukemia while somewhat less myelosuppressive agents may be more successful in patients with solid tumors.

Summary

Adriamycin is now firmly established as a drug with a very broad spectrum of antitumor activity. It has had a major impact on the therapy of sarcomas. The dose response effect in this tumor is steep and combinations which compromise the dose of adriamycin too greatly are showing inferior results. In lung and breast cancer combinations with adriamycin have been extensively tried. The FAC Regimen in breast cancer has given excellent results at the M.D. Anderson Hospital. The inclusion of adriamycin in combinations has had an impact in the poor prognosis histologies of non-Hodgkin's lymphomas. The CHOP regimen is one of the best developed to date for diffuse histiocytic lymphomas. In the leukemias adriamycin is probably equivalent to daunorubicin which has been more extensively used in this country. A new analog called Rubidazone has shown good activity in AML with a smooth induction and its incorporation into combination with Ara-C, vincristine and prednisone in a regimen called ROAP is being investigated. Adriamycin in complex with DNA has been clinically evaluated, but at this time, no advantage for this approach can be demonstrated.

References

1. Aur, R. J., Simone, J. V., Pratt, C. B.: Successful Remission Induction in Children with Acute Lymphocytic Leukemia at High Risk for Treatment Failure. Cancer, **27** 1332–1336 (1971).
2. Benjamin, R. S., Burgess, M. A., Bodey, G. P., Freireich, E. J.: A Phase I–II Study of Adriamycin-DNA Complex (A-DNA). Proc. AACR and ASCO, **18** 305 (1977).
3. Benjamin, R. S., Baker, L. H., Rodriguez, V. et al.: The Chemotherapy of Soft Tissue Sarcomas in Adults. Proceedings of the 21st Annual Clinical Conference on Cancer, M.D. Anderson Hospital, Houston, Texas: Current Concepts in the Management of Bone and Soft Tissue Sarcomas. Year Book Medical Publishers, Chicago, Ill., 1977, pp. 309–315.
4. Benjamin, R. S., Gottlieb: J. A., Baker, L. O., Sinkovics, J. G.: CYVADIC vs CYVADACT: A Randomized Trial of Cyclophosphamide (CY), Vincristine (V) and Adriamycin (A), plus Decarbazine (DIC) or Actinomycin-D (DACT) in Metastatic Sarcomas. Proc. AACR and ASCO, **17** 256 (1976).
5. Benjamin, R. S., Keating, M. J., McCredie, K. B.: A Phase I-II Trial of Rubidazone in Patients with Acute Leukemia. Cancer Res. **37**: 4623–4628, 1977.
6. Benjamin, R. S., Keating, M. G., McCredie, K. B. et al.: Clinical and Pharmacologic Studies of Rubidazone (R) in Adults with Acute Leukemia. Proc. AACR and ASCO, **17** 72 (1976).
7. Benjamin, R. S., Valdivieso, M., Rodriguez, V. et al.: A Phase I–II Study of Rubidazone in

Patients with Solid Tumors. Proc. AACR and ASCO **18** 143 (1977).

8. Bloomfield, C. D., Brunning, R. D., Kennedy, B. J.: Daunorubicin-Prednisone Treatment of Erythroleukemia. Ann. Intern. Med. **81** 746–750 (1974).
9. Bloomfield, C. D., Brunning, R. D., Kennedy, B. J.: Daunorubicin Therapy in Adult Acute Lymphatic Leukemia. Cancer, **30** 47–55 (1972).
10. Bloomfield, C. D., Brunning, R. D., Theologides, A., et al.: Daunorubicin-Prednisone Remission Induction with Hydroxyurea Maintenance in Acute Non-lymphocytic Leukemia. Cancer **31** 931–938 (1973).
11. Blum, R. H.: An Overview of Studies with Adriamycin (NSC-123127) in the United States. Cancer Chemother. Rep. **6**, (2), 247–251 (1975).
12. Blum, R. H. and Carter, S. K.: Adriamycin, A New Anticancer Drug with Significant Clinical Activity. Ann. Intern. Med. **80**(2), 249–259 (1974).
13. Blumenschein, G. R.: Chemotherapy in the Management of Breast Cancer. In: "Cancer Chemotherapy: Fundamental Concepts and Recent Advances," Proceedings of the 19th Annual Clinical Conference on Cancer, 403–415 (1975). M.D. Anderson Hospital and Tumor Institute, Houston, Texas. Chicago: Year Book Medical Publishers.
14. Blumenschein, G. R., Buzdar, A. U., Tashima, C. K., Hortobagyi, G. N., Gutterman, J. U.: Adjuvant Chemoimmunotherapy of Stage IV (NED) Breast Cancer. In: Adjuvant Therapy of Cancer, S. E. Salman and S. E. Jones, eds. Elsevier/North-Holland Biomedical Press. Amsterdam, 1977, pp. 147–152.
15. Blumenschein, G. R., Montague, E. D., Eckles, N. E., Hortobagyi, G. N., Barker, J. L.: Sequential Combined Modality Therapy for Inflammatory Breast Cancer. Breast, **2**(2), 16–20 (1976).
16. Bonadonna, G., Delena, M., Monfardini, S., Rossi, A., Brambilla, C., Uslenghi, C., Zucali, R.: Combination Usage of Adriamycin (NSC-123127) in Malignant Lymphomas. Cancer Chemotherapy Reports, Part 3, **6**(2), 381–388 (1975).
17. Buzdar, A. U., Blumenschein, G. R., Gutterman, J. U. et al.: Adjuvant Chemoimmunotherapy following Regional Therapy in Breast Cancer. Amsterdam, 1977, pp. 139–146. In: Adjuvant Therapy of Cancer. S. E. Salman and S. E. Jones, eds. Elsevier/North-Holland Biomedical Press.
18. Carey, R. W., Ribas-mundo, M., Ellison, R. R., Glidewell, O., Lee, S. T., Cuttner, J. Comparative Study of Cytosine Arabinoside Therapy Alone and Combined with Thioguanine, Mercaptopurine, or Daunorubicin in Acute Myelocytic Leukemia. Cancer, **36** (5), 1560–1566 (1975).
19. Carter, S. K.: Adriamycin—A Review. J. NCI, 55, 1265–1274 (1975).
20. Carter, S. K., Bachur, N. R., Benjamin, R. S. et al., (eds.): Adriamycin: New Drug Seminars. Cancer Chemotherapy Reports, Part. 3, Vol. **6** (1975).
21. Carter, S. K., Dimarco, A., Ghione, M. et al. (eds.): International Symposium on Adriamycin. Berlin-Heidelberg-New York: Springer 1972.
22. Case, D. C., Jr., Young, C. W., Nisce, L., Lee, B. J., III, Clarkson, B. D.: Eight-Drug Combination Chemotherapy (MOPP and ABDV) and Local Radiotherapy for Advanced Hodgkin's Disease. Cancer Treat. Rep. **60**, 1217–1224 (1976).
23. Chang, P., Wiernik, P., Bachur, N. R., Stoller, R., Chabner, B.: Failure to Predict Response of Acute Non-Lymphocytic Leukemia (ANLL) Using Assays for Deoxycytidine Kinase (K) Cytidine Deaminase (D) and Daunorubicin Reductase (Red.). Proc. AACR and ASCO, **18**, 352 (1977).
24. Cortes, E. P., Holland, J. F., Wang, J. J. et al.: Amputation and Adriamycin in Primary Osteosarcoma. N. Eng. J. Med. **291**, 998–1000, (1974).
25. Cortes, E. P., Ellison, R. R., Yates, J. W.: Adriamycin (NSC-123127) in the Treatment of Acute Myelocytic Leukemia. Cancer Chemother. Rep. **56**(2), 237–243, (1972).
26. Creagan, E. T., Hahn, R. G., Ahmann, D. L., Edmonson, J. H., Bisel, H. F., Eagan, R. T.: A Comparative Clinical Trial Evaluating the Combination of Adriamycin, DTIC, and Vincristine, the Combination of Actinomycin-D, Cyclophosphamide, and Vincristine, and a Single Agent, Methyl CCNU in Advanced Sarcomas. Cancer Treatment Rep., **60**, 1385–1388 (1976).
27. Cuttner, J. Bekesi, J. G., Holland, J. F.: Chemoimmunotherapy of Acute Leukemia Using MER. Proc. AACR and ASCO, **18**, 196, (1977).
28. Daniels, J.: This volume.
29. Eagan, R. T., Ingle, J. N. Frytal, S., Rubin, J. et al.: Platinum-based Polychemotherapy Versus Dianhydrogalactitol in Advanced Non-small Cell Lung Cancer. Cancer Treat. Rep. **61**: 1339–1345, 1977.
30. Einhorn, L., Williams, S., Rohn, R.: Combination Chemotherapy of Refractory Hodgkin's Disease (HD) with Adriamycin (ADR) and CCNU. Proc. AACR and ASCO, **18**: 269 (1977).
31. Ghione, M., Fetzer, J., Maier, H. (eds).: Adriamycin Symposium, Frankfurt/Main, 1974. Berlin-Heidelberg-New York: Springer 1974.
32. Glucksberg, H., Buckner, C. D., Fefer, A., Demarsh, Q., Coleman, D., Dobrow, R. B., Huff, J. Kjobech, C., Hill, A. S., Dittman, W., Neiman, P. E., Cheever, M. A., Einstein, A. B., Thomas, E. D.: Combination Chemotherapy for Acute Nonlymphoblastic Leukemia in Adults. Cancer Chemother. Rep. **59** 1131–1131 (1975).

33. Gottlieb, J. A.: Clinical Trials with Adriamycin A one and in Combination: The American Experience. In: Progress in Chemotherapy; Volume III: Antineoplastic Chemotherapy: Proceedings of the 8th International Congress of Chemotherapy, Athens, 1973, George K. Daikos, ed. Hellenic Society for Chemotherapy, Athens. pp. 564-571 (1974).
34. Gottlieb, J. A., Baker, L. H., O'Bryan, R. M., Sinkovics, J. G., Hoogstraten, B., Quagliana, J. M., Rivkin, S. E., Bodey, G. P., Rodriguez, V., Blumenschein, G. R., Saiki, J. H., Coltman, C., Jr., Burgess, M. A., Sullivan, P., Thigpen, T., Bottomley, R., Balcerzak, S., Moon, T. E.: Adriamycin (NSC-123127) Used Alone and in Combination for Soft-Tissue and Bony Sarcomas. Cancer Chemother. Rep., Part 3, **6**, 271-282 (1975).
35. Green, W., Huffman, D., Wiernik, P. H., Schimpff, S., Benjamin, R., Bachur, N.: High Dose Daunorubicin Therapy for Acute Nonlymphocytic Leukemia: Correlation of Response and Toxicity with Pharmacokinetics and Intracellular Daunorubicin Reductase Activity. Cancer **30**, 1419-1427 (1972).
36. Gutterman, J. U., Cardenas, J. O., Blumenschein, G. R., Hortobagyi, G., Livington, R. B., Mavligit, G. M., Freireich, E. J., Gottlieb, J. A., Hersh, E. M.: Chemoimmunotherapy of Disseminated Breast Cancer—Prolongation of Remission and Survival. Br. Med. J., **2**, 1222-1225 (1976).
37. Haghbin, M., Tan, C., Clarkson, B. D., et. al.: Intensive Chemotherapy in Children with Acute Lymphoblastic Leukemia. Cancer, **33(6)**, 1491-1498 (1974).
38. Holton, C. P., Vietti, T. J., Nora, A. H., et al.: Clinical Study of Daunomycin and Prednisone for Induction of Remission in Children with Advanced Leukemia. N. Engl. J. Med., **280**, 171-174 (1969).
39. Hortobagyi, G., Gutterman, J. U., Tashima, C., et al.: Levamisole in the Chemoimmunotherapy of Metastatic Breast Cancer. Proc. AACR and ASCO, **18**, 351 (1977).
40. Huffman, D. H., Benjamin, R. S., and Bachur, N. R.: Daunorubicin Metabolism in Acute Nonlymphocytic Leukemia. Clin. Pharmacol. Ther. **13**, 895-905 (1972).
41. Hyde, L., Lowe, W. C., Phillips, R. and Wolf, J.: Chemotherapy for Squamous Cell Cancer of the Lung. Proc. AACR and ASCO, **18**, 276 (1977).
42. Jacquillat, C., Weil, M., Gemon-Auclerc, M. D., et al.: Clinical Study of Rubidazone (R.P. 22050), a New Daunorubicin Derived Compound in 170 Patients with Acute Leukemia and Other Malignancies. Cancer, **37**, 653-659.
43. Jaffe, N., Frei, E. III, Traggis, D., et al.: Adjuvant Methotrexate and Citrovorum Factor Treatment of Osteogenic Sarcoma. New Engl. J. Med. **291**, 994-997 (1974).
44. Jones, B., Holland, J. F., Morrison, A. R. et al.: Daunorubicin (NSC-83142) versus Daunorubicin plus Prednisone (NSC-10023) versus Daunorubicin plus Vincristine (NSC-67574) plus Prednisone in Advanced Childhood Acute Lymphocytic Leukemia. Cancer Chemother. Rep. **56**(6), 729-737 (1972).
45. Keating, M. J., Benjamin, R. S., McCredie, K. B., et al.: Remission Induction Therapy with a Rubidazone-Containing Combination (ROAP) in Acute Leukemia. Proc. AACR and ASCO, **18**, 180 (1977).
46. Lindberg, R. D., Murphy, W. K., Benjamin, R. S., et al.: Adjuvant Chemotherapy in the treatment of Primary Soft Tissue Sarcomas—A Preliminary Report. Proceedings of the 21st Annual Clinical Conference on Cancer, M.D. Anderson Hospital and Tumor Institute, Houston, Texas: Current Concepts in the Management of Bone and Soft Tissue Sarcomas. Year Book Medical Publishers, Chicago, Ill. 1977, pp. 343-352
47. Lippmann, M., Zager, R., Henderson, E. S.: High-Dose Daunorubicin (NSC-83142) in the Treatment of Advanced Acute Myelogenous Leukemia. Cancer Chemother. Rep. **56**(6), 755-760 (1972).
48. Livington, R. B., Fee, W. H., Einhorn, L. H. et al.: BACON (Bleomycin, Adriamycin, CCNU, Oncovin, and Nitrogen Mustard) in Squamous Lung Cancer—Experience in Fifty Patients. Cancer, **37**, 1237-1242 (1976).
49. Livingston, R. B. and Moore, T. N.: Combined Modality Treatment of Oat Cell Carcinoma of the Lung. Proc. AACR and ASCO, **17**, 152 (1976).
50. Loh, K. K., Gamble, J. F., Shullenberger, C. C., Fuller, L. M.: Combination Chemotherapy in MOPP Resistant Hodgkin's Disease. Proc. AACR and ASCO, **18**, 267 (1977).
51. Lokich, J. J., Frei, E., Jaffe, N., Tullis, J.: New Multiple Agent Chemotherapy (B-DOPA) for Advanced Hodgkin's Disease. Cancer **38** (2), 667-671 (1976).
52. McCredie, K. B., Bodey, G. P., Burgess, M. A., Gutterman, J. U., Hester, J. P., Rodriguez, V. and Freireich, E. J.: The Management of Acute Leukemia in Adults. Cancer Chemotherapy: Proceedings of the 19th Annual Clinical Conference on Cancer, M.D. Anderson Hospital and Tumor Institute. pp. 173-186 (1975). Chicago: Year Book Medical Publishers.
53. McCredie, K. B., Hewlett, J. S., Gehan, E. A. and Freireich, E. J.: Chemoimmunotherapy of Adult Acute Leukemia (CIAL). Proc. AACR and ASCO, **18**, 127 (1977).

54. McKelvey, E. M., Gottlieb, J. A., Wilson, H. E., et al.: Hydroxyldaunomycin (adriamycin) Combination Chemotherapy in Malignant Lymphomas. Cancer, **38**, 1484–1493 (1976).
55. Minow, R. A., Benjamin, R. S. and Gottlieb, J. A.: Adriamycin (NSC-123127) Cardiomyopathy—An Overview with Determination of Risk Factors. Cancer Chemotherapy Rep., Part **3**, 6, 195–202 (1975).
56. Minow, R. A., Benjamin, R. S., Lee, E. T., Gottlieb, J. A.: Adriamycin Cardiomyopathy: Risk Factors. Cancer, **39**, 1397–1402 (1977).
57. Murphy, W. K., Benjamin, R. S., Eyre, H. J., et al.: Adjuvant Chemotherapy in Osteosarcoma of Adults. A SWOG Group Study. In: Adjuvant Therapy of Cancer, S. E. Salmon and S. E. Jones, eds. Esevier/North-Holland Biomedical Press. Amsterdam, 1977, pp. 399–406.
58. Omura, G. A., Vogler, W. R., Lynn, M. J.: A Controlled Clinical Trial of Chemotherapy vs. BCG Immunotherapy vs. No Further Therapy in Remission Maintenance of Acute Myelogenous Leukemia (AML). Proc. AACR and ASCO, **18**, 272 (1977).
59. Paroly, W. D.: Personal Communication of unpublished data from the Western Cancer Study Group.
60. Pizzo, P. A., Henderson, E. S., Leventhal, B. G.: Acute Myelogenous Leukemia in Children: A Preliminary Report of Combination Chemotherapy. J. Pediatrics, **88**, 125–130 (1976).
61. Porzig, K., Robertson, A.: Treatment of Advanced Hodgkin's Disease (HD) with B-CAV Following MOPP Failure. Proc. AACR and ASCO, **18**, 342 (1977).
62. Poth, J. L., Johnson, P. K., George, R. P., Schrier, S. L.: Therapy of Acute Myelocytic Leukemia. Daunomycin contrasted with a Combination of Cytosine Arabinoside and 6-Thioguanine. Calif. Med. **117**(6), 1–11 (1972).
63. Preisler, H. D. Bjornsson, S., Henderson, E. S.: Chemotherapy for Acute Myelocytic Leukemia (AML) with Cytosine Arabinoside (ARA-C) and Adriamycin (ADR). Blood, **48**, 982 (1976).
64. Rodriguez, V., Bodey, G. P., Freireich, E. J.: Increased Remission Rate and Prolongation of Survival in Patients with Soft Tissue Sarcomas Treated with Intensive Chemotherapy on a Protected Environment Antibiotic Program (PEPA). Proc. AACR and ASCO, **18**, 320 (1977).
65. Rodriguez, V., Bodey, G. P., Gutterman, J. U. et al.: Combination Chemotherapy of Adult Acute Leukemia for Remission Induction and Maintenance. In: Therapy of Acute Leukemia. Proceedings of International Meeting. Rome, December 6–8, 1975, pp. 569–577 (1975). Torino: Centro Minerva Medico.
66. Rodriguez, V., Bodey, G. P., McKelvey, E. M., et al.: Combination Chemotherapy (CHOP-BLEO) of Advanced Diffuse Histiocytic Lymphoma (DHL). Proc. AACR and ASCO, **17**, 249 (1976).
67. Rodriguez, V., Cabanillas, F., Burgess, M. A. et al.: Combination Chemotherapy (CHOP-BLEO) in Advanced (Non-Hodgkin's) Malignant Lymphoma. Blood, **49**, 325–333 (1977).
68. Rosen, G., Murphy, M. L., Huvos, A. G., Guiterriz, M., Marcove, R. C.: Chemotherapy, en bloc Resection and Prosthetic Bone Replacement in the Treatment of Osteogenic Sarcoma. Cancer (suppl.) **37**, 1–11 (1976).
69. Rosenbaum, C. and Schoenfeld, D.: Treatment of Advanced Soft Tissue Sarcoma. Proc. AACR and ASCO, **18**, 287 (1977).
70. Rosenthal, D. S. and Moloney, W. C.: The Treatment of Acute Granulocytic Leukemia in Adults. New Engl. J. Med. **286**, 1176–1178 (1972).
71. Schein, P.: This volume.
72. Simone, J. V., Aur, R. J., Husto, H. O., et al.: Combined Modality Therapy of Acute Lymphocytic Leukemia. Cancer, **35**, 25–35 (1975).
73. Staquet, M., Tagnon, H., Kenis, Y., et al. (eds): Adriamycin Review. European Press Medikon, Ghent, Belgium, (1975).
74. Starling, R. A., Berry, D. H., Britton, H. A., et al.: Three Dose Regimens of Adriamycin for Induction of Remission in Acute Leukemia in Children: A Southwest Oncology Group Study. Med. and Pediat. Oncol. **1**, 271–276 (1975).
75. Sutow, W. W., Gehan, E. A., Vietti, T. J., et al.: Multidrug Chemotherapy in Primary Treatment of Osteosarcoma. J. Bone and Joint Surg. **58**: 629–633 (1976).
76. Sutow, W. W., Romsdahl, M. M., Dyment, P. G. and Frias, A. E.: Long-Term Follow-up Evaluation of CONPADRI—I Adjuvant Cheotherapy in Osteosarcoma. Proc. AACR and ASCO, **18**, 127 (1977).
77. Tan, C. T. C., Tan, R.: Adriamycin Combination Chemotherapy in Childhood Hodgkin's Disease—A Six-Year Progress Report. Blood, **48**, 983 (1976).
78. Trouet, A.: Personal communication of unpublished data.
79. Trouet, A., Deprez-de Campeneere, D., De Smedt-Malengreaux, M., Atassi, G.: Experimental Leukemia Chemotherapy with a "Lysosomotrophic" Adriamycin-DNA Complex. Europ. J. Cancer, **10**, 405–411 (1974).
80. Vaughan, W. P., Karp, J. E., Braine, H. G., Burke, P. J.: Prolonged Unmaintained Remission

Following Timed Sequential Chemotherapy of Acute Myelocytic Leukemia. Blood **48**, 982 (1976).

81. WALLACE, H. J., HOLLAND, J. F., GLIDEWELL, O. J., et al.: Therapy of Acute Myelocytic Leukemia. Acute Leukemia Group B studies. In: Therapy of Acute Leukemia, Proceedings of the International Meeting, Rome, Dec. 6–8, 1973 pp. 255–269 (1975). (Torino: Centro Minerva Medico.)
82. WALKER, M. D.: Personal Communication of unpublished data from the Brain Tumor Study Group.
83. WEIL, M., GLIDEWELL, O. J., JACQUILLAT, C. et al.: Daunorubicin in the therapy of Acute Granulocytic Leukemia. Cancer Res., **33**, 921–928 (1975).
84. WEISS, A. J., METTER, G. E., FLETCHER, W. S., et al.: Studies on Adriamycin using a Weekly Regimen Demonstrating its Clinical Effectiveness and Lack of Cardiac Toxicity. Cancer Treat. Rep., **60**, 813–822 (1976).
85. WILSON, H. E., BODEY, D. P., MOON, T. E., et al.: Adriamycin Therapy in Previously Treated Adult Acute Leukemia. Cancer Treat. Rep. **61**: 905–907, 1977.
86. WIERNIK, P. H.: Personal communication of unpublished data from ALGB study.
87. WIERNIK, P. H., SCHIMPFF, S. C., SCHIFFER, C. A., LICHTENFELD, J. L., AISNER, J., O'CONNELL, M. T. FORTNER, C.: Randomized Clinical Comparison of Daunorubicin (NSC-82151) Alone with a Combination of Daunorubicin, Cytosine Arabinoside (NSC-63878), t-Thioguanine (NSC 752) and Pyrimethamine (NSC-3061) for the Treatment of Non-lymphocytic Acute Leukemia. Cancer Treat. Rep., **60**, 41–53 (1976).
88. WIERNICK, P. H. and SERPICK, A. A.: A Randomized Clinical Trial of Daunorubicin and a Combination of Prednisone, Vincristine, 6-Mercaptopurine and Methotrexate in Adult Acute Nonlymphocytic Leukemia. Cancer Res. **32**, 2023–2026 (1976).
89. YATES, J. W., WALLACE, H. J., ELLISON, R. R., HOLLAND, J. F.: Cytosine Arabinoside (NSC-63878) and Daunorubicin (NSC-83142) Therapy in Acute Myelogenous Leukemia. Cancer Chemother. Rep. **57**, 485–488 (1973).

ADDENDUM

Recent data indicate that the high levels of daunorubicin seen following rubidazone administration in our initial studies were due to artifactual production of daunorubicin by in vitro hydrolysis. We cannot state at present whether daunorubicin or rubidazone is the principal plasma species following rubidazone administration. Daunorubicinol levels are indeed lower than with daunorubicin administration.

Clinical Experiences with Aclacinomycin-A

H. FURUE, T. KOMITA, I. NAKAO, I. FURUKAWA, T. KANKO, and T. YOKOYAMA

Aclacinomycin A (subsequently referred to as ACM) is a new anticancer agent of the anthracycline group, and was isolated and purified by Dr. Hamao Umezawa in 1974 from a culture of *Streptomyces galilaeus.* With a chemical structure as shown in Fig. 1, ACM is similar in basic structure to adriamycin (ADM) and daunomycin (DNM), but differs from the latter in that it contains three sugars, rhodosamine, 2-deoxyfucose and L-cinerulose. Basic studies of this compound have revealed the following characteristics of the agent:

1. ACM may be classified among the drugs of the anthracycline group such as DNM and ADM.
2. The LD_{50}s of ACM in mice, rats and hamsters by any route of administration are 2–3 times as high as those of DNM and of ADM (Table 1).
3. ACM differs slightly in anticancer spectrum from DNM and ADM.
4. ACM is taken up by the lungs at high concentrations, and also by the spleen.
5. Both acute and subacute cardiotoxicity of ACM measured in terms of ECG patterns proved far less than that of ADM, being only about 1/15 that of the latter.

As shown in Table 2, ACM treatment was given in a total of 22 cases, consisting of seven cases of gastric carcinoma, one of hepatic carcinoma, one of biliary carcinoma (with pulmonary metastasis), one of colonic carcinoma, four of primary lung cancer (consisting of two of adenocarcinoma, one of squamous cell carcinoma, and one of small cell undifferentiated carcinoma), two of recurrent breast cancer, three of recurrent carcinoma of the cervix uteri, one of recurrent carcinoma of the corpus uteri (endometrial carcinoma), one of adenocarcinoma with the unknown primary focus (as found in autopsy), and one of chronic myelogenous leukemia.

ACM treatment was assessed effective in all cases where the tumor had regressed by not less than 25% in the sum of diameters in two directions.

Dosage Schedule

The treatment was performed using the dosage schedule of 20 mg ACM, i.v., every other day, up to a total dose of not less than 300 mg, and until any objective adverse reactions appeared.

Anticancer Effects

Because our observation is still in the Phase I stage, and also because the dosage schedule of this agent have not been established, it may not be adequate to mention its anticancer

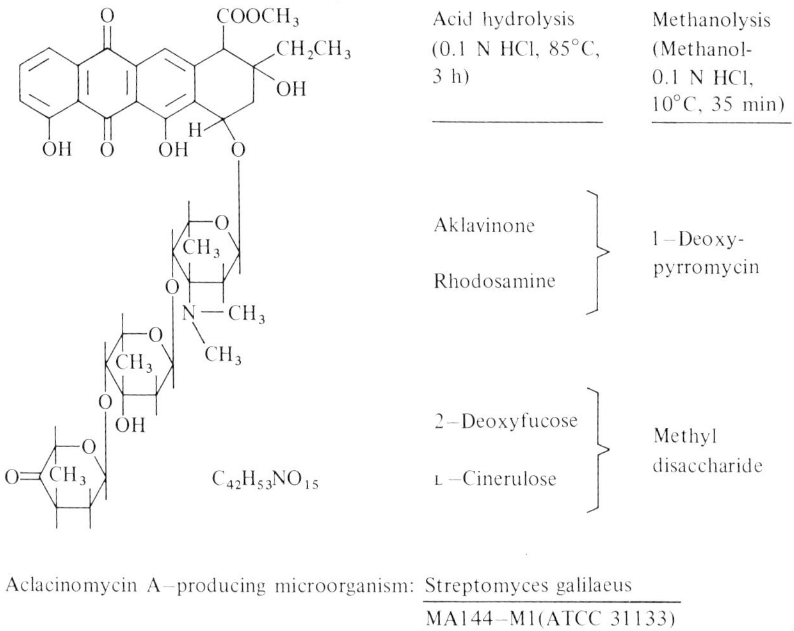

Fig. 1. Structure of aclacinomycin A

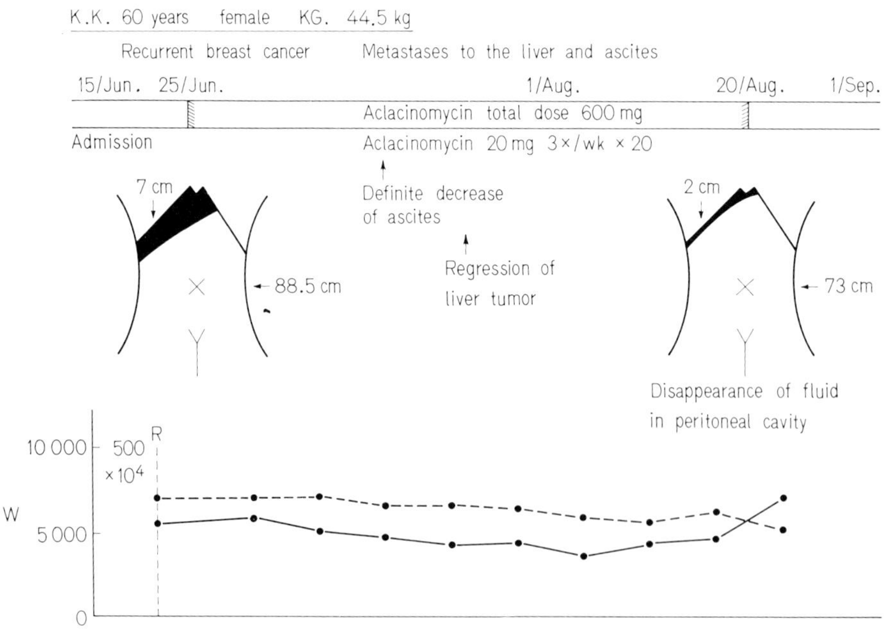

Fig. 2.

activities. However, the agent has apparently proved effective in one case of recurrent breast cancer. In this case, ACM treatment caused regression of hepatic metastoses from 7 cm to 2 cm in the right midclavicular line, and also caused disappearance of ascites (Fig. 2).
Besides this case, slight improvements in objective findings have been seen in five other cases. That is, in one of the cases of gastric carcinoma, a slight regression (less than 25% in size) was seen in the shadow defect of the X-ray finding, associated with an improvement in performance status and definite improvement in subjective symptoms, resulting in the patient's rehabilitation. In another case of gastric carcinoma, severe abdominal pain and ascites were eliminated. In one of the cases of recurrent lung cancer and the case of recurrent endometrial carcinoma (both with many metastatic foci varying in size in the lungs), large foci remained unchanged, but small ones apparently regressed. In the case of chronic myelogenous leukemia, no hematologic improvements were achieved, but splenomegaly regressed definitely (by 3-4 fingerbreadths), associated with improvement of subjective symptoms such as a tensed feeling of the abdomen. In a total of above mentioned six cases, ACM was administered in a total doses of not less than 300 mg, except in the case of CML.

Side Reactions

As shown in Table 3, anorexia developed in four cases, nausea and vomiting in seven, hepersalivation in two, mild alopecia in one, mild leucopenia (below 4000 counts) in four, leucopenia (less than 3000 counts) in one, mild thrombopenia (less than 100,000) in two, thrombopenia (less than 70,000) in one, anemia (below 300×10^4) in five (in all five cases, no bleeding was seen), mild liver disturbances in five, and ECG changes in one out of the 22 cases. No side reactions have developed in seven cases.
Nausea and vomiting was present in seven cases. These side reactions developed with the administration of the initial dose of 20 mg in six of them. They developed 7-8 h after the administration in many cases, and on some occasions persisted for 1-2 days or even longer. In two out of these seven cases, further administration of ACM was discontinued. However, administration of 10 mg of ACM never caused nausea and vomiting in any of our cases.
The relationship between leucopenia and the total doses administered is given in Fig. 3. These side reactions tended to develop with administration of total doses not less than 350 mg. However, recovery of bone marrow supression was seen soon after discontinuation of ACM treatment.
Anemia developed in five cases. In these five cases, neither bleeding nor bone marrow metastases were found, and ACM was also administered in total doses of not less than 300 mg. The hematologic findings of blood samples in the presence of anemia are given in Table 4. The reticulocytes, MCV, HCV, plasmin, serum iron value were not vastly altered: thus iron deficiency anemia was excluded. The anemia recovered soon after discontinuation of ACM therapy.
Liver disturbances occurred in five cases (including one case with the proven hepatic metastasis); however, they were transient and became normal on withdrawal of the treatment. The incidence of liver disturbances was high in the cases treated with total doses of not less than 300 mg ACM. Details of the liver disturbances are presented in Table 5. γ-GPT, LDH, and Al-pase were slightly and transiently elevated. However, elevation of GOT and GPT were insignificant.

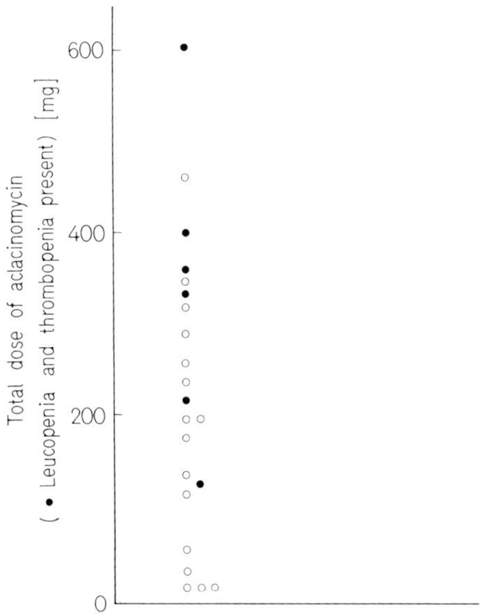

Fig. 3

Conclusions

From our clinical observations with aclacinomycin A, the drug showed anticancer activities in some instances. On the other hand, the side reactions were mild, transient, and all of them were reversible. Our clinical observations with aclacinomycin A warrant further clinical studies.

Summary

Aclacinomycin is a new anthracycline analog of adriamycin and daunomycin. Aclacinomycin contains three sugars. The drug has been studied in 22 cases in a phase 1 type of trial on a schedule 20 mg i.v. every other day up to a total of 300 mg. Toxicity has consisted of myelosuppression, nausea and vomiting, and transient hepatic disturbances. Evidence of clinical activity was observed in several cases including a case of breast cancer and gastric cancer. Although no full patial remissions were recorded, further study is continuing.

Tables

Table 1. LD_{50} of aclacinomycin A, adriamycin and daunomycin

		Aclacinomycin A (mg/kg)	Adriamycin (mg/kg)	Daunomycin (mg/kg)
Mouse	i.p.	27.7	12-14	4-5
(dd)	i.v.	34.1	9-10	17-20
	s.c.	36.0	16-22	—
	p.o.	—	700-760	—
Rat	i.p.	37.5	16-17	8
(Wistar)	i.v.	32.5	12-13	13-15
	s.c.	—	22-24	—
Hamster	i.v.	22.1	—	—

Table 2. Distribution of cases treated with aclacinomycin A

Primary site	No. of cases	Regressors	Responder
Gastric cancer	7	2	
Liver cancer	1		
Bile duct cancer	1		
Colon cancer	1		
Lung cancer	4	1	
Recurrent breast cancer	2		1
Recurrent uterine cancer	3		
Recurrent endometrial cancer	1	1	
Primary unknown adenocarcinoma	1		
Chronic myelogenous leukemia	1	1	
Total	22	5	1

Table 3. Side reactions of aclacinomycin A

Anorexia	4 cases out of 22		
Nausea and vomiting	7		
Hypersalivation	2		
General lassitude	0		
Fever	0		
Alopecia	1		
Leucopenia	5	less than 4000	4 cases
		less than 3000	1 case
Thrombopenia	3	less than 10×10^4	2 cases
		less than 7×10^4	1 case
Anemia	6	less than 300×10^4	
E.C.G. changes	0		
Liver disturbances	5		
Free from side reactions	7		

Table 4. K.K. female, 60 years, recurrent breast cancer, 44.5 kg.

	Aclacinomycin A 600 mg. 16/Jun.	5/Aug.
Hemoglobin	10.9 g/dl	9.0
Erythrocyte	351 $\times 10^4$	285
Reticulocyte	12‰	10
Hematocrit	33.6%	28.2
Mean corpuscular volume	95 μ^3	95
Leucocyte	5300	3900
Thrombocyte	31 $\times 10^4$	24
Plasmin	12 h	12
Fibrinogen	400 mg/dl	380
Serum Fe	98 μg/dl	133
Serum Cu	173 μg/dl	136

Table 5. E.S. 58 years, cancer of the stomach (scirrhus)

	Aclacinomycin treatment (400 mg)				
	June 21st	July 20th	July 25th	Aug 3rd	Aug 17th
Leucocyte	5000	3800	3900	5600	6000
TTT	—	4.4	2.2	4.6	9.5
Bilirubin	1.1 mg/dl	0.7	0.9	0.6	0.6
LAP	19 mu/ml	28	33	18	22
Cholinesterase	0.7 ΔPH	0.7	0.5	0.5	0.8
Al-P	60 mu/ml	45	121	37	50
GOT	12 mu/ml	25	25	15	24
GPT	20 mu/ml	20	7	29	36
LDH	161 mu/ml	163	374	183	188
γ-GTP	—	33	66	23	26
Aldolase	—	2	2	2	3
Fe	96 μg/dl	—	—	—	—
Cholesterol	249 mg/dl	185	162	197	242

Clinical Aspects of Adriamycin in Japan

H. FURUE and T. KOMITA

Adriamycin (ADM) is one of the anticancer agents occasionally used in Japan. There are some reasons why the agent is not so frequently used as in Europe and USA. The first reason is the frequent use of mitomycin C. Because of its potent anticancer effect and broad anticancer spectrum, mitomycin C is one of the most widely used anticancer agents in Japan. The second reason is the intense side reactions of ADM. Especially, the high incidence of severe alopecia restricts the wide use of this agent. Table 1 shows the side reactions of ADM that have developed in 810 cases recently treated with single administration of ADM in Japan. Side effects on the digestive system, alopecia and bone marrow toxicity are considerably frequent, and cardiotoxicities such as tachycardia, ECG change, arrhythmia are also frequent.

Nevertheless, ADM has proved to exert excellent anticancer effects. The results of ADM treatment are summarized by us as shown in Table 2 and Table 3. The criteria for evaluation of anticancer effects and response rate vary slightly from author to author; however, the treatment has proved effective (with definite tumor regression) in 31 out of 92 cases of gastric cancer. There have also been 27 responders to ADM treatment among 84 cases of lung cancer, 15 responders among 46 cases of malignant lymphomas. Thus, ADM has proved never less effective than the other currently available anticancer drugs.

Recent clinical uses of ADM in Japan that call for attention are cited as below;

1. Treatment of cancer in childhood.
2. Treatment of osteosarcoma.
3. Intrapleural application.
4. Local application in the treatment of bladder cancer.
5. Intra-arterial infusion.
6. Combination chemotherapy.

In these fields of ADM treatment, favorable clinical effects have been also reported.

ADM has been given with various dose schedules. The dose schedules of ADM therapy (i.v. administration) that have been employed by the leading research workers in Japan are given in Table 4.

a) A dose of 10 mg is administered every other day.
b) A dose of 20–30 mg daily is administered for 2 or 3 consecutive days, and the treatment is repeated at 3-week intervals.
c) A single dose of 60 mg is administered at 3-week intervals.

With any dose schedule, the total dose for each treatment does not exceed 2 mg/kg. There is no unanimously supported conclusion in Japan as yet on the dose schedule of ADM. Compared with the dose schedules employed in Europe and America, the agent is commonly used in relatively small doses in Japan. The results of a recent comparative clinical studies by the Tokyo Cancer Chemotherapy Co-operative Study Group also have shown that consecutive administration of small doses is more effective than intermittent administration of median doses. In a study by this group in which eight daily administration of 10 mg were compared with two consecutive administrations of 40 mg ADM, the former gave a higher response rate and a less incidence of alopecia and bone marrow toxicities, as shown in Table 5, and 6.

In i.a. administration of ADM, dose schedule of 5 mg daily application and 30 mg repeated at 3-week intervals are the common use (Table 7).
The intrapleural administration of ADM is also performed using a single dose of 10–100 mg.
The local administration of ADM in the treatment of bladder cancer is also effective. 60 mg ADM is dissolved in 30 ml saline solution and is infused into the bladder. The patient is instructed to urinate 1 h later. This schedule is repeated six times at 2-week intervals. Favorable tumor response have been seen in 36 out of 50 cases so treated by Dr. Niijima (Table 8).
Combination chemotherapy has also been studied intensively in Japan. Combination chemotherapy with ADM and 5-FU is most common, but attempts have also been made at using this agent in combination with mitomycin C, with carbazilquinone, or with OK-432 or even with vinca alkaloids and ifosphamide as shown in Table 9.
It may be said that the clinical studies of ADM has become active gradually in Japan, too.

Summary

Adriamycin has not been as extensively evaluated in Japan as in some other countries. This is due both to the widespread use of mitomycin C and importantly to the alopecia caused by adriamycin being particularly disturbing to Japanese patients. Japanese studies have shown the drug to be highly active in tumors such as stomach cancer (31/92), lung cancer (27/84), and malignant lymphomas (15/46). Combination studies have been mainly with 5-FU although others have also been investigated. Other approaches which have been studied include intraarterial infusion, local application in bladder cancer, intrapleural application and in the treatment of childhood malignancies.

Tables

Table 1. Side reactions of adriamycin
810 cases treated with single administration of adriamycin in Japan.

Side reaction	No. of cases	%
G.I. tract: Nausea and vomiting	249	30.7
Anorexia	228	28.1
Diarrhea	31	3.8
Stomatitis	182	22.4
General lassitude	31	3.8
Fever	77	9.5
Exanthema	7	0.9
Pigmentation	8	1.0
Alopecia	421	52.0
Bone marrow toxicity: Leucopenia	298	36.8
Thrombopenia	117	14.4
Anemia	95	11.7
Cardiotoxicity: Tachycardia	50	6.2
Arhythmia	5	0.6
ECG-change	113	14.0
Liver disturbance	27	3.3
Kidney disturbance	4	0.5
Cystitis	7	0.9
Miscellaneous	46	5.7

Table 2. Response rate of single administration of adriamycin

Authors	No. of cases	Responders	%	
Sakai	17	2	11.8	
TCCSG[a]	55	7	12.7	
Yamamoto	15	2	13.3	
Saito	25	4	16.0	
Ohta	33	6	18.2	
Shimoyama	42	8	19.1	
Furue	10	2	20.0	
Kimura	34	8	23.5	
Takemasa	18	7	23.5	
Hara	57	23	40.4	
Matsunaga	11	5	45.5	
Yamawaki	12	8	66.7	Osteosarcoma
Inuyama	13	5	38.5	Head and neck cancer
Kawakita	4	3	75.0	AML
Ise	29	14	48.3	Cancer of children
Taguchi	12	7	58.3	Intraartery
Sakai	17	6	35.3	Intraartery
Niijima	50	36	72.0	Bladder cancer

[a] TCCSG; Tokyo Cancer Chemotherapy Co-operative Study Group.

Table 3. Response rate of single administration of adriamycin

Tumor site	No. of cases	Responders	%
Stomach cancer	92	31	33.7
Liver cancer	8	1	12.5
Pancreas cancer	6	2	33.3
Colon cancer	22	3	13.6
Head and neck cancer	13	5	38.5
Lung cancer	84	27	32.1
Breast cancer	25	14	56.0
Ovary cancer	9	6	66.7
Bladder cancer	50	36	72.0
Osteosarcoma	12	8	66.7
Neuroblastoma	10	6	60.0
Rhabdomyosarcoma	6	3	50.0
Wilms's tumor	4	1	25.0
Malignant lymphoma	46	15	32.6
AML	7	3	42.9

Table 4. Method of administration of adriamycin

Authors	Method of administration	Interval	Total dose
Shimoyama	10 mg × 4 daily	5-7 days	440-500 mg
	20 mg × 2 daily	5-7 days	500 mg
Takemasa	10 mg every second day		80 mg
Furue	20 mg × 1-3/weekly		100 mg
Saito	10 mg × 4 daily	7 days	
	40-50 mg/m² × 1-2 days	3 weeks	
Sakai	0.4 mg/kg × 3 days	3 weeks	
Hoshino	20 mg × 3 days	3 weeks	
Hara	20 mg × 3 days	3 weeks	
	30 mg × 2 days	3 weeks	
	60 mg × one day	3 weeks	
Inagaki	20 mg/m² × 3 days	3 weeks	500 mg/m²
Ohta	60 mg/m² × one day	3 weeks	
Abe	0.5-0.7 mg/kg × 3 days	1-2 months	600-900 mg
TCCSG[a]	10 mg × 8 days	3 weeks	
	40 mg × 2 days	3 weeks	

[a] TCCSG; Tokyo Cancer Chemotherapy Co-operative Study Group.

Table 5. Effect of adriamycin

Tumor site	10 mg × 8 No. of cases	Responders	40 mg × 2 No. of cases	Responders
Stomach cancer	14	3 (21.4%)	8	0 (0 %)
Lung cancer	4	0 (0 %)	14	4 (28.6%)
Miscellaneous	5	0 (0 %)	10	0 (0 %)
Total	23	3 (13.0%)	32	4 (12.5%)

(Tokyo Cancer Chemotherapy Co-operative Study Group).

Table 6. Side reactions of adriamycin

Side reactions	10 mg × 8 (22 cases)		40 mg × 2 (37 cases)	
Anorexia	7 cases	(31.8%)	8 cases	(25.4%)
Nausea, vomiting	6	(27.3%)	10	(27.0%)
Diarrhea	2	(9.1%)	0	(0 %)
Stomatitis	10	(45.5%)	6	(16.2%)
Alopecia	8	(36.4%)	30	(81.1%)
ECG-change	2	(9.1%)	2	(2.7%)
Leucopenia	8	(36.4%)	21	(56.8%)
Thrombopenia	4	(18.2%)	9	(24.3%)
Anemia	14	(63.6%)	12	(32.4%)

(Tokyo Cancer Chemotherapy Co-operative Study Group).

Table 7. Interaartery administration of adriamycin

Authors	Method of administration	Interval	Total dose
Hattori	5 mg daily for 28 days (one week before operation and 3 weeks after operation)		140 mg
Inokuchi	5 mg daily for 28 days		
Hara	30 mg × 1	3 weeks	
Ohta	30 mg × 1	3 weeks	
Sakai	0.6 mg/kg 2×/week		
Abe	0.5–0.7 mg/kg × 3 days plus 5-GU daily		

Table 8. Local administration of adriamycin

Authors	Method of administration	Interval	
Hattori	10 mg (plus OK 432-10 KE)		Intrapleural
Abe	10–20 mg 1–2×/week		Intrapleural
Takemasa	10 mg × 4 days	one week	Intrapleural
Kimura	30–60 mg		Intrapleural
Shimoyama	40 mg		Intrapleural
	80–100 mg		Intrapleural
Hara	100 mg		Intrapleural
Niijima	60 mg for 1h 3×/week for 2 weeks		Intra urinary bladder

Table 9. Combined administration of adriamycin

Authors	Combination	Dose schedule of ADM
Inokuchi	ADM, 5-FU	20 mg weekly
Shimoyama	ADM, 5-FU	
Kimura	ADM, 5-FU	1.2 mg/kg/3 weeks
Saito	ADM, 5-FU, ACNU	30 mg/m^2/6 weeks
Hara	ADM, 5-FU, MMC	0.8 mg/kg/4 weeks
Hoshino	ADM, 5-FU, MMC	Modification of Cooper's method
Taguchi	ADM, 5-FU, CQ	40 mg/1–2 weeks
Takemasa	ADM, Ft-207, endoxan	40 or 80 mg
Ohta	ADM, 1/2 MFC	1.2 mg/kg/3 weeks
Abe	ADM, BCG, OK 432	0.5–1.0 mg/kg × 3 days
Hattori	ADM, Ok 432	Intrapleural
Kimura	ADM, VCR, Z 4942	0.5 mg/kg weekly or
	ADM, VCR, Z 4942, steroids	0.5–1.2 mg/kg/3 weeks

Clinical Investigations of Neocarzinostatin in Japan

I. KIMURA

Introduction

Neocarzinostatin (NCS) was isolated in 1964 by Dr. N. Ishida of Tohoku University. The agent was found in the culture filtrate of the F-41 strain of *Streptomyces carzinostaticus* from soil of Sendai city. NCS is an acid polypeptide (Fig. 1) with a molecular weight of 10,700, structured from 109 known natural amino acids [8, 11].

The agent was found to have an antitumor effect on a wide spectrum of experimental tumors [2, 5, 8, 14]. Investigation of the NCS mode of action in *Sartina lutea* and HeLa cells revealed: inhibition of DNA synthesis at the "switch-on point" between late G1 and S phase, inhibition of cell division, and DNA degradation at high dosage [3, 4, 12, 15].

In 1971, clinical trials of NCS were started in Japan. The phase I study was not completed but preliminary data is available. The phase II study is presently underway in various malignant tumor patients.

```
1
Ala-Ala-Pro-Thr-Ala-Thr-Val-Thr-Pro-Ser-Ser-Gly-Leu-Ser-Asp-

16
-Gly-Thr-Val-Val-Lys-Val-Ala-Gly-Ala-Gly-Leu-Gln-Ala-Gly-Thr-

31                  37
-Ala-Tyr-Asp-Val-Gly-Gln-Cys-Ala-Ser-Val-Asn-Thr-Gly-Val-Leu-

46                                      56
-Trp-Asn-Ser-Val-Thr-Ala-Ala-Gly-Ser-Ala-Cys-Asx-Pro-Ala-Asn-

61
-Phe-Ser-Leu-Thr-Val-Arg-Arg-Ser-Phe-Glu-Gly-Phe-Leu-Phe-Asp-

76                              84                  89
-Gly-Thr-Arg-Trp-Gly-Thr-Val-Asx-Cys-Thr-Thr-Ala-Ala-Cys-Gln-

91
-Val-Gly-Leu-Ser-Asp-Ala-Ala-Gly-Asp-Gly-Glu-Pro-Gly-Val-Ala-

106
-Ile-Ser-Phe-Asn
```

Fig. 1. Primary structure of neocarzinostatin. (From MEIENHOFER et al. [11])

Preclinical Investigations

Effects on Experimental Tumors

NCS efficacy was found in Sarcoma 180, Ehrlich tumor, L1210 leukemia, Yoshida sarcoma, and rat ascitic hepatomas (AH-13, AH-44, AH-66, AH-66F, AH-414, and AH-7974) [2, 5, 8, 14] In Yoshida sarcoma the maximum tolerable dose was more than 0.5 mg/kg and the minimum effective dose was 0.01 mg/kg. The chemotherapy index was greater than 50. In Yoshida sarcoma strain resistant to anticancer agents, NCS did not show a cross resistance to cyclophosphamide, busulfan, thio-TEPA, 6-mercaptopurine, and 5-fluorouracil [7]. In L1210 leukemia the maximum tolerable dose was 1 mg/kg, the minimum effective dose was 0.25 mg/kg, and the chemotherapy index was 4. There was no cross resistance between this agent and antimetabolites such as methotrexate and cytosine arabinoside [5].

Pharmacokinetics

NCS concentrations in rabbit blood were bioassayed by Fujita et al. [6] after i.v. injection (Fig. 2). At 2.5 min after injection, a very high NCS concentration was present. A rapid decrease followed and a tenth of the initial concentration was present at 15 min. No NCS was detected at 120 min after injection.

In the same study, NCS was distributed at high concentrations in the kidneys, skin, stomach, pancreas, lungs, and muscles. The distributions in the lungs and skin were similar to those of bleomycin which is also a polypeptide anticancer agent. The high distributions in the pancreas and stomach suggest NCS effectiveness in tumors at these sites. The agent was also distributed at high concentrations in cancer cells of ascitic tumors.

The urinary excretion of i.v. administered NCS was examined in mice by Toriyama and Koyama [16] (Fig. 3). At 30 min, 60% of NCS was excreted and 77.5% was excreted within 5 h after injection. The excretion was mainly from the kidneys, liver excretion was low.

NCS inactivation was observed in vitro in tissue homogenates of the liver, kidneys, testes, intestines, and spleen. NCS inactivation was not as clear in the lungs, serum, and skin [6]. These results were also similar to those of bleomycin.

Clinical Investigations

Effects on Leukemia

NCS effectiveness in acute leukemia induction chemotherapy was initially reported by our group in 1972 and a later study has confirmed the initial results [10]. Moreover, we have undertaken many investigations in search of the most effective combination chemotherapy using NCS.

a) Single Administration of NCS

There were 51 known acute leukemia cases treated with NCS in Japan between June 1972 and December 1973. These patients were treated in special hospitals that conduct leukemia chemotherapy. Table 1 shows the details on the treated patient population. NCS was administered at 2–3 mg/day in 500 ml 5% glucose solution by drip infusion for 4 consecutive days, followed by a rest interval of 7–10 days. This course was repeated until remission was obtained.

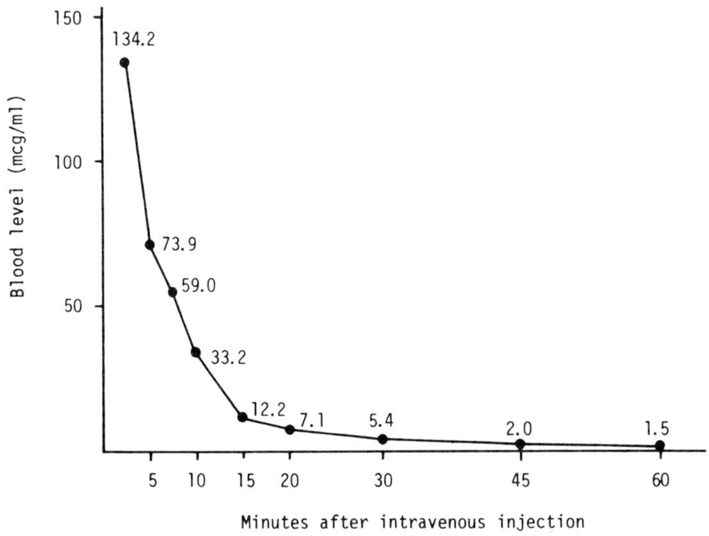

Fig. 2. NCS blood levels in rabbits after intravenous injection of 20 mg/kg NCS. (From FUJITA et al. [6])

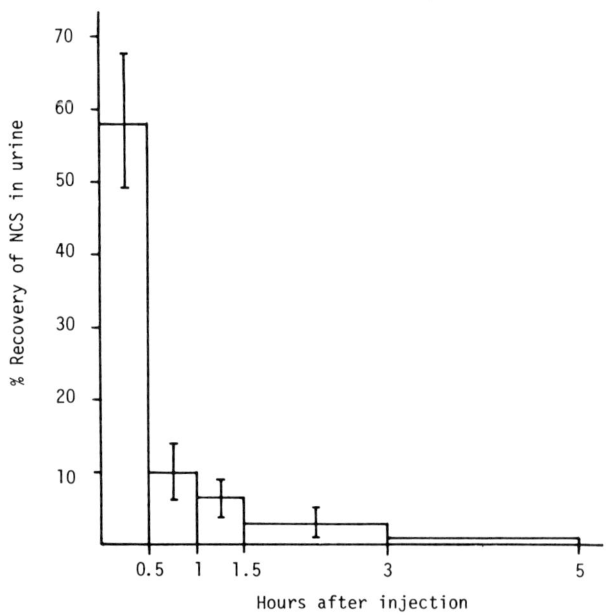

Fig. 3. Urinary excretions of NCS in mice after intravenous injection of 10 mg NCS/kg. Each column represents the average of five mice. The vertical bars are standard deviations. (From TORIYAMA and KOYAMA [16])

Of these 51 cases, complete remission (CR) was obtained in nine cases, partial remission (PR) in nine cases, and no remission in 33 cases. Table 2 shows the results according to type of acute leukemia. The nine CR cases included four patients in old age, one with acute promyelocytic leukemia, and three with acute monocytic leukemia that are considered highly intractable. Seven of these CR cases had not received any previous cancer chemotherapy. A total dose of 10-28 mg NCS (9-98 days administration) was required until CR was reached. The remission duration was 15-250 days (median 70 days).

Our own experience with 18 of these cases showed CR in seven cases and PR in four cases (61.1% remission rate). In our cases, changes in peripheral blood counts were evaluated at the endpoint of the first course of NCS chemotherapy and at the time of CR (Fig. 4). An abrupt decrease of leukemic cells was noted in all but two cases whereas a remarkable drop in platelet counts was noted in only one case. The platelet counts were at the normal range by remission in all cases. In bone marrow, however, some cases showed no remarkable decreases in leukemic cells despite the remarkable decrease in nucleated cell counts (Fig. 5). These cases proved to be intractable and great difficulty was encountered in inducing remission. Only minimum effects were noted on erythropoiesis and granulopoiesis.

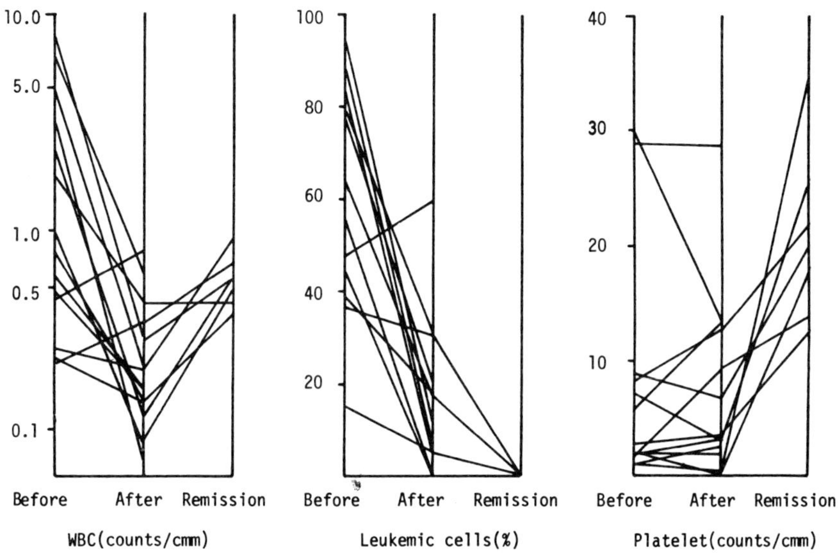

Fig. 4. NCS effects on peripheral blood of leukemia patients

Table 3 summarizes the side effects. Mild abdominal symptoms such as anorexia, nausea, and vomiting were the most frequent side effects. Mild abnormalities in liver function were noted in nine cases, but the cause may have been serum hepatitis, rather than NCS. In our patient group the longest period of NCS treatment in a single patient was 64 injections. A total of 3500 injections were administered and only one case developed shock symptoms. This case recovered after routine treatment.

As an acid polypeptide, NCS has been shown to have antigenicity, suggesting that some patients may form antibody to NCS. This possibility prompted us to conduct an investigation for anti-NCS antibody. A total of 65 peripheral blood samples were obtained from 43 patients at different periods in the NCS chemotherapy schedule. Evaluations were conducted by the passive hemoagglutination test and the passive cutaneous anaphylaxis reaction. No positive findings suggestive of anti-NCS antibody formation were obtained in the samples.

b) NCDP Combination Therapy

25 acute leukemia patients (age range 13-68; 15 males, 10 females), hospitalized in our clinic between October 1974 and June 1975 were treated by NCDP therapy (Table 4). The

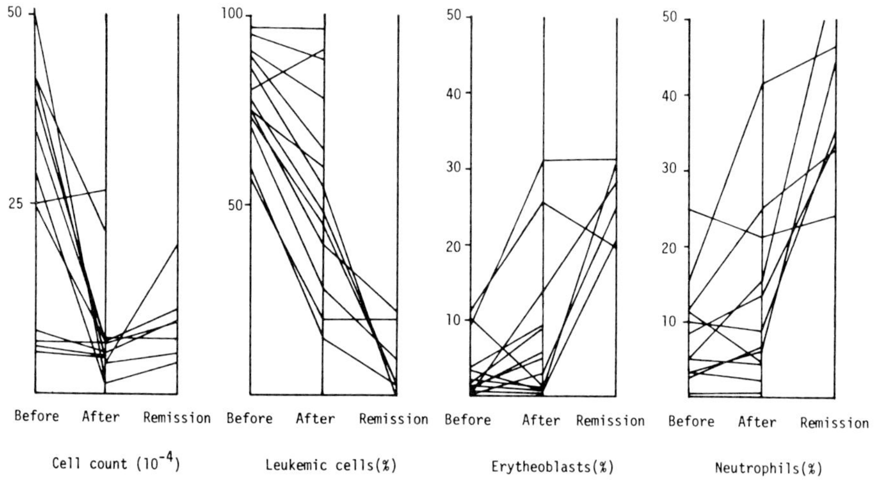

Fig. 5. NCS effects on bone marrow of leukemia patients

combination included: NCS at 0.04 mg/kg/day, cytosine arabinoside at 1.2–1.6 mg/kg/day, daunorubicin at 0.6–0.8 mg/kg/day, and prednisolone at 1.0–1.5 mg/kg/day. The treatment period was for 4 consecutive days, with a rest interval of 7–14 days. This protocol course was repeated in cycles until remission was obtained.

The initial induction series induced CR in 11 and PR in two of 14 cases (Table 5). The two PR cases subsequently became CR with vincristine replacing daunorubicin in the protocol. Induction treatment of relapsed cases produced CR in six and PR in one of 11 cases (63.5%).

Effects on Cancer

Table 6 shows the clinical trial results with NCS on eight kinds of solid tumors, including cancer of the stomach, pancreas, and urinary bladder.

a) Cancer of the Stomach [1]

NCS was usually administered at a daily dose of 3–4 mg by i.v. drip infusion or one shot i.v. injection, with a total dose of 30–100 mg. An objective response (evaluated as 1-A or 1-B by Karnofsky's criteria) was noted in 12 of 141 evaluated cases.

b) Cancer of the Pancreas [9]

NCS was usually administered at a daily dose of 2–3 mg for 15 days by i.v. drip infusion. The schedule was repeated in 1–3 cycles, resulting in a total dose of 30–120 mg. Tumor regressions were noted in 10 of 68 evaluated cases. These results indicate that NCS is a comparatively effective drug in cancer of the stomach and pancreas. The optimal rate of administration, dose level and administration schedule remain to be investigated in further detail.

c) Cancer of the Urinary Bladder [13]

Sakamoto et al. [13] conducted NCS studies in the urinary bladder. A daily NCS dose of 1 mg was administered for 7 consecutive days on 15 cases with histologically proven papillary transitional cell carcinoma. These schedule was repeated 1–4 times, resulting in a total dose of 7–28 mg. Apparent positive responses were confirmed endoscopically in 10 of 15 cases. These investigators also bioassayed the tissue concentration of NCS in the urinary bladder following i.v. NCS injection in rabbits in which bilateral ureteral fistulae were performed. They confirmed that the urinary bladder NCS concentration was significantly lower in rabbits with ureteral fistulae than in controls. Furthermore, after infusing radioactive NCS in the urinary bladder of rabbits with ureteral fistulae formation, these investigators succeeded in recovering high level of radioactive NCS from ureter. From 30% to 50% of recovered NCS had the original NCS molecular weight. These investigators deduced that, in a normal state, NCS exerts an effect not only through blood but also through urine in the urinary bladder. Clinical trials of NCS have also been performed on other solid tumors such as cancer of the esophagus, colorectal cancer, hepatoma, cancer of the lung, and malignant lymphoma, but no definite conclusions can be drawn at present because of the absence of clear response criteria. Furthermore, better controlled trials are needed.

d) Side Effects in Solid Tumors

Side effects were evaluated in 434 patients placed on NCS treatment for malignant solid tumors such as cancer of the stomach and pancreas (Table 7). Hematologic examination revealed a decrease of leukocyte counts to less than 4000/cmm in 33.6% of cases and a decrease in platelet counts to less than 100,000/cmm in 16.6% of cases. Gastrointestinal symptoms such as anorexia (17.3%) and nausea and/or vomiting (16.4%) were noted; fever was noted in 14.3% of cases. Rare side effects included stomatitis, exanthema, abnormal liver function, and hypotension. Anaphylactic shock was not encountered.

Conclusions

Investigations on cancer therapy with NCS in Japan indicate that the present usefulness of the drug is mainly for acute leukemia. The results are preliminary but relatively consistent and similar positive results are expected in investigations presently underway. The side effects of the drug were mainly marrow suppression and gastrointestinal disturbances.

Summary

Neocarzinostatin (NCS) is an antibiotic from streptomyces carzinostaticus which inhibits DNA synthesis. Clinical trials in Japan began in 1971. NCS is active against S-180, Ehrlich tumor, L1210, Yoshida sarcoma, and a range of ascitic hepatomas. In rabbits NCS is distributed at high concentrations in the kidney, skin, stomach, pancreas, lung, and muscles. The high distribution in the pancreas and the stomach suggested possible effectivness in human tumors at these sites. In clinical studies NCS has been shown to be active against acute leukemia. As a single agent 9 out of 51 obtained a CR with 9 more achieving a PR. Anorexia, nausea, and vomiting were the most frequent side effects. NCS has been tried in combination with Ara-C, daunorubicin and prednisolone and CR was seen in 11 out of 14. In stomach cancer responses of some kind were observed in 12 out of 141 cases, while in the case of pancreatic tumors there were 10 out of 68.

Tables

Table 1. Characteristics of 51 acute leukemia patients treated with NCS

Sex	
Male	28
Female	23
Age	7–74 (median 37)
Type of leukemia	
AML	29
APL	4
AMoL	11
ALL	7
Previous therapy	
Yes	21
No	30

Table 2. NCS effects in 51 acute leukemia patients

Type of leukemia	No. of cases	Response		Response rate (%)
		CR	PR	
AML	29	4	4	27.5
APL	4	1	1	50.0
AMoL	11	3	4	63.7
ALL	7	1	—	14.3
Total	51	9	9	35.3

Table 3. NCS side effects in acute leukemia patients

Side effects	Percentage
Anorexia	50
Nausea	42
Vomiting	12
General fatigue	12
Fever	10
Exanthema	4
Palpitation	4
Hepatic impairment	17
Bleeding tendency	2
Shock symptoms	2

Table 4. Characteristics of 25 acute leukemia patients treated with combination of NCS, cytosine arabinoside, daunorubicin and prednisolone (NCDP).

Sex	
Male	15
Female	10
Age	13–68 (median 41)
Type of leukemia	
AML	10
APL	3
AMoL	4
ALL	6
Previous therapy	
Yes	11
No	14

Table 5. NCDP therapy effects on acute leukemia

Type of leukemia	No. of cases	CR	PR	NR
Previously untreated				
AML	9	7	2	—
APL	2	2	—	—
AMoL	3	2	—	1
Total	14	11 (78.6)	2 (14.3)	1 (7.1)
Previously treated				
AML	3	2	—	1
APL	1	—	—	1
AMoL	1	—	—	1
ALL	6	4	1	1
Total	11	6 (54.5)	1 (9.1)	4 (36.4)

Numbers in parentheses are percentages.

Table 6. NCS effects on various types of malignancy

Disease	No. evaluated	No. of responders	Response rate (%)
Stomach cancer (1)	141	12[b]	8.5
Pancreatic cancer (9)	68	10	14.7
Urinary bladder cancer (13)	15	10	66.7
Esophagal cancer	6	1[a]	
Colorectal carcinoma	12	6[a]	
Hepatoma	8	5[a]	
Lung cancer	9	2[a]	
Malignant lymphoma	2	1[a]	

[a] Response criteria indefinite.
[b] Cases evaluated as 1-A or 1-B by Karnofsky's criteria.

Table 7. NCS side effects in 434 patients with solid tumors

Side effects	Percentage
Leukopenia (<4000/cmm)	33.6
Thrombopenia (<10^5/cmm)	16.6
Anorexia	17.3
Nausea/vomiting	16.4
Stomatitis	2.3
Exanthema	3.2
Fever	14.3
Abnormality in liver function tests	1.4
Hypotension	0.2

References

1. Aneha, Y., Kikuchi, K., Kanno, H., Kunii, Y.: Clinical trails of neocarzinostatin on stomach cancer. Proceedings of 14th Congress of Japan Society for Cancer Therapy, p. 257 (1976) (in Japanese).
2. Brander, W. T.: Neocarzinostatin (NSC-69856): An antitumor antibiotic effective against L1210 in mice. Cancer Chemother. Rep. **50** (1, 2), 79–84 (1966).
3. Ebina, T., Ishida, N.: Inhibition of formation of microtubular paracrystals in HeLa-S3 cells by neocarzinostatin. Cancer Res. **35**, 3705–3709 (1975).
4. Ebina, T., Otsuki, K., Seto, M., Ishida, N.: Specific G2 block in HeLa-S3 cells by neocarzinostatin. Eur. J. Cancer **11**, 155–158 (1975).
5. Fujimoto, S., Inagaki, J., Horikoshi, N., Kuraishi, Y., Hoshino, A., Amo, H., Kato, T., Ota, K.: Antitumor effects of neocarzinostatin in L1210 mouse leukemia: Cross-resistance and combination chemotherapy. Cancer and Chemother. **1**, 851–860 (1974) (in Japanese).
6. Fujita, H., Nakayama, N., Sawabe, T., Kimura, K.: *In vivo* distribution and inactivation of neocarzinostatin. Jap. J. Antibiot. **23**, 471–478 (1970) (in Japanese).
7. Hoshino, A., Kato, T., Amo, H.: Unpublished data.
8. Ishida, N., Miyazaki, M., Kumagai, K., Rikimaru, M.: Neocarzinostatin, an antitumor antibiotic of high molecular weight: Isolation, physicochemical properties and biological activities. J. Antibiot. (Tokyo) **18**, 68–76 (1965).
9. Ishii, K., Nakamura, K.: Neocarzinostatin in the treatment of pancreatic cancer: Results of cooperative study. Cancer and Chemother. **1**, 433–442 (1974) (in Japanese).
10. Kitajima, K., Kamimura, O., Hiraki, K.: Neocarzinostatin: A new chemotherapeutic approach to acute leukemia. Acta Haematol. Jap. **37**, 316–323 (1974).
11. Meienhofer, J., Maeda, H., Glaser, C. B., Czombos, J., Kuromizu, K.: Primary structure of neocarzinostatin, an antitumor protein. Science **178**, 875–876 (1972).
12. Ono, Y., Watanabe, Y., Ishida, N.: Mode of action of neocarzinostatin: Inhibition of DNA synthesis and degradation of DNA in Sartina lutea. Biochim. Biophys. Acta **119**, 46–58 (1966).
13. Sakamoto, S., Ogata, J., Ikegami, K.: Chemotherapy of urinary bladder carcinoma with neocarzinostatin. Igaku-No-Ayumi **101**, 87–90 (1977) (in Japanese).
14. Sato, H., Ichimura, H.: Effects of neocarzinostatin on rat ascitic hepatomas. Igaku-No-Ayumi **74**, 499–500 (1970) (in Japanese).
15. Sawada, H., Tatsumi, K., Sasada, M., Shirakawa, S., Nakamura, T., Wakisaka, G.: Effect of neocarzinostatin on DNA synthesis in L1210 cells. Cancer Res. **34**, 3341–3346 (1974).
16. Toriyama, K. and Koyama, Y.: Unpublished data.

Neocarzinostatin: Initial Clinical and Pharmacologic Studies in the United States

R. L. COMIS, T. GRIFFIN, V. RASO, and S. J. GINSBERG

Introduction

Neocarzinostatin (NCS) is a protein antitumor antibiotic isolated from *Streptomyces carzinostaticus*, var 41. The drug is a polypeptide consisting of 109 amino acids (m.w. 10,700) linked by two disulfide bridges. The amino acid sequence has been determined by MEINHOFFER [9]. NCS is the highest molecular weight antitumor antibiotic currently in clinical trials.

Since its discovery in 1965 by ISHIDA [5], antitumor activity has been demonstrated in a variety of animal tumor systems including L1210, Erlich's ascites carcinoma, SN-36 leukemia, and B_{16} melanoma. No significant schedule dependency has been demonstrated in animal tumor studies [3]. Large animal toxicology studies performed at the National Cancer Institute (U.S.A.) revealed a steep dose/toxicity relationship. The highest nontoxic dose on a single dose schedule was 0.2 mg/m^2, and the lethal dose was 0.8 mg/m^2. No "toxic dose low" was demonstrable, i.e., a dose which produced reversible toxicity and double the dose produced no lethality. The dose limiting toxicity in beagle dogs was an irreversible interstitial nephritis [13].

NCS has undergone extensive clinical evaluation in Japan since 1967 [7]. Over 400 patients have been treated and antitumor activity has been reported in acute leukemia and a variety of solid tumors. The most commonly employed i.v. doses have ranged from 0.04-0.06 mg/kg/d × 4-5, with courses repeated every 7-10 days. Toxicities were reportedly mild employing this dose schedule. The incidence of leukopenia ($< 4 \times 10^3$ cells/mm^3) ranged from 16%-32% and thrombocytopenia ($< 100 \times 10^3/mm^3$) 12%-16%. No dose limiting toxicity was apparent from the Japanese studies.

The mechanism of action of NCS is unknown. The drug has been shown to inhibit DNA > RNA > protein synthesis [12]. In addition to the inhibition of DNA synthesis manifested by decreased [H^3]-thymidine uptake, it causes DNA single and double strand breaks in vitro and may interfere with DNA template activity [1]. Cytokinetic studies employing HeLa S_3 and Chinese hamster ovary cells have shown that NCS is most active in the G_2 phase of the cell cycle [14, 4].

There is controversy over whether it is necessary for intact drug to enter cells to obtain cytocidal and growth inhibitory effects. Autoradiographic studies employing tritiated NCS incubated with L1210 cells indicate that the radiolabel enters cells [8]. In these experiments, considerable NCS degradation occurred during incubation, raising questions whether intact drug or fragments gained entry. Recently, LAZARUS et al. have reported a series of experiments employing NCS covalently bound to agarose beads. The data indicate that NCS may exert its DNA inhibitory and cytocidal effects by a membrane action, independent of direct cellular entry [6].

NCS has been of interest to investigators in the United States because of its animal and human antitumor activity, reported lack of significant myelotoxicity, unique structure, and possibly unique mechanism of action. Phase I clinical trials were initiated in the United States in early 1976. The dose schedules employed in these initial evaluations have included single dose, 5-day continuous infusion, weekly, and daily × 5 i.v. push regimens. Clinical and pharmacologic data generated from investigations performed at the Sidney Farber Cancer Institute, Boston and the Upstate Medical Center, Syracuse will be described in detail.

Materials and Methods

Phase I Clinical Study

Previously treated patients, or patients for whom no current therapy is of known benefit, were selected for therapy. Pretreatment laboratory investigations including a complete blood count and platelet count, BUN, electrolytes, creatinine, creatinine clearance, urinalysis, liver function tests, and EKG were performed on all patients. Patients were required to have a white blood count ⩾ 4000 cells/mm^2, platelet count ⩾ 100,000/mm^3, and normal renal and hepatic function. Complete blood count and platelet counts were obtained weekly after treatment. Renal and hepatic function tests were performed at 3-week intervals or prior to each treatment.

The drug employed was produced by Kayaku Antibiotics Research Co., Ltd. and obtained through the Investigation Drug Branch, Division of Cancer Treatment, of the U.S. National Cancer Institute. Vials (2 ml) containing 2000 units neocarzinostatin dissolved in an acetic acid-sodium acetate buffer, pH 5.0, were employed. For the purpose of comparison between Japanese and American clinical data, 1000 units = 1 mg. The drug was administered by rapid i.v. injection daily for 5 consecutive days. The starting dose was 500 units/m^2 (0.5 mg/m^2). Doses were escalated in some patients receiving repeat courses. Initially, 5-day courses were repeated every 14–21 days, but because of delayed toxicity most patients received repeat courses every 28–35 days.

Pharmacology

Serum levels were measured by radioimmunoassay, the details of which have been previously reported [11]. A double antibody technique was employed, using a rabbit antibody directed against purified NCS, a sheep anti-rabbit globulin directed against the FC fragment of rabbit gammaglobulin, and [I^{125}]-labeled NCS. No free tyrosine groups are available for iodination. Therefore, the drug was radiolabeled by acylation of the protein with an [I^{125}]-labeled N-hydroxysuccinimide ester of 3-(4-hydroxy-phenyl) propionic acid according to the method of Bolton and Hunter [2].

The drug was administered by rapid i.v. injection over 1 minute to three patients treated with 1500 u/m^2 and six patients treated with 2250 u/m^2. Serum samples (5 ml) were obtained prior to injection, at 2 min, at 5-min intervals from 5–20 min, every 30 min until 2 h had elapsed and then hourly for a total of 4–6 h. Urine was collected in 4-hour aliquots. Appropriate biologic samples were collected and immediately stored at −4°C.

Results

Phase I Study

Table 1 shows the patient characteristics and evaluability rates. Approximately 80% of all patients had some form of prior therapy, with the majority having had prior chemotherapy exposure. Eight patients were inevaluable for toxicity because of death, unrelated to therapy, within 4 weeks.

The incidence of myelotoxicity at each dose level for all evaluable patients and courses is presented in Table 2. The first dose level, 500 u/m², is about 30% of the lower dose (0.04 mg/kg) used in Japanese studies. No significant myelotoxicity or constitutional effects were noted before reaching a dose of 1500 u/m², which approximates a dose of 0.04 mg/kg. A progressive decrease in platelet count was observed with doses ranging from 1500–2250 u/m². Severe thrombocytopenia occurred in some patients at each dose level above 1000 u/m². Thus a 50% dose escalation, from 1000 to 1500 u/m², yielded significant thrombocytopenia in some patients.

Since cumulative toxicity has been encountered with NCS, the myelotoxicity data has been analyzed for the first course of therapy (Table 3) as well as all courses. Thrombocytopenia was encountered on the first course of therapy in 50% of patients treated with 2000 and 2500 u/m². Table 4 shows the incidence of myelotoxicity for all evaluable patients and courses, as well as the median nadir and day of nadir encountered at doses of 1500–2250 u/m². Leukopenia was delayed and moderate to severe when it occurred. There was no apparent relationship between dose and the white blood cell nadir or range of nadirs (0.7–2.9 × 10³ cells/mm³). Thrombocytopenia occurred later than leukopenia, with the median day of nadir ranging from 25–28 days. The platelet count ranged from 10–90 × 10³/mm³ and was not dose dependent. Because of the delayed myelotoxicity, courses of NCS were repeated every 35 days.

Prior chemotherapy significantly increased the incidence of leukopenia and thrombocytopenia (Table 5). No myelotoxicity was encountered in thriteen courses administered to previously untreated patients at doses of 1500–2000 u/m². A 12.5% escalation in dose to 2250 u/m² was associated with significant thrombocytopenia in four of six patients.

Cumulative myelotoxicity occurred in eight of 15 patients treated with multiple courses of NCS. Cumulative toxicity was defined as: a) an increasing depth of blood count depression when the initial dose was repeated, or b) a similar degree of myelotoxicity with a reduced dose of drug. Cumulative toxicity was manifested by severe and protracted thrombocytopenia in most patients. Nine of eighty patients evaluable for toxicity developed severe and protracted thrombocytopenia. Two of the nine patients had no prior chemotherapy. Four of nine died of causes unrelated to thrombocytopenia before platelet recovery. Those patients who recovered had significant platelet suppression for 2–3 months. Bone marrow examination in three such patients revealed decreased megakaryocytes.

The constitutional side-effects of neocarzinostatin administered on this schedule were manageable (Table 6). The majority of patients treated at doses of ⩾ 2000 u/m² experienced a shaking chill 30–60 min after drug administration which lasted approximately 30 min. The rigor occurred only on the first day of drug administration and could be prevented with diphenhydramine pretreatment. Temperature elevation (⩾ 101°F) was unusual. Nausea and vomiting was mild. Hypotension occurred soon after drug administration in two cases. Both episodes responded to intravenous diphenhydramine, steroids and fluid administration. One patient was retreated without recurrence of the signs. No renal or hepatic toxicity was documented.

Table 7 shows the objective response data for evaluable patients. Objective response was defined as a ⩾ 50% shrinkage in the sum of the products of a measurable lesion, without progression of any other lesion. For malignant hepatomegaly, a ⩾ 30% reduction in the span of the liver below the costal margin with associated stabilization or improvement in liver function tests was required. One of 17 responses was noted in lung cancer, this being an anaplastic, non-oat cell, tumor. Three of 16 responses were seen in gastrointestinal cancer with two of two responses in hepatoma and a probable response in carcinoma of the pancreas demonstrated by computerized axial tomography (CAT) scan lasted approximately 6 weeks. One of eight patients with melanoma responded and two of two responses were seen in malignant lymphoma. There have been two of 10 responses in refractory acute leukemia, one of five in lymphoblastic leukemia and one of five in acute myelogenous leukemia.

OHNUMA has reported another recently completed Phase I study [10]. Two dose schedules were employed: a) a 2-hour single dose infusion; b) a 5-day continuous i.v. infusion. Employing the 2-hour infusion, doses of 3000–4500 u/m² were associated with constitutional side effects which were felt to be dose-limiting including flushing, tachycardia, hypotension and hyperpyrexia. No significant myelosuppression was seen at either dose. No attempts at employing diphenhydramine or steroids before therapy were made. Employing the 5-day continuous infusion, significant myelosuppression was encountered at doses of 3000–12,500 u/m². Out of 26 patients, 20 exhibited leukopenia (WBC < 4500 cells/mm³) and 19 out of 25 patients developed platelet counts of < 100,000/mm³. The maximally tolerated dose for the 5-day continuous i.v. infusion was 6000 u/m²/day for previously untreated patients and 4500 u/m²/day for previously treated patients. Employing these two schedules of administration, renal toxicity manifested by transient increases in blood urea nitrogen (BUN) or creatinine were reported in 11 of 43 patients. Renal or hepatic dysfunction did not preclude therapy in any patient. No responses were seen in a variety of solid tumors. A complete remission occurred in one patient with acute myelogenous leukemia treated on the continuous infusion schedule.

Pharmacology

Fig. 1 shows the standard displacement curve for the radioimmunoassay. No nonspecific binding or inhibition was detected when standards assayed in serum, plasma, bile, CSF, or urine were compared to buffer. The level of sensitivity of the assay is 1 ng or 1×10^{-13} moles.

Fig. 2 and 3 show the decay curves for those patients treated at a dose of 1500 u/m² and 2250 u/m², respectively. The actual data points are represented by the different symbols while the curve is that defined by a two compartment model fitting the sum of two exponentials. For the 1500 u/m² dose, the excretion half-life of the drug, or $t\frac{1}{2}\beta$, was 16,43 and 236 min, respectively. The patient with the prolonged drug excretion phase had a creatinine clearance of 25 ml/min. Decay curves from four representative patients treated with 2250 u/m² are presented in Fig. 3. Again, the blood levels decreased in a biexponential manner. The $t\frac{1}{2}\beta$ ranged from 40–107 min, with a mean of 72 min. The half-life of the distribution phase, $t\frac{1}{2}\alpha$, was very rapid ranging from 6–13 min.

Table 8 presents the pertinent clinical and pharmacologic data for both doses. There was no obvious relationship between creatinine clearance and the $t\frac{1}{2}\beta$ for creatinine clearances of 48–102 ml/min. One patient having a significantly decreased creatine clearance (25 ml/min) was treated with a dose of 1500 u/m². This patient had a $t\frac{1}{2}\beta$ three times greater than the average of 72 min seen at the 2250 u/m² dose. Patients R.M. and R.C. had normal serum creatinine, but no creatinine clearances were performed. The estimated renal clearance was obtained by multiplying the calculated total drug clearance by the percent of the total dose excreted in the urine. With a decreased estimated renal clearance, the drug/renal clearance

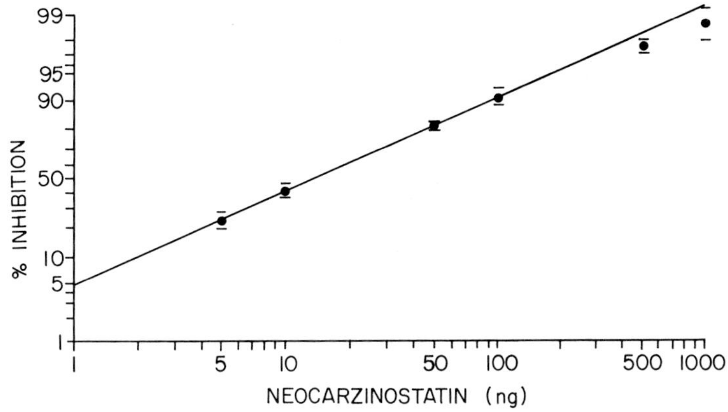

Fig. 1. Standard displacement curve showing the inhibition of binding of [I^{125}]-labeled NCS to specific rabbit antiserum by purified NCS

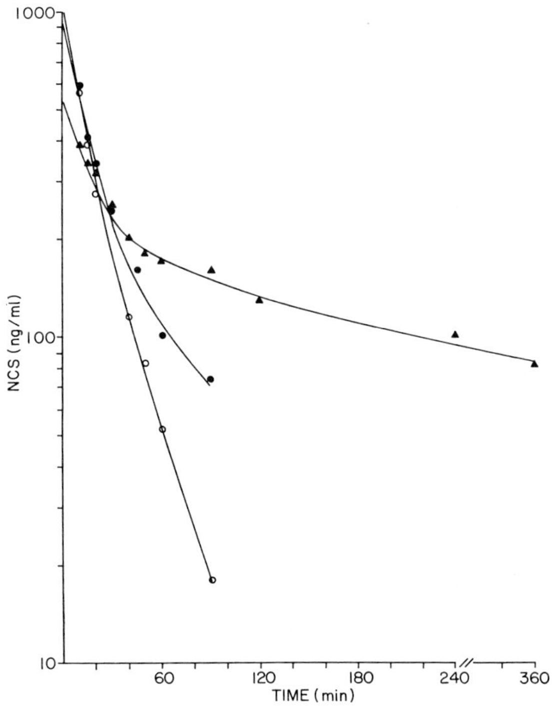

Fig. 2. Serum decay surves of patients treated with 1500 u/m^2. Symbols represent actual data points. The solid curve represents the computed curve drawn by fitting the actual data to an equation describing the sum of two exponentials (two compartment model)

ratio tends to increase, possibly representing an increase in nonrenal clearance mechanisms. Although complete drug metabolism studies are not available, no drug was detected in the bile of one patient assayed after a bolus injection of neocarzinostatin.

Immunochemically intact drug was rapidly excreted in the urine (Table 9), with 75% of the

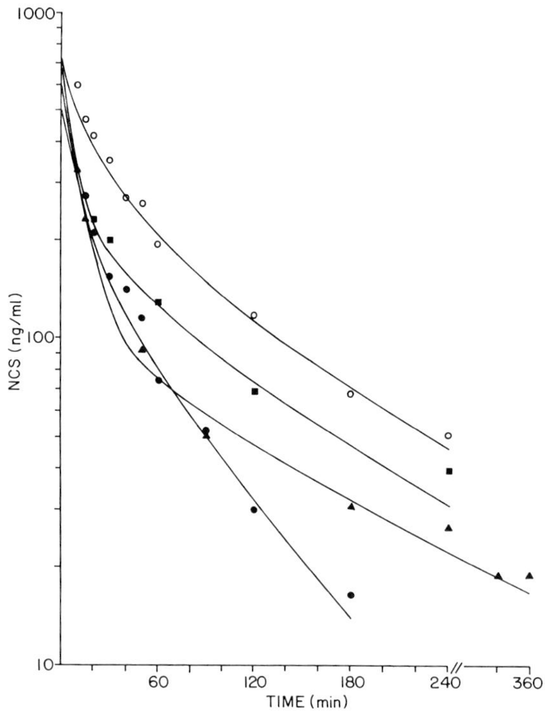

Fig. 3. Serum decay curves of four patients treated with 2250 u/m². Symbols represent actual data points. The solid curve represents the computed curve drawn by fitting the actual data to an equation describing the sum of two exponentials (two compartment model)

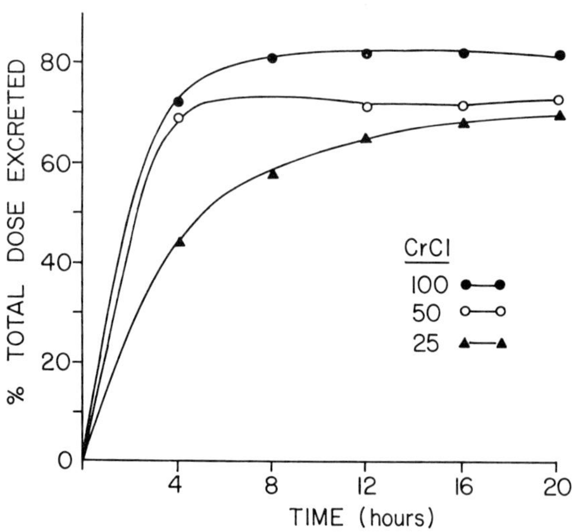

Fig. 4. The % of the total dose excreted per four-hour aliquot of urine. Drug was assayed by radio-imunoassay as described in materials and methods and reference 11

administered dose excreted in 24 h. Fig. 4 presents the percentage of the total dose excreted over time for patients with creatinine clearances of 25, 50 and 100 ml/min, respectively. Employing 4-hour collection times, delayed drug excretion was apparent in the patient with the creatinine clearance of 25 ml/min. No significant difference in urinary excretion time was apparent for the patients with the 50 and 100 ml/min clearances, under these conditions.

The calculated volume of the central compartment, V_1, and the apparent volume and distribution (VD) of the drug for both doses is also presented in Table 8. The average value of the central compartment for the 1500 u/m² dose was 2.8 liters or approximately 5% of body weight. The apparent volume of distribution ranged from 6%-19%, with a mean of 12%. The average volume of distribution for the 2250 u/m² dose was 11 liters or 17% of total body weight, approximating extracellular fluid volume. The calculated volume of the central compartment was 5 liters or 7%, approximating total blood volume.

Although the drug is apparently distributed in the extracellular fluid volume, analysis of three serous effusions yielded no detectable drug after bolus injection. This is probably a result of its rapid disappearance from the blood after bolus injection.

Protein binding and metabolism studies have recently been initiated using radiolabeled neocarzinostatin incubated in normal human serum for 4 h at 37°C (Fig. 5). No significant protein binding was demonstrated under these conditions. It has subsequently been shown that the elution pattern for iodinated neocarzinostatin incubated in phosphate buffered saline is the same as presented in this figure. This implies that no significant in vitro metabolism occurs under these conditions.

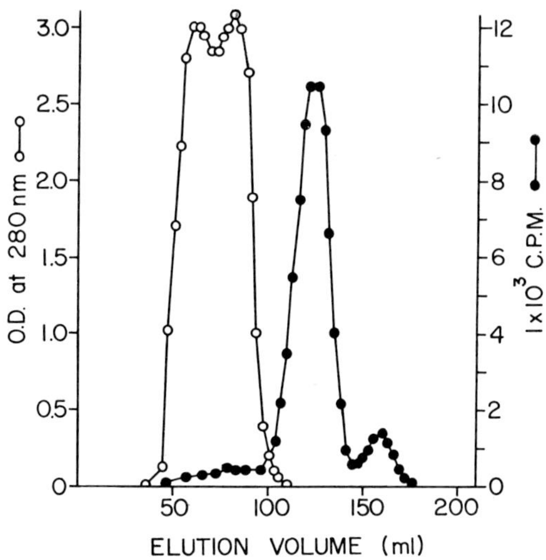

Fig. 5. Elution of [I^{125}]-NCS incubated in normal human serum for 4 h from a G100 Sephadex column, ph 7.4, equilibrated with isotomic phosphate buffered saline; o—o optical density at 280 nm; ●—●[I^{125}]-NCS

Summary and Conclusions

Phase I Study

Myelosuppression, predominantly thrombocytopenia, is the dose-limiting toxicity of neocarzinostatin administered by i.v. injection daily × 5 days. Myelosuppression seen at doses of 2000–2250 u/m²/d × 5 is somehwat unpredictable, since only 50% of patients develop significant depression of blood counts. Also, thrombocytopenia can be cumulative and occasionally protracted. Prior therapy significantly increases the incidence of significant leukopenia and thrombocytopenia. The recommended dose on the daily × 5 day schedule is 1500 u/m² for previously treated patients and 2250 u/m² for previously untreated patients.
Constitutional side-effects including a vigorous rigor, mild temperature elevation, nausea and vomiting have not been dose limiting. The rigor can be prevented in most instances by the administration of diphenhydramine prior to drug administration. No consistent or significant renal or hepatic toxicity has been encountered with the drug.
Preliminary results indicate that the drug may have some activity in acute leukemia, undifferentiated lung cancer, malignant melanoma, lymphoma and hepatoma. Further Phase II testing is necessary to determine the significance of these observations.

Pharmacology

After bolus injection, neocarzinostatin has a rapid elimination half-life. The mean half-life after a dose of 2250 u/m² is 72 min (range 42–107). Immunochemically intact drug is rapidly excreted in the urine. Within the first 4 h, 58% of the total dose is excreted and 75% is excreted within the first 24 h. Delayed serum elimination and urinary excretion has been observed in one patient with a creatinine clearance of 25 ml/min, whereas no significant difference in serum or urinary elimination has been detected in patients with creatinine clearances ranging from 48–102 ml/min. The apparent volume of distribution of the drug is 11 liters (17% body weight) approximating the extracellular fluid volume. Because of the relatively rapid elimination half-life, and the reported G_2 phase specificity, clinical and pharmacologic studies are now being performed employing a 5-day continuous infusion.

Tables

Table 1. Neocarzinostatin phase I study: Patient characteristics

Patients Entered	88
Evaluable Patients	
Toxicity	80
Response	53
Prior Chemotx:	73%
Prior XRT:	65%

Table 2. Neocarzinostatin: Hematologic effects

Dose (u/m²/d ×5)	No. evaluable patients	No. evaluable courses	Hematologic effects: WBC ×10³ Median nadir	WBC ×10³ Range	PLT ×10³ Median nadir	PLT ×10³ Range
500	4	4	6.9	(5.6-8.9)	276	(198-311)
1000	3	3	7.5	(5.6-9.1)	187	(124-424)
1500	14	14	5.3	(1.2-8.7)	182	(16-359)
2000	28	44	4.6	(0.7-10.2)	116	(11-290)
2250	32	52	4.1	(0.8-9.2)	102	(10-370)

Table 3. Neocarzinostatin Myelotoxicity: First course of therapy

Dose (u/m²/d×5)	Myelotoxicity: WBC < 3 × 10³	PLT < 100 × 10³
1500	2/14	3/14
2000	3/28	14/28
2250	7/30	15/30

Table 4. Neocarzinostatin: Hematologic toxicity

Dose (u/m²/d × s)	No. patients	No. courses	Nadir (median) Cells × 10³	Day
		WCB < 3.0 × 10³		
1500	2/14	2/14	1.2	20
2000	5/28	7/44	2.0	20
2250	9/32	8/02	1.8	20
		PLT < 100 × 10³		
1500	3/14	3/14	42	27
2000	14/28	20/44	62	28
2250	16/32	16/52	41	25

Table 5. Neocarzinostatin myelotoxicity: Effects of prior chemotherapy

Dose (u/m²/d × 5)	Prior chemotherapy: WCB	Prior chemotherapy: PLT	No prior chemotherapy: WBC	No prior chemotherapy: PLT
1500	2/11	3/11	0/3	0/3
2000	3/17	14/17	0/11	0/11
2250	6/24	11/24	1/6	4/6
Total	11/52	28/52	1/20	4/20

Table 6. Neocarzinostatin: non-myelosuppressive toxicities

	Toxic courses		
Dose ($u/m^2/d \times s$)	Rigor + temp.	Vomiting	Hypotension
500–1000	0/10	0/10	0/10
1500	4/13	1/13	0/13
2000	10/20	8/20	0/20
2250	24/59	19/59	2/59

Table 7. Neocarzinostatin: Phase I objective response

Disease	No. Responders/No. Evaluable	
Lung	1/17	
G.I.	3/16	
hepatoma		2/2
pancreas		1/4[a]
colon		0/13
gallbladder		0/1
G.U.	0/6	
kidney		0/4
bladder		0/2
Melanoma	1/8	
Sarcoma	0/6	
Lymphoma	2/2	

[a] By CAT (computerized axial tomography) scan.

Table 8. Neocarzinostatin. Pharmacokinetic data

			Clearance (ml/min)				Volumes			
							V_1		V_D	
Patient	Total dose (u)	$t_{\frac{1}{2}}\beta$ (min)	CrCl	Drug	Renal[a]	Drug/renal	Liters	% Body wt.	Liters	% Body wt.
						1500 u/m^2				
E.M.	1800	16	48	96	69	1.37	1.2	3.5	2.3	6.8
R.M.	2400	43	—	91	—	—	2.4	4.0	5.6	10.0
J.B.	2400	236	25	33	23	1.43	4.3	7.0	11.3	19.0
					2250 u/m^2					
V.J.	3600	40	69	168	—	—	3.9	6.9	9.6	17
B.P.	3800	45	101	223	187	1.22	7.4	9.2	14.7	18
R.M.	3500	78	—	115	—	—	3.9	6.9	13.1	22
R.C.	3600	79	—	107	—	—	3.6	5.7	12.2	19
M.M.	3800	83	50	83	52	1.30	5.4	8.0	10.6	16
G.Z.	3600	107	102	159	130	1.20	3.6	6.0	5.8	11
Mean		72					5.1	7.0	11.0	17

[a] Estimated renal clearance = $CL_D \times$ % Total dose excreted.

Table 9. Urinary excretion of NCS by radioimmunoassay

Time (h)	% Total dose	
	Mean	Range
0-4	57.6	43-72
4-8	9.8	8.6-14
8-12	4.4	1.0-9.4
12-16	2.3	0.2-6.3
16-20	1.0	0.1-1.7
20-24	<1.0	
24 h excretion	75.1	(69-82.4)

References

1. Beerman, T. A., Goldberg, I. H.: DNA strand scission by the antitumor protein neocarzinostatin. Biochem. Biophys. Res. Commun. **59**, 1254-1261 (1974).
2. Bolton, A. E., Hunter, W. M.: The labeling of proteins to high specific radioactivities by conjugation to a ^{125}I-containing acylating agent. Biochem. J. **133**, 529-539 (1973).
3. Bradner, W. T., Hutchinson, D. J.: Neocarzinostatin (NCS-69856): an antitumor antibiotic effective against ascitic leukemia L1210 in mice. Cancer Chemother. Rep. **50**, 79-84, (1966).
4. Ebina, T., Ohtsuki, K., Seto, M., Ishida, N.: Specific G2 block in Hela-S3 cells by neocarzinostatin. Eur. J. Cancer **11**, 155-158 (1975).
5. Ishida, N., Ishii, K., Kitajami, K., Hiraki, K., Kikuchi, M.: Clinical evaluation of antitumor protein neocarzinostatin. Prog. Chemotherapy **3**, 927-940 (1965).
6. Lazarus, H., Raso, V., Samy, T. S. A.: Neocarzinostatin-a protein antibiotic with unusual properties. Proc. Am. Assoc. Cancer Res. **17**, 107 (1976).
7. Legha, S. S., Van Hoff, D. D., Slavik, M., Muggia, F. M.: Neocarzinostatin (NSC-157365) a new cancerostatic compound. Cancer (in press).
8. Maeda, H., Aikawa, S., Yamashita, A.: Subcellular fate of protein antibiotic neocarzinostatin in culture of a lymphoid cell line from Burkitt's lymphoma. Am. Res. **35**, 554-559 (1975).
9. Meinhofer, J., Maeda, H., Glaser, C. B., Kuromizu, K.: Primary structure of the antitumor protein neocarzinostatin. Science. **178**, 875-876 (1972).
10. Ohnuma, T., Nogeive, C., Cuttner, J., Holland, J. F.: Initial clinical studies with neocarzinostatin (NCS). Proc. Am. Soc. Clin. Oncology **18**, 332 (1977).
11. Raso, V., Samy, T. S. A.: Radioimmunoassay of neocarzinostatin, an anti-tumor protein. Cancer Res. **36**, 4378-4381 (1976).
12. Sawada, H., Tatsumi, K., Masataka, S., Shirakawa, S., Nakamura, T., Gyoichi, W.: Effect of neocarzinostatin on DNA synthesis in L1210 cells. Cancer Res. **34**, 3344-3346 (1974).
13. Schaeppi, W., Menninger, F., Fleishman, R. W., Bogden, A. E., Schein, P. S., Cooney, D. A.: Toxicity of neocarzinostatin (NSC-69856): an antitumor antibiotic with radiomimetic and antigenic characteristics. Cancer Chemother. Rep. pt. 3. 5(1), 43-54 (1974).
14. Tobey, R. A.: Different drugs arrest cells at a number of distinct stages in G_2. Nature **254**, 245-247 (1975).

Synthetic Analogs of Antitumor Drugs Under Development in Japan

Y. SAKURAI

Synthetic studies on new antitumor drugs in Japan are being mostly oriented to search for new analogs of the known antitumor drugs, although a few compounds having original chemical structure are also under investigation.

Analogs of Nitrosourea

Prior to the introduction of antitumor activity of streptozotocin, some trials were started in Japan to find a water-soluble analog of BCNU or CCNU by replacing part of the molecule by a basic chemical group. In the course of this study, Arakawa succeeded in preparing a pyrimidine derivative of nitrosourea, 1-(4-amino-2-methylpyrimidine-5-yl)methyl-3-(2-chloreothyl)-3-nitrosourea (ACNU: NSC D245382), which, as the hydrochloride, is soluble in water. Antitumor activity of ACNU on various experimental tumors has already been reported in detail by ARAKAWA et al. [4, 6]. On mouse leukemia L1210, a single i.p. injection of 25 mg/kg on day 1 showed 440% ILS with 60% long survivors. Also, increase of life-span 10 i.p. injections of 10 mg/kg on every other day gave 363%. ACNU was also effective against intracerebrally inoculated L1210, giving 140% ILS after a single oral adminstration of 20 mg/kg. The metabolic degradation of ACNU in vivo is indicated in Fig. 1. ACNU at present is still in the stage of clinical evaluation [8]. The main clinical side-effects seem to be myelotoxicity but nausea and vomiting were less frequent than with methyl-CCNU.

Stimulated by the information from the United States of the interesting property of chlorozotocin, various derivatives of nitrosourea having a sugar moiety have been investigated. Among them, GANU (NSC D254157) and MCNU (NSC D270516) are now ready for Phase I clinical study in Japan. The former was synthesized by SUAMI [17, 18], and biologically tested AOSHIMA and SAKURAI [1]. The latter was prepared by IWASAKI, et al. [15] (Fig. 2).

The antitumor effect and myelotoxocity of GANU and chlorozotocin (DCNU) were compared by AOSHIMA, et al. [1]. The results are indicated in Table 1. SCHEIN, et al. [11] also referred to the biologic and biochemical behavior of GANU in their recent publication, with slight different results from the data in Table 1. According to Aoshima, myelotoxicity of these two compounds was found to be similar to one another, both being far milder than BCNU (Fig. 3).

MCNU has been extensively studied by IWASAKI, et al. [15]. A characteristic behavior of this compound is that it exhibited nearly the same effect on L1210 by oral administration as by i.v. injection of the same dose (Fig. 4). Comparative data of MCNU on L1210 and its acute toxicity with other nitrosourea compounds are indicated in Tables 2 and 3.

A few years ago, methyl-CCNU was introduced into Phase I study in Japan by the aid of NCI. Since then, there have been many attempts to carry out clinical chemotherapy trials on stomach cancer by combination protocols with 5-FU and methyl-CCNU. However, the side-effects, especially subjective ones such as nausea and vomiting, occurred frequently and

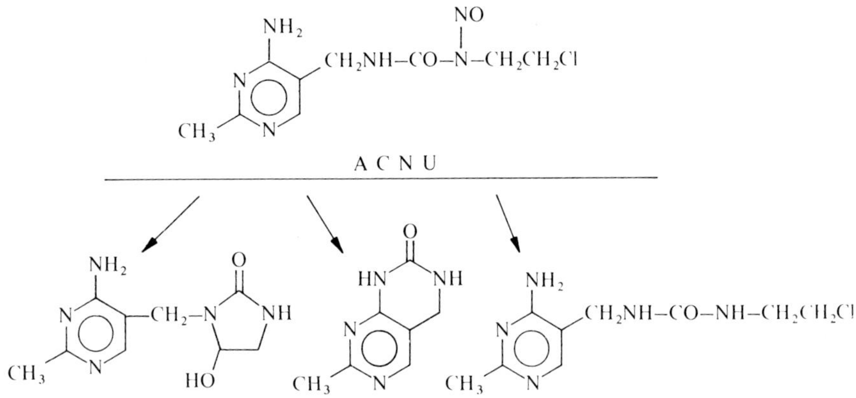

Fig. 1. Metabolites of ACNU in rat urine. Maximum tolerated dose of ACNU was given i.v. to Wistar rats. The metabolites were detected by TL-chromatography in the urine collected during the 24 hours following injection of ACNU

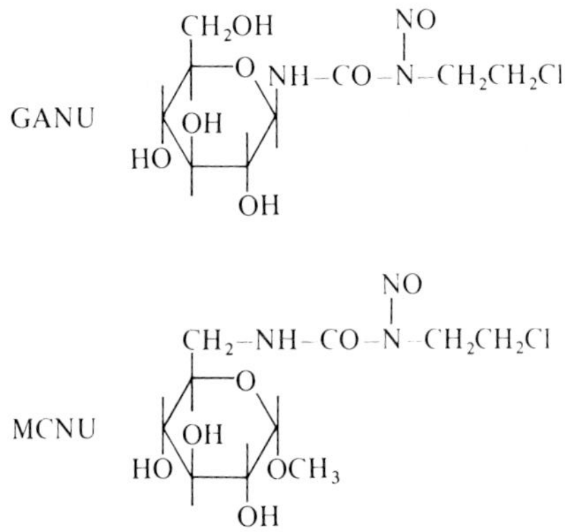

Fig. 2. Chemical structures of GANU (NSC D254157) and MCNU (NSC D270516)

hindered wide use of this protocol. From this point of view, the development of water-soluble and less toxic analogs has been emphasized.

Besides the two analogs mentioned above, a few analogs of nitrosourea are now in the stage of experimental investigation. For instance, Suzuki, et al. [20] prepared a series of alkylene-bis-nitrosoureas which have no 2-chloroethyl group but still showed a strong antitumor activity on L1210 and rat ascites hepatoma AH13. Of the series, 1, l'-ethylenebis(1-nitrosourea) (EBNU) was most effective and its chemical reactivity in vivo was closely studied by Suzuki et al. [19] (Table 4).

EBNU and its series compounds may be expected to effect cross-linking alkylation on a target molecule of the cell. Table 4 shows a preliminary screening result of the series of compounds.

Analogs of Alkylating Agents

A series of bis-methanesulfonate of aminoglycols were preapred as the analogs of myleran by Sakurai, et al. in 1965 [9, 10]. Among those compounds, bis(3-mesyloxypropyl)-amine

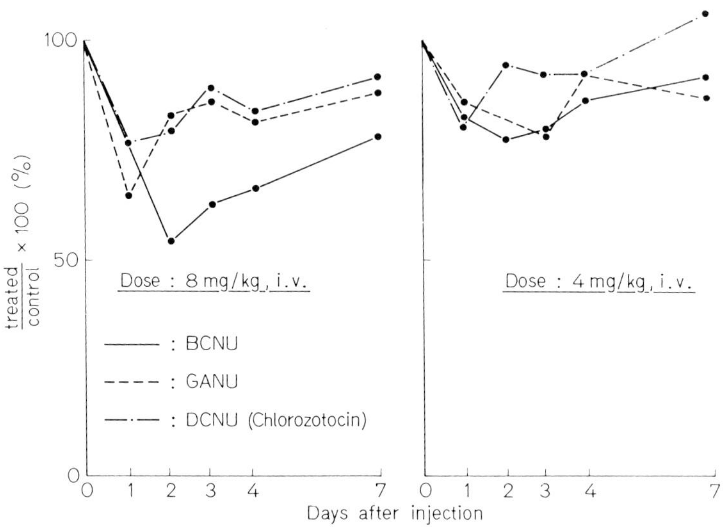

Fig. 3. Effect of GANU, chlorozotocin, and BCNU on the bone marrow cellularity of rats.
*Total nucleated cells in the femur bone marrow were (1.1 ± 0.2) × 10^8/femur in normal Donryu rats (♀, 8–9 weeks)

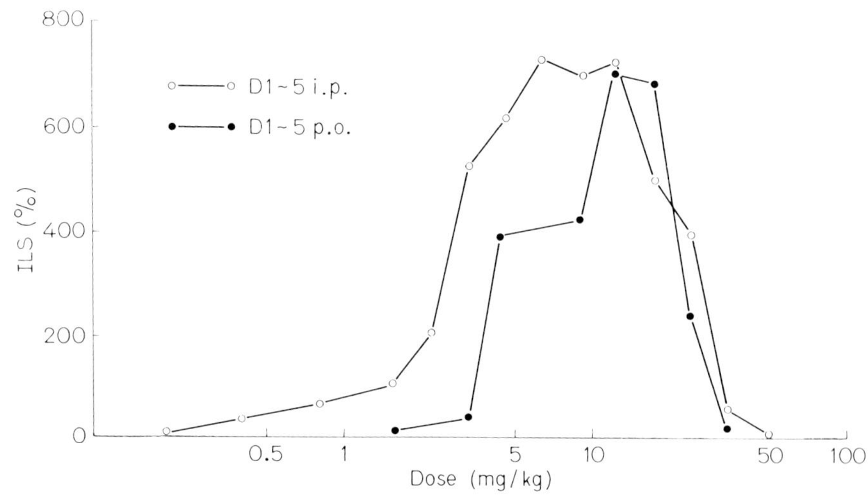

Fig. 4. Dose Response of MCNU on L1210 by i.p. and p.o. Administration

hydrochloride (NSC 102627) exhibited a strong effect on L1210 and other rodent tumors, contrary to myleran. The antitumor spectrum on the series of rat ascites hepatoma was also quite different from that of the known derivatives of nitrogen mustard. From these facts, it was expected that this compound might have a clinical utility different from myleran; but the results of clinical trials in Japan so far collected were rather similar to myleran and its related compounds.

The studies of active metabolites of cyclophosphamide in vivo have been extensively pursued by many workers for past years. 4-Hydroxy cyclophosphamide was pointed out by CONNORS et al. [7] to be one of the active intermediates which might exist in an aqueous solution in equilibrium with aldophosphamide. TAKAMIZAWA [22] first synthesized 4-hydroperoxy-cyclophosphamide, which was reduced by triphenyl phosphine into 4-hydroxy-cyclophosphamide, to identify the properties of this intermediate. It was reported that this 4-hydroxy derivative proved to be very active against L1210, and later that the 4-hydroperoxy-derivative was similarly active against L1210, supposedly through reduction in vivo to the 4-hydroxy-derivative. Nine analogs of 4-hydroperoxy-cyclophosphamide were reported in 1976 by TAKAMIZAWA et al. [23], among which 4-hydroperoxy-ifosfamide (No. 40497) has been investigated in the most detail.

As for aziridine derivatives, 2, 5-bis(1-aziridinyl)-3-(2-carbamoyloxy)-1-methoxyethyl)-6-methyl-1, 4-benzoquinone (carbazilquinone) was introduced by ARAKAWA et al. [5] in 1973. This drug was clinically tested by SAITO, et al. [21] and is now available for clinical use in Japan.

Analogs of Antimetabolites

Other lines of analog study have been developed in Japan in the field of metabolite antagonists. 2, 2'-Anhydro-1-β-D-arabinofuranosylcytosine hydrochloride (cyclocytidine) was prepared by Kohjin Co., Ltd., and biologically studied in detail by KURETANI and HOSHI [14], and HIRAYAMA [13]. This compound once attracted our interest in that it was effective on L1210 even by oral administration, but this was not the case in clinical trials. However, its clinical efficacy by i.v. injection proved to be comparable to the parent nucleoside. It was claimed that the effect lasted longer than the parent compound after i.v. administration, possibly owing to the fact that cyclocytidine is not a substrate of cytidine deaminase. On the other hand, a few untoward side-effects of cyclocytidine were reported: temporary depression of the blood pressure immediately after injection and pain on the parotis. A new protocol, a modification of DCMP (daunorubicin, cytosine arabinoside, 6-mercaptopurine riboside, and predonisolone), is now being tested in Japan for the treatment of acute leukemia, in which cytosine arabinoside is replaced by cyclocytidine.

The other analog of cytosine arabinoside is N^4-behenoyl-cytosine arabinoside which has been studied by SAKURAI et al. [2, 3] in collaboration with Asahi Chemical Industry Co., Ltd. N^4-stearoyl-cytosine arabinoside was mingled by chance, in the course of random screening in our Chemotherapy Center, with the samples from the company. N^4-acetyl-cytosine arabinoside was prepared by FOX et al. [25] in 1968 and was reported to have only a poor activity on L1210. Conversely the N^4-stearoyl derivative was found to have a strong activity against L1210 and also against some types of mouse tumor. From this finding, a series of N^4-acylated cytosine arabinosides were synthesized and tested on L1210 (Table 5).

As reported by Fox, the analogs with short fatty acid chains did not exhibit excellent activity, but the effect increases with increasing chain length. Maximum effectiveness was attained by palmitoyl or stearoyl derivatives. However, these analogs were only barely soluble in water. We tried to find some water-soluble analogs by substituting a hydroxyl group at the 5-position of the sugar with anionic or cationic groups (Table 6). But, unfortunately, most of these water-soluble analogs showed more or less hemolytic action on the erythrocytes with manifestation of greater toxicity to the host animal than the insoluble analogs. Therefore, we are at present mainly studying N^4-behenoyl-1-β-D-arabinofuranosylcytosine dissolved in an aqueous solution containing a detergent named HCO-60. The behenoyl analog formed a stable solution most easily with this detergent and yet maintained its excellent antitumor

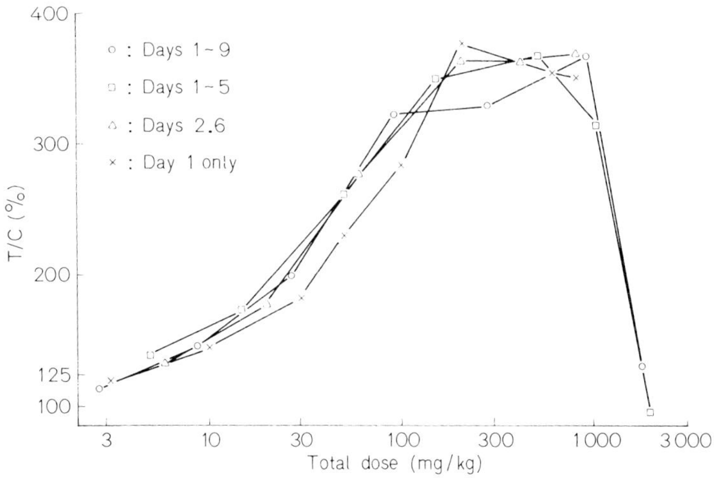

Fig. 5. Effect of N^4-Behenoyl-1-β-D-arabinofuranosyl-cytosine on L1210 by various Dose Schedules

activity. A characteristic property of this analog was that its effect on L1210 was manifested independently of the dose schedule, divided or single, provided the same total dose was given. It was quite a different finding from the parent compound (Fig. 5).

This new analog was effective against B16 melanoma and Lewis lung carcinoma, but not effective against the cytosine arabinoside-resistant line of L1210 nor against most rat tumors, similar to the parent nucleoside.

Another focus of interest in the analog study in Japan is chemical modification of 5-FU. 5-FU is still one of the major tools for the treatment of stomach cancer, which is the cancer of the highest incidence in Japan. Several years ago, FT-207 was introduced into Japan from USSR. The first trial in Japan of the compound by i.v. injection resulted in rather poor evaluation, but later its oral administration gained a better reputation. Encouraged by this fact, various analogs of 5-FU, especially of masked type, have been synthesized by UNEMI, et al. [24]. Among them, 1,3-bis(tetra-hydro-2-furanyl)-5-flouro-2,4-pyrimidinedione (FD-1) attracted the interest of the clinical field in Japan. FD-1 showed antitumor effect on the solid forms of sarcoma 180, Ehrlich carcinoma, and Walker 256 nearly as strongly as FT-207. However, the effect on L1210 was not remarkable, just as FT-207 (Table 7).

The comparative experiments on the fate of FD-1 and FT-207 in vivo showed that the level of active metabolite, 5-FU, in plasma was far higher and longer-lasting in the case of FD-1 than FT-207 after oral administration of 0.6 mmole of either compound. The tetrahydrofuranyl group at the 3-position of pyrimidinedione is split off first in vivo, because FT-207 is found as the primary metabolite in plasma.

Acute toxicity (LD_{50}) of FD-1 by oral administration was 2664 mg/kg on mice and 1730 mg/kg on rats, while that of FT-207 was 820 mg/kg on mice and 1220 mg/kg on rats. Detailed experimental data on the pharmacokinetics of this compound will be presented by FUJITA [12].

Analogs of Platinum Complex

Kidani et al. [16] have synthesized many platinum complexes. They successfully separated dichloro-(1,2-diamino-cyclohexane)Pt II complex into the purified cis and trans forms. The latter was again resolved into two optical isomers, trans-**l**- and trans-**d**-forms. According to the results of screening with L1210, the trans-**l**-form was the most potent, giving 379% T/C with a daily dose of 12.5 mg/kg by two i.p. injections on days 1 and 5. The trans-**d**-form gave 291% T/C by the same dose schedule. The antitumor effect of the cis-form was weaker than the both of the trans-forms. In summary, it is noteworthy that the conformation of the platinum complexes seemed to have a great influence on their antitumor activity.
To find the less toxic analogous complexes, Kidani prepared new analogs by replacing two chlorine atoms by dicarboxylates such as oxalate, malonate, or methyl-malonate. Of these complexes with mixed ligand, oxalo(trans--l-diamino-cyclohexane)Pt II complex was noticeable because of its very strong antitumor activity on P388 mouse leukemia, giving 188% T/C at a dose of 6.25 mg/kg and 152% at 3.12 mg/kg.

Comments

In the development of new analogs of antitumor agents, there are still some problems in methodology of screening. For instance, analogs of nitrosourea are apt to exhibit a very high activity on L1210 or P388 that is unimaginable in cases of other types of compounds. This high ILS does not necessarily predict the corresponding grade of clinical effectiveness, and for all that, we have to make a choice of one compound among numerous candidates by the ILS value. FT-207 is another example. It showed only a poor effect on L1210 when compared with any of the nitrosourea derivatives, while it exhibited an undeniable effect on human cancer. It would be difficult to make a rational conclusion, especially in cases of masked type compounds, using a limited number of animal tumors. We have felt the need of some new tools and systems for the comparative evaluation of analogs of every type of antitumor agents.

Summary

Synthetic studies on new antitumor drugs in Japan are mainly oriented toward analogs of known active structures. In the nitrosourea area ACNU, a pyrimidine analog of CCNU, is currently under clinical investigation and has myelosuppression as a side effect. Nitrosoureas with a sugar moiety are of great interest and two compounds called GANU and MCNU are now ready for phase I study in Japan. Among new alkylating agents are included a series of bis-methanesulfonate of aminoglycols, an analog of cyclophosphamide called 4-hydroperoxy-cyclophosphamide, and aziridine derivatives which include the now commercially available carbazilquinone. In the antimetabolite field cyclocytidine is an analog of arabinosyl cytosine which has been extensively studied. A newer analog called N^4-behenoyl-cytosine arabinoside is now being studied experimentally. In the fluorinated pyrimidine area Ftorafur has been extensively studied and a new compound FD-1 is of interest.

Tables

Table 1. Comparison of the effect of GANU and DCNU on L1210

		GANU			DCNU		
Route	Dose (mg/kg)	Body wt. change[a]	MST[b]	T/C (%)	Body wt. change[a]	MST[b]	T/C (%)
	3.6	-0.6	⩾17.8	⩾237 (1/5)	-1.2	15	182
	5.4	-1.2	16.6	221	-1.0	⩾19.8	⩾241 (1/5)
i.p.	8.9	0.0	17.4	232	-0.8	⩾28.0	⩾341 (4/5)
	13.3	-1.2	⩾28.2	⩾376(4/5)	-1.8	⩾31.0	⩾378 (5/5)
	20	-2.0	⩾27.0	⩾360 (3/5)	-2.4	⩾19.8	⩾241 (1/5)
	30	-2.4	⩾15.0	⩾200 (1/5)	-4.0	8.6	104
	3.6	-0.4	11.8	143	+0.4	10.6	129
	5.4	-1.0	13.6	165	-0.6	13.0	158
i.v.	8.9	-1.0	11.6	141	-1.0	15.0	182
	13.3	-2.0	12.2	148	-2.2	15.8	192
	20	-2.6	10.0	121	-3.4	13.0	158
	30	-4.8	8.0	97	-4.6	7.4	90
	3.6	0.0	12.0	146	+0.9	8.0	97
	5.4	-1.4	12.8	156	+0.6	9.4	114
oral	8.9	-1.2	13.8	168	+0.4	9.2	112
	13.3	-1.2	14.0	170	0.0	10.2	124
	20	-1.6	15.4	187	+0.8	9.0	109
	30	-3.0	9.6	117	0.0	8.6	104

L1210 cells (10^5/mouse) were inoculated i.p. into each group of 5 mice. The drug was injected i.p. or i.v., or given orally on days 1 and 5 after the inoculation. Numbers in parentheses show 30-day survivors. a) Body weight change shows the difference of the body weight measured on days 1 and 5. b) MST = mean survival time in days. MST of the untreated control and in the group treated i.p. with GANU was 7.5 days and in other groups was 8.2 days.

Table 2. Comparative effect of nitrosourea analogs on L1210

Treatment	Agent	Dose in ILS_{30} mg/kg	Optimal dose mg/kg	Max. ILS (60-day survivors)	Therapeutic ratio[a]
D 1-5 i.p.	MCNU	0.36	12.5	>722 (6/6)	34.7
	DCNU	0.65	6.3	>622 (5/6)	9.7
	GANU	0.4	6.3	>427 (4/6)	15.8
	CCNU	2.0	18	>689 (6/6)	9.0
	ACNU	1.3	18	>650 (6/6)	13.8
D 1-5 p.o.	MCNU	2.5	18	>679 (6/6)	7.2
	DCNU	—	100	18 (0/6)	—
	GANU	2.6	6.3	76 (0/6)	2.9
	CCNU	3.5	35	>567 (6/6)	10.0

[a]Therapeuric ratio = optimal dose/dose in ILS_{30}.

Table 3. LD_{50} Acute toxicity (mg/kg)

	Rat		Mouse	
	i.v.	p.o.	i.v.	p.o.
ACNU	47	124	65	106
GANU	10	21	20	33
MCNU	32	50	44	49

Table 4. Effect on L1210 of alkylene-bis-nitrosourea compounds. Structure of alkylene-bis-nitrosourea compounds:

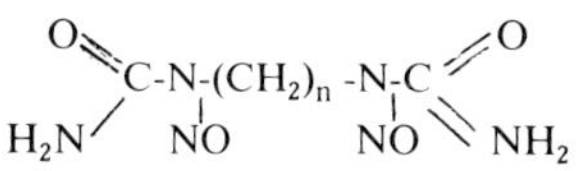

n	Dose (mg/kg)	T/C
2	100	>362
3[a]	25	>226
4[a]	25	>278
5	50	163
6	100	186
7	100	171
8	400	165
9	200	134
10	400	112

Injections were carried out on days 2 and 5 except the cases denoted by [a], in those cases days 1, 5, and 9.

Table 5. Effect of N^4-substituted 1-β-D-arabinofuranosyl-cytosine on L1210 by i.p. injections on days 2 and 6

R (N^4-)	T/C%		
Acyl groups	100 mg/kg	200 mg/kg	400 mg/kg
Butyryl	131	131	139
Valeryl	133	171	191
Caproyl	125	133	150
Caprylyl	123	127	163
Capryl	159	188	284
Lauroyl	177	272	296
Myristoyl	211	191	90
Pentadecanoyl	246	309	91
Palmitoyl	361	242	78
Margaroyl	405	152	99
Stearoyl	329	123	111
Nonadecanoyl	298	260	134
Arachidoyl	313	363	329
Behenoyl	241	298	342
Oleoyl (cis-9-$C_{17}H_{33}$CO)	218	214	109

Table 6. Effect of N^4-, 5'-disubstituted 1-β-arabinofuranosylcytosine on L1210 by i.p. injections on days 2 and 6

R(N^4-) Acyl groups	$R^{6}{}_{5}{\leftarrow}^{7}$	T/C%		
		100 mg/kg	200 mg/kg	400 mg/kg
Stearoyl	Phosphate	321	362	104
Palmitoyl	Sodium-phosphate	221	296	129
Stearoyl	Sodium-phosphate	250	313	200
Behenoyl	Sodium-phosphate	204	221	204
Stearoyl	3', 5'-diphosphate	263	337	293
Stearoyl	Sodium-succinate	232	275	215
Stearoyl	Sodium-glutarate	190	266	0
Stearoyl	Diethyl-glycinate	275	321	125
Stearoyl	Diethylaminopropriate	305	345	106

Table 7. Antitumor effect of FD-1 and FT-207 on Ehrlich carcinoma (solid form) by oral administration. (host mice: ddY)

	Dose (mmole/kg) day 1–7	Body wt. change (g)	Tumor wt. (g)	T/C
Control	—	+5.1	0.56±0.21	—
FD-1	0.05	+7.4	0.35±0.13	0.63
	0.15	+4.5	0.28±0.12	0.50
	0.45	+4.0	0.22±0.14	0.39
FT-207	0.45	+2.4	0.26±0.16	0.46
5-FU	0.08	+5.9	0.32±0.22	0.58

References

1. Aoshima, M., Sakurai, Y.: Comparative studies on the antitumor activity and the bone marrow toxicity of 1-(β-D-glucopyranosyl)-3-(2-chloroethyl)-3-nitrosourea and 2-[3-(2-chloroethyl)-3-nitrosoureido]-D-glucopyranose. Gann **68**, 247–250 (1977).
2. Aoshima, M., Tsukagoshi, S., Sakurai, Y., Ohishi, J., Ishida, T., Kobayashi, H.: Antitumor activity of newly synthesized N^4-acyl-1-β-D-arabinofuranosylcytosine. Cancer Res. **36**, 2726–2732 (1976).
3. Aoshima, M., Tsukagoshi, S., Sakurai, Y., Ohishi, J., Ishida, T., Kobayashi, H.: N^4-Behenoyl-1-β-D-arabinofuranosylcytosine as a new potential antitumor agent. Cancer Res. **37** (in press) (1977).
4. Arakawa, M., Shimizu, F.: Effect of 3-(amino-2-methyl-5-pyrimidinyl)-1-(2-chloroethyl)-nitrosourea hydrochloride on lymphoid leukemia L1210. Gann **66**, 149–154 (1975).
5. Arakawa, M., Nakao, H., Aoki, T.: Effect of carbazilquinone on transplantable and primary tumors in mice. Gann **61**, 535–539 (1970).
6. Arakawa, M., Shimizu, F., Okada, N.: Effect of 1-(4-amino-2-methylpyrimidin-5-yl)methyl-3-(2-chloroethyl)-3-nitrosourea hydrochloride on leukemia L1210. Gann **65**, 191 (1974).
7. Connors, T. A., Cox, P. J., Farmer, P. B., Foster, A. B., Jarman, M.: Some studies of the active intermediates formed in the microsomal metabolism of cyclophosphamide and isophosphamide. Biochem. Pharmacol. **23**, 115–129 (1974).
8. COOPERATIVE STUDY GROUP OF PHASE I STUDY ON ACNU: Phase I study of 1-(4-amino-2-methyl-5-pyrimidinyl)methyl-3-(2-chloroethyl)-3-nitrosourea hydrochloride (ACNU). Jap. J. Clin. Oncology **6**, 55–62 (1976).

9. El-merzabani, M. M., Sakurai, Y.: A new alkylating agent effective to experimental tumors resistant to nitrogen mustard. Gann **56**, 589–594 (1965).
10. El-merzabani, M. M., Sakurai, Y.: Anticancer activity of methanesulfonic acid esters of aminoglycols against mouse leukemia L1210. Gann **58**, 199–203 (1967).
11. Fox, P. A., Panasci, L. C., Schein, P.: Biological and biochemical properties of 1-(2-chloroethyl)-3-(β-D-glucopyranosyl)-1-nitrosourea (NSC D 254157), a nitrosourea with reduced bone marrow toxicity. Cancer Res. **37**, 783–787 (1977).
12. Fujita, H., Ogawa, K., Kato, A., Kitazato, K., Yasuda, A., Kimura, K.: Pharmacokinetics of new masked type fluorinated pyrimidines; FD1 FD2 and FDx. Proc. Jap. Cancer Assoc., The 35th Annual Meeting, p. 123 (1976).
13. Hirayama, H., Sugihara, T., Hamada, F., Kanai, T., Hikita, J., Araki, Y., Kuretani, K., Hoshi, A.: Distribution and excretion of cyclocytidine in monkeys, dogs, and rats. Gann **65**, 153–161 (1974).
14. Hoshi, A., Kanzawa, F., Kuretani, K.: Antitumor activity of cyclocytidine in a variety of tumors. Gann **63**, 353–360 (1972).
15. Iwasaki, M., Sekido, S., Ninomiya, K., Sekine, J., Ueno, S., Nagamatsu, Y., Kimura, G.: Antitumor activities of 3-methyl-α-D-glucopyranos-6-yl)-1-(2-chloroethyl)-1-nitrosourea. Gann **67**, 137–139 (1976).
16. Kidani, Y., Inagaki, K., Tsukagoshi, S.: Examination of antitumor activities of platinum complexes of 1,2-diamino-cyclohexane isomers and their related complexes. Gann **67**, 921–922 (1976).
17. Machinami, T., Kobayashi, K., Hayakawa, I., Suami, T.: Synthesis of sugar derivatives of N-alkyl-N-nitrosourea. Bull. Chem. Soc. Jap. **48**, 3761–3762 (1975).
18. Machinami, T., Nishiyama, S., Kikuchi, K., Suami, T.: Synthesis of (2-chloroethyl)-nitrosourea derivatives of carbohydrate. Ibid. **48**, 3763–3764 (1975).
19. Morimoto, K., Yamaha, T., Nakadate, M., Suzuki, I.: Biochemical studies on 1,1-ethylenebis (1-nitrosourea) (EBNU). I. Degradation of EBNU in mild conditions. Chem. Pharm. Bull. (Tokyo) **25**, 151–157 (1977).
20. Nakadate, M., Anzai, M., Suzuki, I., Ishidate, Jr., M., Odashima, S.: Carcinostatic effect of 1, 1'-polymethylenebis-(1-nitrosourea) on AH 13 and L-1210 cells. Gann. **64**, 415–416 (1973).
21. Saito, T., Ogira, S., Wakui, A., Yokoyama, M., Takahashi, H., Himori, T., Kudo, T., Maezawa, S., Ujiie, S., Sugawara, N.: Clinical experience with a new anticancer agent, carbazilquinone (NSC-134679). Cancer Chemother. Rep. **57/1**, 447–457 (1973).
22. Takamizawa, A., Matsumoto, S., Iwata, T., Katagiri, K., Tochino, K., Yamaguchi, K.: Studies on cyclophosphamide metabolites and their related compounds. II. Preparation of an active species of cyclophosphamide and some related compounds. J. Am. Chem. Soc. **95**, 985–986 (1973).
23. Takamizawa, A., Yamaguchi, K., Shiratori, O., Kasai, H., Uchida, N., Satoh, H., Ichikawa, H.: Relationship between antitumor activity and functional groups of 4-hydroperoxy-cyclophosphamide (40487) analogues. Proc. Jap. Cancer Ass., The 35th Annual Meeting, p. 117 (1976).
24. Unemi, N., Yasumoto, M., Morita, K., Kajihara, M., Toide, H.: Antitumor effects of new 5-FU derivatives. Proc. Jap. Cancer Ass., The 35th Annual Meeting, p. 132 (1976).
25. Wempen, I., Miller, N., Falco, E. A., Fox, J. J.: Syntheses of some N^4-substituted derivates of 1-β-D-arabinofuranosyl-cytosine and 5-fluorocytosine. J. Med. Chem. **11**, 144–148 (1968).

New Anticancer Antibiotics under Development and Clinical Evaluation in the National Cancer Institute

M. SLAVIK

The Division of Cancer Treatment, National Cancer Institute, maintains a high interest and strong commitment to the development and clinical evaluation of anticancer antibiotics.
The fermentation development is expected to yield new active compounds preferably with novel structure and mode of action, which subsequently, when synthesized, could lead to the second generation of synthetics or fermentation analogs with higher clinical therapeutic index. Thus, effective, accurate and adequate evaluation of the results from the clinical studies using investigational anticancer antibiotics and high quality feedback to the fermentation program is the essential prerequisite for its successful function.
This paper will discuss selected antitumor antibiotics under development or early clinical evaluation by the National Cancer Institute. In order to avoid unnecessary overlap and duplication we have limited ourselves to the compounds not discussed by others at this symposium. In spite of this limitation, we hope to have enough examples to demonstrate a variety of interesting features in the clinical evaluation and development of fermentation products.

New Antitumor Antibiotics under Clinical Evaluation

Among the investigational antitumor antibiotics currently under clinical evaluation are anguidine (NSC 141537), piperazinedione (NSC 135758), and pyrazofurin (NSC 143095).
Anguidine (NSC 141537) is the principle phytotoxic compound produced by the parasitic fungus *Fusarium Equiseti* [3]. Structurally, diacetoxyscirpenol [8, 9], it represents a unique structure among compounds with antitumor activity. Although its mode of action has not yet been fully elucidated, it appears that anguidine (similarly to Fusarenon-x isolated from *Fusarjum Nivale* [28]) primarily inhibits protein synthesis. Protein inhibition, irreversible after 30 min of exposure of 10^{-7}M anguidine to HeLa cells, has been reported by GROLLMAN [15], while only partial inhibition of DNA synthesis and no inhibition of RNA synthesis was achieved. Anguidine was selected for clinical studies because of its antitumor activity in vivo against P388 leukemia, L1210 leukemia, AKR leukemia, and B16 melanoma in mice. However, the clinical interest in this drug has been recently stimulated by its activity against transplantable dimethylhydrazine-induced colon carcinoma in mice [7]. In two Phase I studies [24, 17], the daily x 5 intravenous schedule was explored and the starting dose of 0.1–0.2 mg/m^2/day × 5 escalated up to 6.0 mg/m^2/day × 5 [17] and 7.5 mg/m^2/day × 5, respectively [24]. Hypotension, chills, fever, and CNS changes which included hallucination, confusion, and irratic behaviour were reported, in doses above 4.5 mg/m^2/day × 5, when anguidine was given by rapid i.v. administration [17]. Myelosuppression becomes dose limiting in absence of other toxicities when anguidine is given by 4–8 hour infusion [17]. The recommended dose for Phase II studies appears to be 4.5 mg–5.0 mg/m^2/day × 5 by 4-hour i.v. infusion [17]. Stabilization of disease in patients with large bowel cancer reported in

Phase I studies and true therapeutic synergism when anguidine is administered to mice in combination with 5-FU in colon adenocarcinomas [7] are two principle reasons for clinical enthusiasm, which however, remains to be proven in the ongoing clinical studies.

2,5 Piperazinedione, 3,6-bis (5-chloro-2-piperidyl)-dihydrochloride (NSC 135758) was isolated from a fermentation broth of *Streptomyces Griseoluteus* by Gitterman et al. [13]. The structure was deducted from chemical and physical evidence by Arison and Beck [1].

The biologic effects of piperazinedione include inhibition of growth of human tumors in the chick embryo [13] and of transplantable mouse neoplasms in vivo [35].

Elegant studies on the mode of action [36, 4, 30] revealed that piperazinedione prevents progression of tumor cells in culture through S phase to mitosis, produces accumulation of cells with G_2 phase DNA content, and causes inhibition of DNA but not RNA or protein synthesis in adenocarcinoma 755 cells in culture [36]. Chemical evidence for alkylating activity of piperazinedione was obtained by demonstrating its reaction with 4-(p-nitrobenzyl) pyridine [4]. These results suggest that piperazinedione acts as an alkylating agent. However, findings on piperazinedione selective inhibition of DNA synthesis in L1210 cells resistant to cyclophosphamide as well as on its in vivo antitumor against L1210 strains resistant to cyclophosphamide or BCNU [30] promote this antibiotic to a compound with unique mode of action.

In Phase I studies, various schedules were studied including a single dose repeated every 3 weeks [14], weekly schedules [2], and daily × 5 schedules [29]. The bone marrow toxicity is dose limiting and affected both granulocytes and platelets. The nadir of the white blood cells occured at 17 days (median) with median 7 days duration, while the nadir for platelets was reached at 16 days and lasted 12 days. The Phase I studies suggested activity against malignant melanoma (two partial remissions in 16 patients) and chronic myelogenous leukemia blast crisis (two partial remissions in two patients) [14]. Although the doses originally recommended for Phase II studies were 12–15 mg/m^2 every 3 weeks for solid tumors and 24 mg/m^2 i.v. for leukemic patients [14], subsequent clinical experience resulted in recommendation to decrease the dose to 9 mg/m^2/i.v. every 3 weeks, particularly in patients previously treated with chemotherapy. The therapeutic doses recommended for the repeated dose schedules are 3 mg/m^2/day × 5 in solid tumors and 5 mg/m^2/day × 5 in leukemia [29]. Piperazinedione is currently under evaluation in Phase II clinical studies in various solid tumors and lymphoproliferative diseases. Not surprisingly, it was found inactive in advanced squamous cell carcinoma of the lung [22]. However some preliminary results reported to the Investigational Drug Branch suggest piperazinedione activity in patients with various solid tumors and lymphoproliferative diseases resistant to previous combination chemotherapy, including alkylating agents.

In summary, piperazinedione represents another fermentation product with new structure and interesting mode of action open to further structure activity relationship studies. Non-cross-resistance with two classes of alkylating agents has been demonstrated in experimental animals and, if confirmed clinically, would increase its clinical appeal.

Pyrazofurin (NSC 143095) is one of three active c-nucleosides isolated from the broth filtrates of *Streptomyces Candidus* [11, 37]. The biologic effects of pyrazofurin include limited antifungal activity in vitro, suppression of growth of vaccina, herpes, measles, rhino, and influenza viruses in tissue culture and activity against vaccinia virus in vivo [33, 16]. Its effect against Friend leukemia virus [10] led to the evaluation of its activity against experimental animal tumors in vivo, which revealed complete inhibition of growth of Walker carcinosarcoma 256, and more than 50% inhibition of growth of mammary carcinoma 755, Gardner lymphosarcoma and x5563 plasma cell myeloma [34]. However the drug is inactive against P388 and L1210 leukemia in mice [34].

The principle biochemical effect of pyrazofurin is in profound inhibition of de novo pyrimidine synthesis [12]. Pyrazofurin is phosphorylated by adenosine kinase to pyrazofurin-

5-phosphate [20], which is a potent inhibitor of orotidylate decarboxylase, an enzyme converting orotidine-5-phosphate (OMP) to uridine-5-phosphate (UMP).
As a result of this block, precursors are cumulated in tissues and elevated levels of orotic acid and orotidine are found in the rat, dog, rabbit [16], and human [16, 27] after administration of pyrazofurin. Pyrazofurin-5-phosphate is further converted to the corresponding diphosphate and triphosphate by nonspecific kinase [20].
Clinical pharmacology studies conducted by OHNUMA et al. 1976 [27] revealed that after i.v. bolus of pyrazofurin 200–300 mg/m^2, the drug was cleared from serum with an initial half-life of 4–16 min and second one of 20–29 min. Urinary excretion of free drug was less than 10% in 5 days. However, results from another study using [^{14}C]-labeled drug [26] are not in agreement with previous findings. Bolus i.v. injections of 3 mg labeled pyrazofurin/kg were given to two patients with advanced cancer. There was a triphasic plasma decay of radioactivity with plasma half-life of 6 and 4 min for the initial phase, 24 and 22 h for the middle phase, and 114 and 180 h for the terminal phase. Plasma and renal clearances (63 ml/min) were identical in both patients and most of the radioactivity appeared in the urine within 14 days, while fecal excretion was less than 3% of the administered dose [26].
Although controversial in results, both studies recommend intermittent weekly schedules. In Phase I studies, various i.v. schedules were explored including daily × 5, single intermittent, weekly [16], and 24-hour infusion [27]. Toxicities observed in Phase I studies include dose-limiting stomatitis, mild nausea, vomiting, anemia, leucopenia and thrombocytopenia, erythema with bullous formation [16, 27]. Therapeutic i.v. doses recommended for Phase II studies include 100 mg/m^2 weekly and 240 mg/m^2 every 3 weeks.
Pyrazofurin is currently under clinical evaluation in Phase II studies. Although preliminary reports are suggesting inactivity in major solid tumors including lung cancer, large bowel cancer, and breast cancer, some responses may hint its activity in Hodgkin's [16], and non-Hodgkin's lymphomas.
In summary, pyrazofurin represents a fermentation product with new nucleoside structure and unique mode of action which, in inhibition of orotidylate decarboxylate [6], resembles 6-azauridine but in some aspects differs from it. Pyrazofurin is not only a much stronger inhibitor of this enzyme [6] but, unlike 6-azauridine and other pyrimidine nucleosides, is phosphorlated by adenosine kinase. Synergistic effect with other pyrimidine nucleoside analogs, particularly 5-azacytidine has generated clinical interest and will be explored in treatment of acute myeloblastic leukemia [5]. Pyrazofurin also deserves clinical evaluation in diseases in which 6-azauridine has revealed significant activity including mycosis fungoides, polycythemia vera, throphoblastic malignancies and psoriasis [31, 32].

New Antibiotics under Development

Lymphosarcin (NSC 208642), *michicarcin* (NSC 191959) and *5-isoxazolacetic acid* (NSC 163501) are three fermentation products under development in the National Cancer Institute. Having been recommended to proceed through additional animal experiments toward the clinical stage, they are of interest to the clinical oncologist as potential candidates for clinical studies.
Lymphosarcin (NSC 208642) is a fermentation product of *Streptomyces murinus*, which has an unidentified polyene structure. It revealed activity in Friend erythroleukemia in vitro and against P388 leukemia and B16 melanoma in mice in vivo [25].
Michicarcin (NSC 191959) is a polypeptide of molecular weight 10,000–30,000 isolated from fermentation of *Streptomyces species.* Like lymphosarcin it is active in Friend

erythroleukemia in vitro and against P388 leukemia and B16 melanoma in vivo when given in daily schedules. Both compounds are undergoing studies on elucidation of structure, mode of action, and physicochemical properties in order to become feasible for further preclinical testing [25].

Isoxazolacetic Acid (NSC 163501) L-(α S-5-S)-Amino-3-chloro-4,5-dihydro-5-isoxazolacetic acid is a fermentation product of *Streptomyces sviceus*, discovered by HANKA [18] and structurally defined by MARTIN [23]. Its antimicrobial spectrum includes *Bacillus subtilis* and *Escherichia coli* and four fungi: *Saccharomyces pastorianus*, *Pencillium Oxalicum*, *Candida albicans* and *Saccharomyces cerevisiae.* Antimicrobial activity of isoxazolacetic acid against *Bacillus subtilis* can be reversed by histidine and to a lesser extent by deoxyinosine [19]. Studies on mode of action revealed, that isoxazolacetic acid inhibits the utilization of L-glutamine by L-asparagine synthetase both in vitro and in vivo. In L1210 cell culture it inhibits DNA synthesis and produces an arrest of cell cycle progression in G or early S phase, which can be counteracted by glutamine [21]. Thus isoxazolacetic acid represents an antitumor antibiotic of unique structure, which acts as an antimetabolite of histidine in microbial and of glutamine in cell culture. Its in vivo activity against P388 and L1210 leukemia in mice has been well defined [19] and the drug is getting ready for toxicity studies in high experimental animals.

Conclusion

In this paper, six new antibiotics with antitumor activity were discussed in order to illustrate some interesting features in the development and clinical evaluation of new anticancer antibiotics.

Three fermentation products which are still under development, represent a group with tremendous width from structurally simple histidine analog to complex molecules of polyene antibiotic and high molecular weight polypeptide. Although waiting for more preclinical testing, necessary for their safe and effective introduction in clinical studies, they already are attracting the interest of the clinical oncologist.

Three antibiotics under clinical evaluation, anguidine, piperazinedione and pyrazofurin, although heterogenous in structures and mode of action, share one fascinating feature. Each of them represents a drug with an entirely new structure and new mode of action, which has not been clinically studied before. One would like to know how this uniqueness correlates with their therapeutic effect. Unfortunately, in spite of the fact that all of them were introduced in clinical studies 2–4 years ago, sufficient results are not yet available to draw any definite conclusion about their usefulness in cancer treatment. This should emphasize the need for efficient and rational clinical evaluation of new antibiotics. Significant activity confirmed clinically in a drug with novel structure and/or mode of action should stimulate structure-activity studies and a rational search for structural or functional analogs and ultimately result in development of drugs with better therapeutic index.

Close cooperation between the clinical oncologist and the fermentation and organic chemist insuring constant feedback from clinical studies should be rewarding for both, ultimately for the clinician, who is in desperate need for innovation and progress in order to save his patients' lives. New drugs which may be discovered by fermentation are not an unreasonable subject of this hope.

References

1. Arison, B. H., Beck, J. L.: The structure of compound 593A—A new antitumor agent. Tetrahedron **29**, 2743–2746 (1973).
2. Bjornsson, S. E., Henderson, E. S.: Phase I trial of crystalline antibiotic. Proc. Am. Soc. Clin. Oncol. in Proc. Am. Ass. Cancer Res. Abstract No. 1188 **16**, 268 (1975).
3. Brian, P. W., et. al.: Phytotoxic compounds produced by Fusarium equiseti. J. Exp. Botany **12**, 1 12 (1961).
4. Brockman, R. W., Shaddix, S. C., Williams, M. S., Struck, R. F.: Studies with 2,5-piperazinedione, 3,6-bis (5-chloro-2-piperidyl)-dihydrochloride. II. Effects on macromolecular synthesis in cell culture and evidence for alkylating activity. Cancer Treat. Rep. **60**, 1317–1324 (1976).
5. Cadman, E. C., Eiferman, F.: Sequential pyrazofurin and 5-azacytidine: A synergistic chemotherapeutic combination. Clin. Res. **406** A, (1977).
6. Cadman, E. C., Dix, D. E., Hill, S. C., Handschumacher, R. E.: Pyrazofurin: Biochemical and clinicopharmacological studies. Proc. AACR ASCO. Abstr. No. 832 **17**, 208 (1976).
7. Corbett, T. H., Griswold, D. P.: Treatment of colon adenocarcinomas with anguidine NSC 141537 and anguidine +5-FU (NSC 19893). Proc. AACR ASCO Abstr. No. 457 **18**, 115 (1977).
8. Dawkins, A. W.: Phytotoxic compounds produced by Fusarium equiseti. Part II. The chemistry of diacetoxyscirpenol. J. Chem. Soc. [Org] **12**, 115–123 (1966).
9. Dawkins, A. W., Grove, J. F., Tidd, B. K.: Diacetoxyscirpenol and some related compounds. Chem. Comm **2**, 27–28 (1965).
10. DeLong, D. C., Baker, L. A., Gerzon, K., Gutowski, G. E., Williams, R. H., Hamill, R. L.: Inhibition of Friend leukemia virus-induced splenomegaly by pyrazomycin. Proc. of the Seventh International Congress of Chemotherapy, Prague, Czechoslovakia (1971).
11. Gerzon, K., Williams, R. H., Hoehn, M., Gorman, M., DeLong, D. C.: Pyrazomycin, A C-nucleoside with antiviral activity. Second International Congress on Heterocyclic Chemistry. Montpellier, France, 131 (July, 1969).
12. Gerzon, K., DeLong, D. C., Cline, J. C.: C-nucleosides: Aspects of chemistry and mode of action. Int. Pure Applied Chem. **28**, 489–497 (1971).
13. Gitterman, C. O., Rickes, E. L., Wolf, D. E., et al.: The human tumor-egg host system. IV. Discovery of a new antitumor agent compound 593 A. J. Antibiot. **23**, 305–310 (1970).
14. Gottlieb, J. A., Freireich, E. J., Bodey, G. P., Rodiquez, V., McCredie, K. B., Gutterman, J. U.: Preliminary clinical evaluation of piperazinedione a new crystalline antibiotic. Proc. Ass. Cancer Res. **16**, 86 (1975).
15. Grollman, A. P.: Personal communication.
16. Gutowski, G. E., Sweeney, M. J., DeLong, D. C., Hamill, R. L., Gerzon, K.: Biochemistry and biological effects of the pyrazofurins (pyrazomycins): Initial clinical trial. Ann. N.Y. Acad. Sci. **255**, 544–551 (1975).
17. Haas, C., Goodwin, W., Leite, C., Stephens, R., Hoogstraten, B.: Phase I study of anguidine (diacetoxyscirpenol NSC 141537). Proc. AACR ASCO Abstr. C-120 **18**, 296 (1977).
18. Hanka, L. J., Dietz, A.: U-42,126, a new antimetabolite antibiotic: production, biological activity, and taxonomy of the producing microorganism. Antimicrob. Agents Chemother. **3**, 425–431 (1973).
19. Hanka, L. J., Martin, D. G., Neil, G. L.: U-42,126, a new antitumor antimetabolite. Antimicrobial reversal studies and preliminary evaluation against mouse leukemia L1210 *in vivo*. Can. Chemother. Rep. Part 1, **57**, 141–148 (1973).
20. Jakubowski, A., Lehman, C., Moyer, J., Handschumacher, R. E.: Pyrazofurin: Nucleotide interconversions by adenosine kinase and nucleotide kinase. Proc. AACR ASCO **18**, 865 (1977).
21. Jayaram, H. N., Cooney, D. A., Bono, W. H., Neal, G.: L-[S 5S]-amino-3-chloro-4,5-dihydro-5-isoxazolacetic acid (NSC 163501)—A new antitumor antibiotic with the properties of an antagonist of L-glutamine. Proc. AACR ASCO Abstr. No. 291 **16**, 73 (1975).
22. Koons, L. S., Bellet, R., Mastrangelo, M. J.: Piperazinedione (NSC-135578) chemotherapy for advanced squamous cell cancer of the lung. Proc. AACR ASCO Abstract No. 132 **18**, 299 (1977).
23. Martin, D. G., Duchamp, D. J., Chidester, C. G.: The isolation, structure and absolute configuration of U-42,126, a novel antitumor antibiotic. Tetrahedron Lett. No. **27**, 2549–2552 (1973).
24. Murphy, W. K., Livingston, R. B., Gottlieb, J. A., Burgess, M. A., Rawson, R. W.: Phase I evaluation of anguidine. Proc. AACR ASCO **17**, 358 (1976).
25. Natural Products Branch, N.C.I.: Unpublished results.
26. Nelson, R. L., Dyke, W. R., Crabtree, R. E., Zahir-Zafarzai, M.: Clinical pharmacokinetics of pyrazofurin—A new antitumor agent. Proc. AACR ASCO Abstr. 209 **18**, 53 (1977).
27. Ohnuma, T., Roboz, J., Shapiro, M., Holland, J.: Clinical and pharmacologic studies with pyrazofurin. Proc. AACR ASCO Abstr. No. 736 **17**, 184 (1976).

28. OHTSUBO, K., KADES, P., MITTERMAYER, C.: Polyribosomal breakdown in mouse fibroblast (L-cells) by Fusarenon-x, a toxic principle isolated from Fusarium nivale. Biochim. Biophys. Acta **287**, 520–525 (1972).
29. PRATT, C., RIVERA, G., SHANKS, E.: Phase I-II evaluation of piperazinedione in children with cancer. Proc. Am. Ass. Cancer Res. **16**, 82 (1975).
30. SCHABEL, F. M. JR., TRADER, M. W., LASTER, W. R. JR., SHADDIX, S. C., BROCKMAN, R. W.: Studies with 2,5-piperazinedione, 3,6-bis (5-chloro-2-piperidyl)-dihydrochloride. III. Biochemical and therapeutic effects in L1210 leukemias sensitive and resistant to alkylating agents: Comparison with melphalan, cyclophosphamide and BCNU. Cancer Treat. Rep. **60**, 1325–1333 (1976).
31. SLAVIK, M.: Pharmacodynamics of 6-azauridine 2'-3'-5' triacetate with the special interest to new clinical indications. Ph.D. Dissertation Theses, Czechoslovak Academy of Sciences, Prague (1969).
32. SLAVIK, K., ELIS, J., RASKOVA, H.: Therapeutic effects of 6-azauridine triacetate in psoriasis. Pharmacol. Clin. **2**, 120–125 (1970).
33. STREIGHTOFF, F. J., NELSON, J. D., CLINE, J. C., GERZON, K., HOEHN, M., WILLIAMS, R. H., GORMAN, M., DELONG, D. C.: Antiviral activity of pyrazomycin. Ninth Conference on Antimicrobial Agents and Chemotherapy, Washington, D.C. p 8 (Octo., 1969).
34. SWEENEY, M. J., DAVIS, F. A., GUTOWSKI, G. E., HAMILL, R. L., HOFFMAN, D. H., POORE, G. A.: Experimental antitumor activity of pyrazomycin. Cancer Res. **33**, 2619–2623 (1973).
35. TARNOWSKI, G. S., SCHMID, F. A., HUTCHISON, D. J., et al.: Chemotherapeutic effects of compound 593 A (NSC 135758) on mouse leukemias and some transplanted animal tumors. Cancer Chemother. Rep. **57**, 21–27 (1973).
36. WHEELER, G. P., BONO, V. H., BOWDON, B. J., ADAMSON, D. J., BROCKMAN, R. W.: Studies with 2,5-piperazinedione 3,6-bis (5-chloro-2-piperidyl)-dihydrochloride. I. Cell kinetic and biologic effects in cultured L1210 human epidermoid No. 2 and adenocarcinoma 755 cells. Cancer Treat. Rep. **60**, 1307–1316 (1976).
37. WILLIAMS, R. H., GERZON, K., HOEHN, M., GORMAN, M., DELONG, D. C.: Pyrazomycin, A novel carbon-linked nucleoside. (Abstract MICR 38). Am. Chem. Soc. Meeting, (Sept., 1969).

Clinical Evaluation of New Antitumor Antibiotics

F. M. Muggia

In the field of antimicrobial antibiotics, the initial discovery of several active compounds was followed by an era of exploration of modifications on the basic structures. These modifications, in the case of the penicillins, led to changes in pharmacology, important improvements in the therapeutic index and, later, to dramatic changes in the therapeutic spectrum. Similar developments are occurring and may be expected to increase rapidly among the antitumor antibiotics. From relatively minor modifications, it is likely that we shall witness bolder structural alterations of currently active antibiotics based on additional understanding of mechanisms of action.

With the success of the parent compounds, daunomycin and adriamycin, the anthracyclines lead the list of antibiotics with new analogs currently being advanced for clinical evaluation. How effectively are we dealing with the clinical evaluation of these agents? Analysis of the problems associated with the clinical assessment of various anthracyclines will constitute a major topic for discussion. I shall also comment on the evaluation of other families of antitumor antibiotics, such as the actinomycins and bleomycins, that may be emerging for clinical trials. Finally, I will present an overview of other antitumor antibiotics that have been in clinical use and analyze some features unique to their evaluation.

Anthracyclines (Fig. 1)

Although the therapeutic success of the anthracyclines has stimulated analog development, evaluation of daunomycin and adriamycin has been incomplete and cannot be expected to provide the clinical feedback necessary for more rational drug development. In the leukemias and neuroblastoma, where daunomycin was first reported to have antitumor activity, adriamycin has seemed to perform equally well (Table 1) but adequate comparative trials of the two agents have not been performed. In the lymphomas and those solid tumors where adriamycin plays a major role, the evaluation of daunomycin has been insufficient for determining clinical activity [27]. The clinical toxicity of the two agents is qualitatively identical (Table 2).

The major effort in introducing new anthracyclines has been to seek agents retaining the therapeutic efficacy of adriamycin, but with a better therapeutic index. Specifically, the search has been primarily directed to agents with diminished cardiotoxicity. Efforts to establish with certainty a lesser cardiotoxic anthracycline have been hampered by the insensitivity of clinical detection and lack of comparability of various preclinical models. Preliminary claims of other noteworthy toxicologic or pharmacologic modifications in newly introduced anthracyclines include: smoother induction of remission in acute leukemia by rubidazone [4]; activity of carminomycin [26] by the oral route; and, the absence of alopecia and lesser cardiotoxicity with aclacinomycin A [9] and carminomycin [5]. However, many of these claims must be substantiated by additional clinical experience and demonstration of retained efficacy will be of paramount importance.

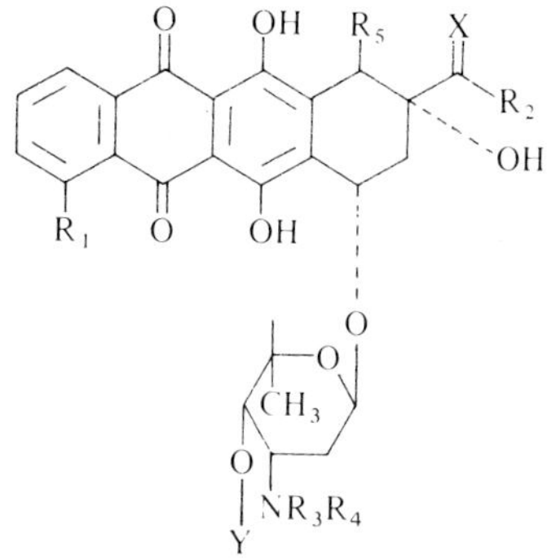

	R_1	R_2	R_3	R_4	R_5	X	Y
Adriamycin	OCH_3	CH_2OH	H	H	H	O	H
Daunomycin	OCH_3	CH_3	H	H	H	O	H
Rubidazone	OCH_3	CH_3	H	H	H	NNHCOO	H
AD 32	OCH_3	CH_2 $OCOC_4H_9$	H	$COCF_3$	H	O	H
Carminomycin	OH	CH_3	H	H	H	O	H
Aclacinomycin A	OH	CH_3	CH_3	CH_3	$COOCH_3$	2H	†

† 2-deoxyfucose/L-cinerulose.

Fig. 1. General structure of anthracyclines

Recently, two anthracyclines, 4'-epi-adriamycin [7] and AD32 [14], have been advanced for clinical use because of an expanded antitumor spectrum or significant improvement in activity in preclinical systems. As with the other compounds being tested, a demonstration of efficacy will have to be coupled with careful toxicologic monitoring.

Table 3 summarizes the clinical studies that are in progress or planned in the initial evaluation of rubidazone, which has recently been introduced in the United States. The rationale for clinical trial was the impression of greater therapeutic index in acute leukemia and the possibility of diminished cardiotoxicity in animal models. However, it should be noted that, although the total dose to cardiotoxicity may be much higher than with daunomycin or adriamycin, the important parameters are the *number of conventional courses leading to high risk of cardiotoxicity and the assessment of risk of cardiomyopathy at each cumulative dose level* [28]. The initial experience at M.D. Anderson Hospital (R Benjamin, personal communication) indicates that cardiotoxicity is common following rubidazone use in patients who have had previous anthracycline treatment. Thus, caution must be exercised in allowing a proliferation of clinical studies before this risk is adequately assessed. This is the reason for the small number of rubidazone studies initially planned, including a study accurately determining its efficacy vis-a-vis adriamycin in advanced breast cancer. It should be noted that rubidazone represents a rather small modification in structure and, in fact, is metabolized to daunomycin (R. Benjamin, this symposium). The approach to other newer anthracyclines may vary considerably but comparative studies of efficacy will be important.

Similar comments apply to complexes or concomitant drug therapy introduced to overcome cardiotoxicity, such as adriamycin-DNA complexes [2] and adriamycin with vitamin E [20].

A final aspect in the evaluation of anthracyclines encompasses the monitoring of cardiotoxicity. More sophisticated techniques, such as endomyocardial biopsy, are being introduced in the hope of providing an accurate prospective assessment of risk [8]. This technique, coupled with other established approaches including analysis of easily available EKG voltage [18], echocardiography [21], systolic time intervals [22], and QKd determinations [11], hopefully will lead to early establishment of the cardiotoxic potential of the anthracyclines. The basic questions concerning any technique used in these studies include: (a) Does the drug cause detectable abnormalities? (b) Do the detectable abnormalities predict clinical cardiomyopathy? (c) Do they predict the time for stopping use of the drug? At present, no single technique answers all these questions.

Actinomycins (Fig. 2a and b)

Initial studies in the 1950s which identified the clinical usefulness of actinomycin D also included analogs with changes in the peptide portion of the molecule [25]. Actinomycin D was selected because of its superior therapeutic index, in spite of considerable toxicity that includes gastrointestinal intolerance, hematopoietic depression, and mucoenteritis.

Modifications in the basic actinomycin structure have recently been tested for possible introduction into clinical use. These alterations include not only changes in the chromophore [19], but also in the amino acids of the peptide portion of the molecule [15, 17]. Several compounds retaining the considerable experimental antitumor spectrum of actinomycin D [10] have been synthesized. One derivative (Pip 1 β, Fig. 2B) retains activity in the P388 leukemia system, while showing more activity in B16 melanoma although on a molar basis it is 10 times less potent than actinomycin D (R. K. Johnson, personal communication).

Introduction of an actinomycin analog into clinical trial may be warranted, particularly if its toxic effects in the GI tract and marrow of large animals are different from the parent compound. The aim of studies with this family of antibiotics would not be to remove actinomycin D from its well deserved place in choriocarcinoma, germ cell tumors, and Wilms tumor, but to expand the therapeutic spectrum to the many solid tumors where actinomycin D exhibits hints of efficacy. Unfortunately, the unpleasant side effects of actinomycin D and competition with many newer agents deserving evaluation, have rendered studies with the parent compound impractical. However, a new analog of actinomycin D would receive favourable attention for testing in a variety of tumors (Table 4). It should be noted that actinomycin D has broad cross-resistance with adriamycin and vincristine [13] and analog testing should take this into consideration.

Bleomycins

Analogs of bleomycin offer several challenging possibilities which have been noted in other papers (Umezawa, Matsuda this symposium). The effectiveness of bleomycin in certain tumor types correlates somewhat with its preferential localization in tissues of lymphoid and epidermal origin. New analogs are being introduced which circumvent the susceptibility of the peptides to hydrolysis by membrane-related hydrolases [6]. Such hydrolase-resistant bleomycin analogs would be expected to have altered sites of localization and, consequently, changes in antitumor spectrum.

Another prevailing rationale of analog development is related to efforts to circumvent the pulmonary toxicity of bleomycin. Therefore, alterations in pulmonary localization are being

Actinomycin D

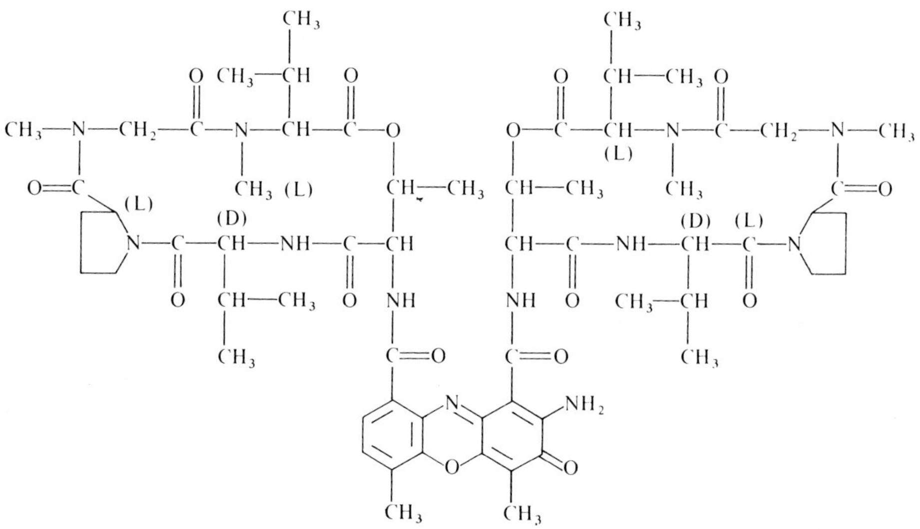

Fig. 2A. Actinomycin D

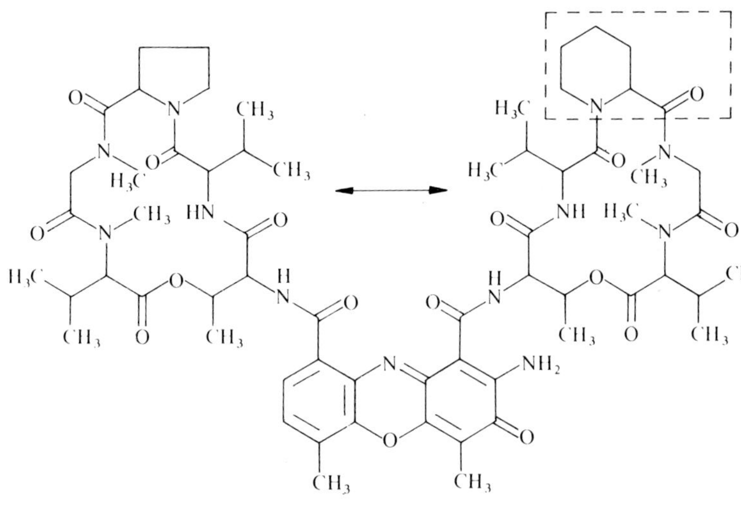

Fig. 2B. Actinomycin Pip-1β (NSC-107660)

sought. With a well-established rationale for introducing bleomycin analogs of different tissue localization into clinical trial, these agents should be treated as new ones for evaluation in tumors where bleomycin has been relatively or absolutely ineffective.

Another worthwhile area of study, both for these agents and the actinomycins, would be analogs having variable radiosensitizing properties.

Other Antitumor Antibiotics

A number of other antibiotics, including two families of analogs, have been under clinical investigation (Table 5). Data on some agents has also ben summarized in a recent review [23]. Porfiromycin is an analog of mitomycin C but there is no convincing evidence of a broader or different antitumor spectrum, and nothing to substantiate a claim for lesser toxicity [12]. In the second family of compounds, the dose-limiting toxicities show interesting variations but these currently have limited clinical applicability. Chromomycin A_3 exhibits predominantly renal toxicity, whereas the major toxicity of mithramycin is hepatic and hematologic [24].

Pyrazofurin, tubercidin, and 5-azacytidine are interesting antibiotics with nucleoside structures. Pyrazofurin is a much more potent inhibitor of orotidylic decarboxylase than the synthetic 6-azauridine. A synthetic derivative of 5-azacytidine, dihydro-5-azacytidine hydrochloride [3], is being advanced for clinical trial on the basis of greater stability in aqueous solutions. This is important since infusions of the drug retain antitumor activity while circumventing unpleasant gastrointestinal effects.

Streptozotocin, a methyl nitrosourea derivative, is an antitumor antibiotic that has been a major influence on the rational synthesis of other nitrosoureas. Its clinical effectiveness and lack of marrow toxicity led to the synthesis of chlorozotocin [1], a glucosated chloroethyl nitrosourea recently introduced into clinical trial. Azotomycin is a glutamine antagonist with mechanism of action similar to 6-diazo-5-oxo-L-norleucine (DON) [16]. Both the antibiotic and the synthetic have undergone relatively inadequate evaluation, compounded by the exhaustion of the azotomycin supply [29]. A similar problem has hampered trials with piperazinedione.

Conclusions

As with the antimicrobial antibiotics, a number of antitumor antibiotics have been introduced into clinical trials and proven to have unique activity spectra and patterns of toxicity. We are currently in the midst of intensive drug development to extend the effectiveness of some of these agents and modify their toxic properties through a variety of structural alterations.

As with other analog studies, a number of problems in the design of clinical trials have been identified. These include mainly the difficulties encountered in conducting comparative studies of single agents in most tumor types. Another problem area is the lack of clearly identified preclinical rationales for advancing drugs into clinical trials. If clear rationales could be established, studies might be better tailored to testing a specific idea. Table 6 compares the reasons behind the introduction of the antibiotic analogs covered earlier. The rationale of bleomycin analog development has been much clearer than that for the anthracyclines so far introduced into the clinic. Actinomycins present another rationale, i.e., reexamination of the antitumor spectrum for both the parent compound and the analog.

Many problems are unique to antitumor antibiotic testing (Fig. 3). Unquestionably, increasing technology has made possible practical yields of semisynthetic derivatives that will greatly enhance analog development. The versatility of these agents is just beginning to be exploited. Refinements in our clinical studies must keep pace with this advancing technology.

MANY POSSIBLE ANALOGS

VARIABILITY IN STRUCTURE ACCORDING TO STRAIN

COMPLEX STRUCTURES
Difficulties With Pharmacologic Studies and Metabolic Fate

ANTIGENICITY
May Evoke Reactions—Variable and Rapid Turnover

LOSS OF STRAIN
Interruption of Studies—Inadequate Evaluation

EXPENSE
Consideration in Drug Selection

Fig. 3. Problems in testing antitumor antibiotics

Summary

The clinical evaluation of new antibiotics and their analogs requires detailed analysis with respect to the best therapeutic strategy.
In the case of anthracycline, diminished cardiac toxicity is as important an aim as increased activity. In the evaluation of cardiac toxicity the most important parameter must be the time to toxicity rather than the total dose. The new endomyocardial biopsy technique may be helpful in the study of analogs such as rubidazone, carminomycin and AD32. Actinomycin D analogs are also of interest, since this drug is part of several curative regimens, but its use has been limited by its severe acute toxicity. In the case of bleomycin, analogs with diminished pulmonary toxicity should be sought.

Tables

Table 1. Clinical activity of anthracyclines

Tumor type	Daunomycin	Adriamycin
ANLL (adult)	+	+
ALL (adult)	NE	+
ANLL (childhood)	+	NE
ALL (childhood)	+	+
Neuroblastomas	+	+
Reticulum cell sarcoma	NE	+
Lymphosarcoma	NE	+
Hodgkin's disease	NE	+
Thyroid	NE	+
Breast	NE	+
Pediatric solid tumor	NE	+
Bladder	NE	+
Sarcoma	NE	+
Lung	NE	+
Testicular	NE	+
Ovary	NE	+
Colon	NE	-
Melanoma	NE	-
Head and neck	NE	-
Brain	NE	-

+ Active - Inactive NE Not evaluable
ANLL: Acute nonlymphocytic leukemia.
ALL: Acute lymphocytic leukemia.

Table 2. Clinical toxicity of the anthracyclines

Toxicity	Daunomycin	Adriamycin
Dose limiting		
Myelosuppression	+	+
Congestive heart failure	+	+
Other		
Gastrointestinal	+	+
Mucositis	+	+
Alopecia	+	+
EKG changes	+	+
Phlebitis/cellulitis	+	+
Skin rash, fever, chills	+	+

Table 3. Protocols utilizing rubidazone

Institution	Phase	Schedule	Disease
M. D. Anderson	I-II	Single dose	Leukemia
Mayo	I	Single dose	Solid tumors
Memorial	I	Q D × 3	Solid tumors[a], leukemia[a]
Wayne State	II	Single dose	Breast[b], lung, colon
SWOG 7633	II	Single dose	Acute leukemia CMLBT[c]
SWOG 7625	II	Single dose + DTIC	Bone sarcomas, mesotheliomas
SWOG 7626	II	Single dose + VCR + Ara-C + prednisone (ROAP)	Acute leukemia[d]

[a] Childhood.
[b] Comparative study versus adriamycin.
[c] CMLBT: Chronic myeloid leukemia, blastic transformation.
[d] Patients ≥ 50 years of age.
SWOG: Southwest Oncology Group.

Table 4. Suggested Phase II studies with an actinomycin analog

Tumor type	Analog treatment
Melanoma	Single agent versus combination with DTIC
Soft tissue sarcoma	Single agent in adriamycin failures
	Single agent in untreated patients
Lung cancer	Single agent in non-small cell
	Combination with DTIC in small cell
Colon cancer	Single agent in 5-FU failures
	Single agent in untreated patients
Breast cancer	Single agent, preferably in patients not treated with adriamycin

Table 5. Miscellaneous antitumor antibiotics—toxicity and efficacy

Antibiotic	Major toxicity	Efficacy
Mitomycin C-porfiromycin	Hematopoietic Local GI	Various solid tumors
Chromomycin A_3-mithramycin	Renal Hepatic[a] Hematopoietic[a]	Embryonal carcinoma of testes[a]
Streptonigrin	Hematopoietic	Lymphomas (?)
Streptozotocin	Renal GI	Islet cell tumors, carcinoid
Tubercidin	Renal Local	Islet cell tumors (?)
Piperazinedione	Hematopoietic	Not established
Azaserine	Hematopoietic GI	Leukemia (?)
Azotomycin	Hematopoietic GI	Colon (?)
Neocarzinostatin	Hematopoietic Fever	Acute leukemia
Pyrazofurin	Mucositis	Leukemia (?), lymphomas (?)
5-Azacytidine	Hematopoietic GI	Acute leukemia

[a] Mithramycin only. GI: Gastrointestinal.

Table 6. Rationale for current analogs of antitumor antibiotics

Rationale	Analog family		
	Anthracyclines	Bleomycins	Actinomycins
Pharmacologic (altered distribution)	–	+	–
Toxicologic (decreased toxicity)	+	+	+ (?)
Therapeutic (increased or different spectrum)	+ (?)	+	+

References

1. Anderson, T., McMenamin, M. G., Schein, P. S.: Chlorozotocin, 2-[3-(chloroethyl)-3-nitrosoureido]-D-glucopyranose, an antitumor agent with modified bone marrow toxicity. Cancer Res. **35**, 761–765 (1975).
2. Atassi, G., Tagnon, H. J., Staquet, M.: Comparison of adriamycin (NSC 123127) and DNA-adriamycin complex in the chemotherapy of experimental tumors and metastases. In: E.O.R.T.C. International Symposium on Adriamycin Review. Ghent: European Press Medikon 1975, pp. 70–78.
3. Beisler, J. A., Hepp, P. L., Quinn, F. R., Driscoll, J.S.: 5-Azacytidine decomposition in aqueous solution: Isolation and characterization of the N-formyl hydrolysis intermediate (Abst. 682). Proc. Am. Assoc. Cancer Res. **18**, 171 (1977).
4. Bernard, J., Jacquillat, C. L., Boiron, M., Weil, M., Geman, M. F., Izrael, V., Schaison, G., Delobel, J.: Observations de leucémies aigues. Essai de traitement pour un dérivé semi-synthétique de la daunorubicine. Nouv. Presse. Med. **1**, 2149–2152 (1972).

5. BORISOV, V. I., LIPATOV, A. M., PEREVODCHIKOVA, N. I., et al.: Results of a cooperative clinical study of a new cancer chemotherapy antibiotic, carminomycin. Submitted to *Antibiotiki* (1976).
6. CARTER, S. K., ICHIKAWA, T., MATHE, G., UMEZAWA, H. (eds.): Fundamental and Clinical Studies of Bleomycin. Gann Monograph on Cancer Research No. 19. Tokyo: University of Tokyo Press 1976.
7. DIMARCO, A., CASAZZA, A. M., GAMBETTA, R., SUPINO, R., ZUNINO, F.: Relationship between activity and amino sugar stereochemistry of daunorubicin and adriamycin derivatives. Cancer Res. **36**, 1962-1966 (1976).
8. FRIEDMAN, M. A., BOZDECH, M. K., BILLINGHAM, M., RIDER, A.: Adriamycin cardiotoxicity in humans: Serial physiologic studies and endomyocardial biopsy. Clin. Res. **25**, 407A (1977).
9. FURUE: H.: Phase I trial with aclacinomycin A. Proc. Jap. Cancer Assoc., 35th Annual Mtg., Abst. 416, October 1976.
10. GOLDIN, A., JOHNSON, R. K.: Evaluation of actinomycins in experimental systems. Cancer Chemother. Rep. **58**, 63-77 (1974).
11. GRECO, F. A., BRERETON, H. D., RODBARD, D.: Noninvasive monitoring of adriamycin cardiotoxicity by 'Sphygmo-Recording' of the pulse wave delay (QKd interval). Cancer Treat. Rep. **60**, 1239-1245 (1976).
12. HENNEY, J., VON HOFF, D. D., ROZENCWEIG, M., MUGGIA, F. M.: Cancerostatic analogues, the same or different? Clin. Pharmacol. Ther. **21**, 106 (1977).
13. INABA, M., JOHNSON, R. K., GOLDIN, A.: Uptake and retention of ^{3}H-actinomycin in sublines of P388 leukemia resistant to adriamycin and daunorubicin. (Abst. 610) Proc. Am. Assoc. Cancer Res. **18**, 153 (1977).
14. ISRAEL, M., MODEST, E. J., FREI, E.: N-trifluoroacetyladriamycin-14-valerate, an analog with greater experimental antitumor activity and less toxicity than adriamycin. Cancer Res. **35**, 1365-1368 (1975).
15. KATZ, E.: Controlled biosynthesis of actinomycins. Cancer Chemother. Rep. **58**, 83-91 (1974).
16. LIVINGSTON, R. B., VENDITTI, J. W., COONEY, D., CARTER, S. K.: Glutamine antagonists in chemotherapy. Adv. Pharmacol. Chemother. **8**, 57-120 (1970).
17. MEIENHOFER, J.: Synthesis of peptide analogs of actinomycin D (NSC-3053). Cancer Chemother. Rep. **58**, 21-34 (1974).
18. MINOW, R. A., BENJAMIN, R. S., LEE, E. T., GOTTLIEB, J. A.: Adriamycin cardiotoxicity—Risk factors. Cancer **39**, 1397-1402 (1977).
19. MODEST, E. J., SENGUPTA, S. K.: 7-Substituted actinomycin D (NSC-3053) analogs as fluorescent DNA-binding and experimental antitumor agents. Cancer Chemother. Rep. **58**, 35-48 (1974).
20. MYERS, C. E., MCGUIRE, W., YOUNG, R.: Adriamycin: Amelioration of toxicity by α-tocopherol. Cancer Treat. Rep. **60**, 961-962 (1976).
21. RAMOS, A., MEYER, R. A., KORFHAGEN, J., WONG, K. Y., KAPLAN, S.: Echocardiographic evaluation of adriamycin cardiotoxicity in children. Cancer Treat. Rep. **60**, 1281-1284 (1976).
22. RINEHART, J. J., LEWIS, R. P., BALCERZAK, S. P.: Adriamycin cardiotoxicity in man. Ann. Intern. Med. **81**, 475-478 (1974).
23. ROZENCWEIG, M., SLAVIK, M., MUGGIA, F. M., CARTER, S. K.: Overview of early and investigational chemotherapeutic agents in solid tumors. Med. Ped. Oncology **2**, 417-432 (1976).
24. SLAVIK, M., CARTER, S. K.: Chromomycin A_3, mithramycin, and olivomycin: Antitumor antibiotics of related structure. Adv. Pharmacol. Chemother. **12**, 1-30 (1975).
25. TAN, C. T. C., GOLBEY, R. B., YAP, C. L., WOLLNER, N., HACKETHAL, C. A., MURPHY, L. M., DARGEON, H. W., BURCHENAL, J. H.: Clinical experiences with actinomycins D, KS2, and F1 (KS4). Ann. N. Y. Acad. Sci. **89**, 426-444 (1960).
26. VERTOGRADOVA, T. P., GOLDBERG, L. Y., FILIPPOSYANTS, S. T., BELOVA, I. P., STEPANOVA, E. G., SHEPELEVTSEVA, N. G.: Mechanism of the toxic effect of the antitumor antibiotic, carminomycin. Antibiotiki **19**, 50-57 (1974).
27. VON HOFF, D. D., ROZENCWEIG, M., SLAVIK, M., MUGGIA, F. M.: Activity of daunomycin in solid tumors. J. Am. Med. Assoc. **236**, 1693 (1976).
28. VON HOFF, D. D., ROZENCWEIG, M., LAYARD, M., SLAVIK, M., MUGGIA, F. M.: Daunomycin-induced cardiotoxicity in children: A review of 110 cases. Am. J. Med. **62**, 200-208 (1977).
29. VON HOFF, D. D., ROZENCWEIG, M., SOPER, W. T., HELMAN, L. J., PENTA, J. S., DAVIS, H. L., MUGGIA, F. M.: Whatever happened to NSC——? Cancer Treat. Rep. **61**, 759-768 (1977).

Antitumor Antibiotics—Thoughts for the Future

S. K. Carter

The antitumor antibiotics are among the most important drugs available in the armenertarium of the medical oncologist. They stand in the forefront of compounds active against the solid tumors accounting for the majority of cancer deaths. They are, because of this, prime candidates for use in the combined modality protocols which are the major strategic approaches to these tumors. In this approach they are used in conjunction with surgery and radiation therapy to attack residual disease which may remain after these local modalities have eradicated the great bulk of tumor. In addition, the antibiotics will be used in combination with other drugs in order to achieve optimal cell kill with resultant palliation in advanced disease and, if successful, these combinations will also be integrated into combined modality protocols.

As with all other cancer drugs, the killing of neoplastic cells is not accomplished without some toxicity to normal cells. The major toxicities of most drugs involves acute effects on the bone marrow and gastrointestinal epithelium. These acute toxicities are expected and can be easily handled, in most cases, by an experienced oncology team. The greater problem that has to be faced when drugs are used in adjuvant studies is chronic organ toxicities which may cause permanent residual damage with resultant morbidity and/or mortality. Some of the most effective antitumor antibiotics are particularly prone to this problem. These include adriamycin with its cardiac toxicity, bleomycin with its pulmonary toxicity and mitomycin C with its renal toxicity.

As soon as any new drug is shown to have meaningful anticancer activity, work begins on the development of analogs which hopefully increase the therapeutic index of the parent compound. Traditionally, analog development has emphasized evaluation of new analogs in systems designed to elucidate greater efficacy. Some programs look for increased analog activity in the predictive system that initially uncovered the parent structure. Other programs look at a spectrum of tumor systems, searching for analog activity in systems not responsive to the parent drug. These approaches are aimed at developing new drugs which will have increased response rates in responsive tumors to the parent drug and/or a broader spectrum of activity. Recently it has become of concern to drug development programs to look for systems which might predict diminished toxicity, especially of the chronic type as mentioned earlier. Work is on-going evaluating bleomycin analogs which hopefully will have lessened pulmonary toxicity. Similar work is on-going with adriamycin analogs attempting to find less cardiotoxic derivatives.

The predictive ability of systems designed to pick up less toxic analogs of bleomycin and adriamycin have not been proven as yet in the clinic. The therapeutic trial to prove than an analog has diminished chronic toxicity is much more difficult than the trial devised to show increased efficacy. In order to show that an analog of bleomycin has diminished pulmonary toxicity, it would be necessary to treat a large enough number of *responding* patients so that a meaningful dose level would be built up which could make comparison of pulmonary toxicity with bleomycin itself meaningful. The critical comparison with a bleomycin analog would not be the total dose which gave pulmonary toxicity as compared to bleomycin, but the duration of treatment which could be safely given in comparison to bleomycin. For example, if the effective dose of a bleomycin analog was 100 mg/m^2 twice weekly and it gave pulmonary toxicity at a total dose of 1000 mg/m^2 or higher, this would be a more toxic drug than bleomycin. The reason is that you would only give 5 weeks of twice weekly treatment with this new analog as compared to 10 weeks of twice weekly treatment with bleomycin at a dose of 15 mg twice weekly to reach a total dose of 300 mg which has been reported as the critical pulmonary toxic dose level for bleomycin. On a total dose-level analysis, the new analog would appear to be three times *less* toxic than bleomycin but on a duration of treatment analysis it would be two times *more* toxic than bleomycin.

Within the framework of the above toxicology considerations, there is a problem in clinical trial design. Study designs need to be developed where the end-point is the development of a severe chronic toxicity such as bleomycin pneumonitis or pulmonary fibrosis or adriamycin cardiomyopathy. These end-points are not simple to determine and cause problems in terms of informed consent and human subject review committee deliberations. Clinical evaluations of these toxicities are needed which do not require the full-blown and often fatal clinical picture. For bleomycin analog trials we need to develop measurements of pulmonary function which will allow us to evaluate pulmonary damage, if it is occurring, prior to the development of the full-blown clinical manifestation. In the adriamycin analog area we have such a tool already on hand in the endomyocardial biopsy technique described by Daniels et al. from Stanford University at this Symposium.

The Northern California Cancer Program has developed a Multidisciplinary Drug Research Group (MDRG) which will be attempting to develop new anthracycline analog compounds. This MDRG has been described by Dr. Martin Apple at this Symposium. This group has developed a clinical trial strategy for a new anthracycline analog which is one approach to the handling of this clinical situation and which will be described as an illustration.

There are four possible ways in which a new anthracycline analog of adriamycin could show superiority to its parent compound:

1. Increased efficacy in tumors responsive to adriamycin as measured by:
   a) increased complete response rate
   b) increased overall response rate (CR + PR)
   c) increased duration of remission
   d) increased survival
2. Efficacy in tumors unresponsive to adriamycin, e.g., adenocarcinoma of the large bowel, malignant melanoma, renal carcinoma.
3. Diminished acute toxicity as measured by:
   a) decreased leukopenia and/or thrombocytopenia
   b) decreased stomatitis
   c) decreased alopecia
   d) decreased gastrointestinal toxicity
4. Diminished cardiac (chronic) toxicity as measured by:
   a) less cardiac functional damage as measured by noninvasive techniques
   b) less pathologic damage on endomyocardial biopsy
   c) diminished incidence of clinical cardiomyopathy

The clinical strategy of MDRG for evaluating a new anthracycline analog of adriamycin will attempt to evaluate for all four ways in which superiority to the parent compound can be demonstrated.

Proposed Strategy

1. An appropriate initial schedule will be chosen based on a careful evaluation of the preclinical data. Among the preclinical data which will be evaluated are the following:
   a) optimal schedule in the experimental tumors which are responsive to the drug
   b) cell cycle specificity or the lack thereof
   c) toxicology of the drug in rodents and large animals
   d) pharmacology of the drug in experimental animals and correlation with all of the above
   e) appropriate biochemical data

2. An appropriate starting dose level will be chosen from analysis of the animal toxicology data. The most commonly used approach is to take a third of the toxic dose low (minimally toxic dose) of the most sensitive large animal species on a mg/m^2 basis. The safety of this approach in a wide range of drugs, including anthracyclines, has been demonstrated by the retrospective analysis of Goldsmith, Slavik and Carter. Rodent toxicologic data will not be ignored as supported also by the above paper.

3. An appropriate dose escalation procedure will be designed based on analysis of the preclinical data including the steepness of the toxicologic dose response curve. It has been shown by the members of the National Cancer Institute's Phase I working group that, with all drugs analyzed to date, doubling of a completely nontoxic dose can be safely performed. This would enable a more rapid escalation than could be accomplished with a modified fibinocci search scheme approach as originally described by Selawry. Doses will not be escalated in the same patient so as to evaluate the potential for cumulative toxicity at each dose level unless this is not considered in the best interest of the patient.
Pharmacologic determinations will be made at each dose level and, if it is deemed appropriate, on the data obtained, the initial schedule will be modified.

4. The end points of the study will be as follows:
   a) the establishment of a maximally tolerated dose on the schedule tested and a recommended dose level for Phase II evaluation
   b) elucidation of the acute toxicity pattern at all dose levels
   c) elucidation of the pharmacokinetics of the drug in man so as to make correlations with the pharmacokinetics in animals
   d) early indication of the cardiac toxic potential of the drug
   e) early indication of the therapeutic efficacy of the drug, recognizing that patients who are placed on Phase I study often do not have measurable disease and may be extensively pretreated with other modalities and/or drugs

5. A decision will be made concerning whether Phase II study is indicated. Factors mitigating against performing Phase II study would be evidence of toxicity that was unpredictable and/or irreversible. Evidence of cardiac toxicity at low dose levels would be a strong negative factor. Lack of any evidence of antitumor effect would not necessarily mitigate against Phase II evaluation.

Phase II Evaluation

1. An appropriate schedule would be chosen derived from the following:
   a) the Phase I study data
   b) the clinical pharmacology of the drug and its correlation with the preclinical data which led to the choice of the Phase I study schedule

2. An appropriate dose level would be chosen from the Phase I study.
3. A series of tumor types would be chosen for efficacy evaluation from the following mix:
   a) tumors highly responsive to adriamycin, e.g., adenocarcinoma of the breast, soft tissue and bone sarcomas, malignant lymphomas, adult leukemia
   b) tumors moderately responsive to adriamycin, e.g., bronchogenic carcinoma (all cell type), gastric cancer, bladder cancer, prostate cancer, ovary cancer, head and neck cancer, multiple myeloma, pancreatic cancer and carcinoma of the uterus (cervix and endometrium)
   c) tumors unresponsive to adriamycin, e.g., adenocarcinoma of the large bowel, malignant melanoma, renal carcinoma and CNS tumors (gliomas)

4. For each tumor type, an appropriate number of patients will be treated with the new drug in order to make a reasonable assessment of whether efficacy compared to adriamycin appears to be potentially greater or equal which would warrant further (Phase III) study.

5. The study design chosen may be a sequential number of patients placed on study (uncontrolled Phase II) or a controlled comparison against either a standard regimen (with cross-over) or another new drug.

6. All patients will be treated until there is evidence of progressive disease.

7. Cardiac toxicity monitoring will be performed at all dose levels and endomycardial biopsy undertaken at selected dose levels.

8. A decision will be made concerning whether Phase III testing should be undertaken. *This decision will be individually made for each tumor type* based on analysis of the following data:
   a) the response rate (CR + PR/No. treated) compared to data with adriamycin
   b) the duration of response compared to data with adriamycin
   c) the survival of the treated group compared to data with adriamycin
   d) the acute toxicity observed
   e) evidence of cardiac toxicity or lack thereof

The critical factor will *not* be the total dose of new drug that causes evidence of cardiac toxicity compared to adriamycin but the total number of courses or duration of therapy. For example, the total dose of a single course of Rubidazone in AML is 600 mg/m^2. Should rubidazone give cardiac toxicity after three courses, the total dose would be 1.80 gm/m^2. If only total dose is looked at, rubidazone would be one third as cardiotoxic as adriamycin. If total courses to toxicity is looked at, then rubidazone would be three times more cardiotoxic than adriamycin.

   f) There are 27 hypothetical end-points of the Phase II studies for each tumor type which are outlined in Table 1.

It must be remembered that Phase II studies often do not give enough data to make definitive decisions. The end-product of a Phase II study is the decision as to whether further study is indicated which will delineate the role for the drug. What can be readily seen is that if Phase II studies are performed on 10 tumor types there are 270 potential clinical end-points which could be observed.

Role Delineation Studies (Phase III)

1. Assuming a positive Phase III study, further studies in each disease could be as follows:
   a) controlled comparison with adriamycin with enough patients to clearly determine which is the superior drug (classic Phase III study).

Table 1. Hypothetical end-points of Phase II studies

Toxicity[a]	Efficacy[b] ↑	—	↘
Acute↑ Cardiac↑	maybe	no	no
Acute↑ Cardiac—	yes	maybe	no
Acute↑ Cardiac↘	yes	yes	yes
Acute↘ Cardiac↑	maybe	no	no
Acute↘ Cardiac—	yes	yes	maybe
Acute↘ Cardiac	yes	maybe	no
Acute— Cardiac↑	maybe	no	no
Acute— Cardiac—	yes	maybe	no
Acute— Cardiac	yes	yes	maybe

[a] Toxicity
↘ evidence that toxicity could be less than observed for adriamycin
—evidence that toxicity is comparable to adriamycin or there are not enough data to make a meaningful decision.
↑ evidence that toxicity could be more than observed for adriamycin

b) combination of analog with other active drugs against the same responsive tumor. This would first necessitate a Phase I study of the combination and probably a Phase III evaluation.
c) combination with another modality, e.g. radiation therapy, immunotherapy or surgery
d) evaluation of new schedules in order to further enhance the therapeutic ratio

Final Analysis

1. Each tumor type that responds to adriamycin would have, in the final analysis, the same 27 possible end-points as were outlined in Table 1 for Phase II studies. Some end-points would indicate that the analog was superior and the experimental prediction was correct and others would indicate the opposite.
2. For each unresponsive tumor type to adriamycin, the potential end-points would be less and would relate to whether the analog was active or not and how the toxicities compared.

Introduction into Medical Practice

This would test the effect of the drug in the community of Northern California and Northwestern Nevada facilities.

In conclusion, the antitumor antibiotics are among the most important drugs available today to the clinical oncologist. Much work remains to be done to improve their therapeutic indices while the search for new and better compounds goes on. Future drug development will be a balance between the search for new structures, the search for improved analogs of existing known actives, and attempts to improve the therapeutic ratio of the currently utilized drugs. Future development will also be a balance between the search for increased activity and a search for diminished toxicity, especially toxicity to organ systems such as the lung, heart, and kidney. New predictive experimental systems will have to be developed and new clinical trial strategies elucidated.

Recent Results in Cancer Research

Sponsored by the Swiss League against Cancer. Editor in Chief: P. Rentchnick, Genève

For information about Vols. 1—9, please contact your bookseller or Springer-Verlag.

10 NELSON, R. S.: Radioactive Phosphorus in the Diagnosis of Gastrointestinal Cancer.
11 FREEMAN, R. G. and J. M. KNOX: Treatment of Skin Cancer.
12 LYNCH, H. T.: Hereditary Factors in Carcinoma.
13 Tumours in Children, 2nd Edition. Edited by H. B. MARSDEN and J. K. STEWARD.
14 ODARTCHENKO, N.: Production Cellulaire Erythropoïétique.
15 SOKOLOFF, B.: Carcinoid and Serotonin.
16 JACOBS, M. L.: Malignant Lymphomas and Their Management.
17 Normal and Malignant Cell Growth. Edited by R. J. M. FRY, M. L. GRIEM, and W. H. KIRSTEN (Symposium).
18 ANGLESIO, E.: The Treatment of Hodgkin's Disease.
19 BANNASCH, P.: The Cytoplasm of Hepatocytes during Carcinogenesis. Electron- and Lightmicroscopical Investigations of the Nitrosomorpholine-intoxicated Rat Liver.
20 Rubidomycin. A new Agent against Cancer. Edited by J. BERNARD, R. PAUL, M. BOIRON, C. JACQUILLAT, and R. MARAL.
21 Scientific Basis of Cancer Chemotherapy. Edited by G. MATHÉ (Symposium).
22 KOLDOVSKÝ, P.: Tumor Specific Transplantation Antigen.
23 FUCHS, W. A., J. W. DAVIDSON, and H. W. FISCHER: Lymphography in Cancer. With contributions by G. JANTET and H. RÖSLER.
24 HAYWARD, J.: Hormones und Human Breast Cancer. An Account of 15 Years Study.
25 ROY-BURMAN, P.: Analogues of Nucleic Acid Components. Mechanisms of Action.
26 Tumors of the Liver. Edited by G. T. PACK and A. H. ISLAMI.
27 SZYMENDERA, J.: Bone Mineral Metabolism in Cancer.
28 MEEK, E. S.: Antitumour and Antiviral Substances of Natural Origin.
29 Aseptic Environments and Cancer Treatment. Edited by G. MATHÉ (Symposium).
30 Advances in the Treatment of Acute (Blastic) Leukemias. Edited by G. MATHÉ (Symposium).
31 DENOIX, P.: Treatment of Malignant Breast Tumors. Indications and Results.
32 NELSON, R. S.: Endoscopy in Gastric Cancer.
33 Experimental and Clinical Effects of L-Asparaginase. Edited by E. GRUNDMANN and H. F. OETTGEN (Symposium).
34 Chemistry and Biological Actions of 4-Nitroquinolin 1-Oxide. Edited by H. ENDO, T. ONO, and T. SUGIMURA.
35 PENN, I.: Malignant Tumors in Organ Transplant Recipients.
36 Current Concepts in the Management of Lymphoma and Leukemia. Edited by J. E. ULTMANN, M. L. GRIEM, W. H. KIRSTEN, and R. W. WISSLER (Symposium).
37 CHIAPPA, S., R. MUSUMECI, and C. USLENGHI: Endolymphatic Radiotherapy in Malignant Lymphomas. With contributions by G. BONADONNA, B. DAMASCELLI, G. FAVA, F. PIZZETTI, U. VERONESI.
38 KOLLER, P. C.: The Role of Chromosomes in Cancer Biology.
39 Current Problems in the Epidemiology of Cancer and Lymphomas. Edited by E. GRUNDMANN and H. TULINIUS (Symposium).
40 LANGLEY, F. A. and A. C. CROMPTON: Epithelial Abnormalities of the Cervix Uteri.
41 Tumours in a Tropical Country. A Survey of Uganda (1964—1968). Edited by A. C. TEMPLETON.
42 Breast Cancer: A Challenging Problem. Edited by M. L. GRIEM, E. V. JENSEN, J. E. ULTMANN, and R. W. WISSLER (Symposium).
43 Nomenclature, Methodology and Results of Clinical Trials in Acute Leukemias. Edited by G. MATHÉ, P. POUILLART, L. SCHWARZENBERG (Symposium).

44 Special Topics in Carcinogenesis. Edited by E. GRUNDMANN (Symposium).
45 KOLDOVSKÝ, P.: Carcinoembryonic Antigens.
46 Diagnosis and Therapy of Malignant Lymphoma. Edited by K. MUSSHOFF (Symposium).
47 Investigation and Stimulation of Immunity in Cancer Patients. Edited by G. MATHÉ and R. WEINER (Symposium).
48 Platinum Coordination Complexes in Cancer Chemotherapy. Edited by T. A. CONNORS and J. J. ROBERTS (Symposium).
49 Complications of Cancer Chemotherapy. Edited by G. MATHÉ and R. K. OLDHAM (Symposium).
50 Cancer Registry. Edited by E. GRUNDMANN and E. PEDERSEN (Symposium).
51 Gliomas. Current Concepts in Biology, Diagnosis and Therapy. Edited by J. HEKMATPANAH (Symposium).
52 The Ambivalence of Cytostatic Therapy. Edited by E. GRUNDMANN and R. GROSS (Symposium).
53 A. CLARYSSE, Y. KENIS, and G. MATHÉ: Cancer Chemotherapy.
54 Malignant Bone Tumors. Edited by E. GRUNDMANN.
55 MATHÉ, G.: Cancer Active Immunotherapy, Immunoprophylaxis, and Immunorestoration.
56 Lymphocytes, Macrophages, and Cancer. Edited by G. MATHÉ, I. FLORENTIN, and M.-C. SIMMLER (Symposium).
57 Breast Cancer: A Multidisciplinary Approach. Edited by G. ST. ARNEAULT, P. BAND, and L. ISRAËL (Symposium).
58 B. S. SCHOENBERG: Multiple Primary Malignant Neoplasms.
59 Selective Heat Sensitivity of Cancer Cells. Edited by A. ROSSI-FANELLI, R. CAVALIERE, B. MONDOVI, and G. MORICCA.
60 Tumors of the Male Genital System. Edited by E. GRUNDMANN and W. VAHLENSIECK (Symposium).
61 D. METCALF: Hemopoietic Colonies.
62 Tactics and Strategy in Cancer Treatment. Edited by G. MATHÉ (Symposium).
63 Antitumor Antibiotics. Edited by S. K. CARTER, H. UMEZAWA, J. DOUROS, and Y. SAKURAI (Symposium).